ORBAN'S
ORAL HISTOLOGY
AND EMBRYOLOGY

ORBAN'S
ORAL HISTOLOGY AND EMBRYOLOGY

EDITED BY

S. N. Bhaskar, B.D.S., D.D.S., M.S., Ph.D.

Major General, U.S. Army (Retired); formerly Chief, U.S. Army Dental Corps;
Diplomate, American Board of Oral Pathology; Diplomate, American Board of Oral Medicine;
Certificate in Periodontics; Private practice limited to Periodontics,
Monterey and Salinas, California

ELEVENTH EDITION

with 601 illustrations

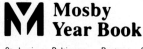

St. Louis   Baltimore   Boston   Chicago   London   Philadelphia   Sydney   Toronto   1990

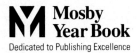

**Mosby
Year Book**

Dedicated to Publishing Excellence

Editor: Robert W. Reinhardt
Assistant Editor: Melba Steube
Project Coordinator: Gina Gay Chan
Designer: David Zielinski

ELEVENTH EDITION

Previous editions copyrighted 1944, 1949, 1953,
1957, 1962, 1966, 1972, 1976, 1980, 1986

Printed in the United States of America

Mosby–Year Book, Inc.
11830 Westline Industrial Drive
St. Louis, Missouri 63146

Orban's oral histology and embryology.—11th ed. / edited by S.N.
   Bhaskar.
        p.   cm.
   Includes bibliographical references and index.
   ISBN 0-8016-0239-4
   1. Mouth—Histology. 2. Teeth—Histology. 3. Embryology,
Human. I. Orban, Balint J. (Balint Joseph). Orban's oral
histology and embryology. II. Bhaskar, S. N. (Surindar Nath).
   III. Title: Oral histology and embryology.
   [DNLM: 1. Stomatognathic System—anatomy & histology.
2. Stomatognathic System—embryology.   WU 101 064]
QM306.07 1991
611'.018931—dc20
DNLM/DLC   90-13634
for Library of Congress   CIP

ISBN 0-8016-0239-4

C/DC 9 8 7 6 5 4 3 2 1

CONTRIBUTORS

GARY C. ARMITAGE, D.D.S., M.S.

Professor and Chairman, Division of Periodontology, University of California, San Francisco School of Dentistry, San Francisco, California

JAMES K. AVERY, D.D.S., Ph.D.

Professor of Dentistry and Anatomy, Department of Oral Biology, The University of Michigan School of Dentistry, Ann Arbor, Michigan

S.N. BHASKAR, B.D.S., D.D.S., M.S., Ph.D.

Major General, U.S. Army (Retired); formerly Chief, U.S. Army Dental Corps; Diplomate, American Board of Oral Pathology; Diplomate, American Board of Oral Medicine; Private Practice limited to Periodontics, Monterey and Salinas, California

*BALDEV RAJ BHUSSRY, B.D.S., D.D.S., M.S., Ph.D.

Formerly Associate Professor and Chairman, Department of Anatomy, Georgetown University Schools of Medicine and Dentistry, Washington, D.C.

ARTHUR R. HAND, D.D.S.

Director, Central Electron Microscopy Facility, Department of Pediatric Dentistry, The University of Connecticut Health Center, Farmington, Connecticut

MALCOLM C. JOHNSTON, D.D.S., M.Sc.D., Ph.D.

Professor of Orthodontics and Anatomy, Schools of Dentistry and Medicine; Senior Scientist, Dental Research Center, University of North Carolina at Chapel Hill, Chapel Hill, North Carolina

SHAKTI P. KAPUR, M.S., Ph.D.

Associate Professor, Department of Anatomy, Georgetown University Schools of Medicine and Dentistry, Washington, D.C.

CHRISTOPHER A.H. MCCULLOUGH, D.D.S., Ph.D., F.R.C.D.(C.)

Assistant Professor of Dentistry, Faculty of Dentistry, University of Toronto, Toronto, Ontario, Canada

ANTONY H. MELCHER, M.D.S., H.D.D., Ph.D., D.Sc.

Professor of Dentistry, Faculty of Dentistry; Associate Dean (Life Sciences), School of Graduate Studies; University of Toronto, Toronto, Ontario, Canada

MOHAMED SHARAWY, B.D.S., Ph.D.

Professor and Chairman, Department of Oral Biology/Anatomy, School of Dentistry; Professor of Anatomy, School of Medicine, Medical College of Georgia, Augusta, Georgia

IRVING B. STERN, D.D.S.

Affiliate Professor of Oral Biology, University of Washington School of Dentistry, Seattle, Washington; Formerly, Professor and Chairman, Department of Periodontology, Tufts University School of Dental Medicine, Boston, Massachusetts; Professor of Periodontics, University of Washington School of Dentistry; Private Practice, Seattle, Washington

*FAUSTINO R. SUAREZ, M.D.

Formerly Assistant Professor, Department of Anatomy, Georgetown University Schools of Medicine and Dentistry, Washington, D.C.

---

*Deceased.

KATHLEEN K. SULIK, Ph.D.

Assistant Professor of Anatomy, Department of Anatomy, University of North Carolina at Chapel Hill, School of Medicine, Chapel Hill, North Carolina

A. RICHARD TEN CATE, B.Sc., B.D.S., Ph.D.

Dean, Faculty of Dentistry, University of Toronto, Toronto, Ontario, Canada

BRANISLAV VIDIĆ, S.D.

Professor, Department of Anatomy, Georgetown University Schools of Medicine and Dentistry, Washington, D.C.

JAMES A. YAEGER, D.D.S., Ph.D.

Professor, Department of Oral Biology, University of Connecticut Health Center, School of Dental Medicine, Farmington, Connecticut

TO

Balint J. Orban

Joseph P. Weinmann

Harry Sicher

Baldev Raj Bhussry

and

Faustino R. Suarez

PREFACE To The Eleventh Edition

During the past few years many changes have occurred in the clinical practice of dentistry. The use of endosseous implants has progressed from an experimental to a widely accepted procedure. New types of alloplastic materials have been developed and are now used routinely in daily practice. Discoveries have been made in the etiology of periodontal disease. Antiplaque agents that help improve the home care of patients have been found. Esthetic dentistry has blossomed and matured and has improved the appearance of hundreds of thousands of Americans. Oral manifestations of acquired immune deficiency syndrome (AIDS) have been studied in more detail, and criteria for their management have been established. New information that assists the practicing dentist in controlling the spread of infection in his office has been made available, and new restorative materials are continuously being developed and perfected for use in our patients.

In all of these advances and in all advances that dentistry will make in the future, the basic scientist has played and will play a major role. Were it not for the dentists who, in addition to dentistry, have devoted time and energy to a variety of basic sciences, such as histology, pathology, bacteriology, immunology, anatomy, physiology, dental materials, and chemistry (to name just a few), progress of dentistry would have been impossible. Dentistry without basic sciences is only a craft but, with a good foundation in these sciences, it is a learned profession.

The eleventh edition of *Orban's Oral*

Histology and Embryology has been written by the same clinicians and scientists and teachers who wrote the tenth edition, and it is presented to the dental student and the graduate dentist with the hope that it will help in understanding the foundations on which daily clinical practice rests.

S.N. Bhaskar

PREFACE To The Tenth Edition

The ultimate test of all dental education is to see how well it prepares the practitioner to serve the patient. No aspect of a dental school curriculum can give greater meaning to a clinical procedure or put it on a more rational foundation than a thorough understanding of basic sciences. An understanding of basic sciences can be the difference between an excellent clinician and one who can treat a patient only as a technician, between a dentist who can lead and one who can only follow, between an innovator and one whose clinical resources are limited and dated.

In the tenth edition of *Orban's Oral Histology and Embryology,* a group of scientists and dentists, varyingly engaged in basic science and clinical research, in teaching dental students and dental practitioners, and in clinical practice of dentistry, have joined together to present the subject with the hope that it will better prepare the student to practice the profession wisely and with confidence.

I record with deep regret that since the publication of the last edition two of my friends and collegues have passed away. Professors Baldev Raj Bhussry and Faustino R. Suarez, both from Georgetown University School of Dentistry, were teachers and researchers of exceptional talents. Their contributions to science and to the development of future generations of dentists will be deeply missed. It is with great respect and gratitude that I add their names to those to whom this edition of the book is dedicated.

S.N. Bhaskar

CONTENTS

---

*Deceased.

ORBAN'S
ORAL HISTOLOGY
AND EMBRYOLOGY

1

DEVELOPMENT OF FACE AND ORAL CAVITY

ORIGIN OF FACIAL TISSUES

DEVELOPMENT OF FACIAL PROMINENCES
    Development of nasal placodes, frontonasal region,
        primary palate, and nose
    Development of maxillary prominences and
        secondary palate
    Development of visceral arches and tongue

FINAL DIFFERENTIATION OF FACIAL TISSUES

CLINICAL CONSIDERATIONS
    Facial clefts
    Hemifacial microsomia
    Treacher Collins' syndrome
    Labial pits
    Lingual anomalies
    Developmental cysts

[handwritten margin note: epiblast = embryo / hypoblast = supp. structures]

This chapter deals primarily with the development of the human face and oral cavity. Consideration is also given to information about underlying mechanisms that is derived from experimental studies conducted on developing subhuman embryos. Much of the experimental work has been conducted on amphibian and avian embryos. Evidence derived from these and more limited studies on other vertebrates including mammals indicates that the early facial development of all vertebrate embryos is similar. Many events occur, including cell migrations, interactions, differential growth, and differentiation, all of which lead to progressively maturing structures (Fig. 1-1). Progress has also been made with respect to abnormal developmental alterations that give rise to some of the most common human malformations (Fig. 1-16). Further information on the topics discussed can be obtained by consulting the references at the end of the chapter.

ORIGIN OF FACIAL TISSUES

After fertilization of the ovum, a series of cell divisions gives rise to an egg cell mass known as the *morula* in mammals (Fig. 1-2). In most vertebrates, including humans, the major portion of the egg cell mass forms the extraembryonic membranes and other supportive structures such as the placenta. The inner cell mass (Fig. 1-2, *D*) separates into two layers, the *epiblast* and *hypoblast* (Fig. 1-2, *E*). Cell marking studies in chick and mouse embryos have shown that only the epiblast forms the embryo, with the hypoblast and other cells forming supporting tissues, such as the placenta. The anterior (rostral) end of the primitive streak forms the lower germ layer, the *endoderm*, in which are embedded the midline notochordal (and prechordal) plates (Figs. 1-2, *F* and 1-3, *A*). Prospective mesodermal cells migrate from the epiblast through the primitive streak to form the middle germ layer, the *mesoderm*.

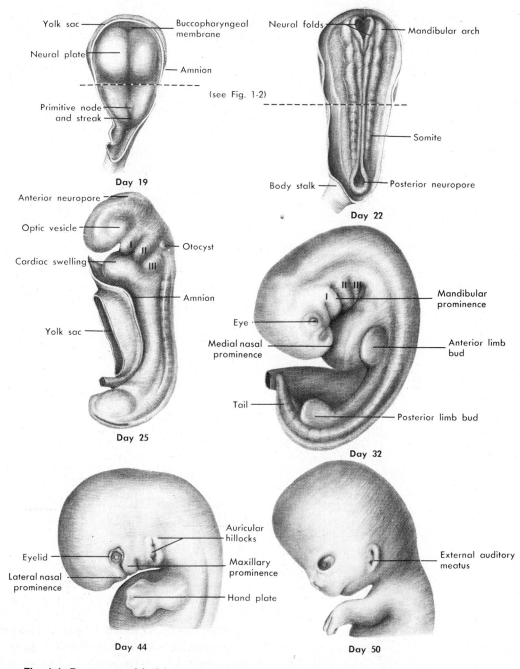

Fig. 1-1. Emergence of facial structures during development of human embryos. Dorsal views of gestational day 19 and 22 embryos are depicted, while lateral aspects of older embryos are illustrated. At days 25 and 32, visceral arches are designated by Roman numerals. Embryos become recognizable as "human" by gestational day 50. Section planes for Fig. 1-2 are illustrated in the upper (days 19 and 22) diagrams.

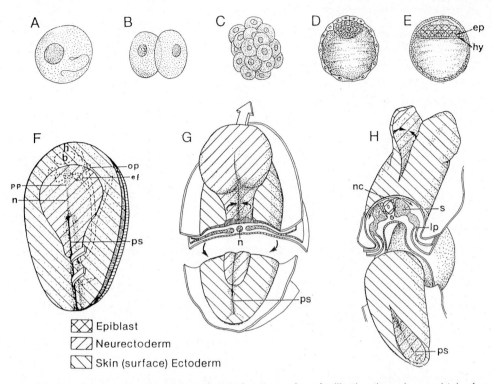

Epiblast
Neurectoderm
Skin (surface) Ectoderm

Fig. 1-2. Sketches summarizing development of embryos from fertilization through neural tube formation. Accumulation of fluid within egg cell mass (morula, *C*) leads to development of blastula *(D)*. Inner cell mass (heavily strippled cells in *D*) will form two-layered embryonic disc in *E*. It now appears that only epiblast *(ep)* will form embryo (see text), with hypoblast *(hy)* and other cell populations forming support tissues (e.g., placenta) of embryo. In *F*, notochord *(n)* and its rostral (anterior) extension, prechordal plate *(pp)*, as well as associated pharyngeal endoderm, form as a single layer. Prospective mesodermal cells migrate (arrows in *F*) through primitive streak *(ps)* and insert themselves between epiblast and endoderm. Epiblast cells remaining on surface become ectoderm. Cells of notochord (and prechordal plate?) and adjacent mesoderm (together termed chordamesoderm) induce overlying cells to form neural plate (neurectoderm). Only later does notochord separate from neural plate *(G)*, while folding movements and differential growth (arrows in *G* and *H*) continue to shape embryo. *h,* Heart; *b,* buccal plate; *op,* olfactory placode; *ef,* eye field; *nc,* neural crest; *so,* somite; *lp,* lateral plate. (Modified from Johnston MC and Sulik KK: Embryology of the head and neck. In Serafin D and Georgiade NG, editors: Pediatric plastic Surgery, vol. 1, St Louis, 1984, The CV Mosby Co.)

Cells remaining in the epiblast form the *ectoderm*, completing formation of the three germ layers. Thus, at this stage, three distinct populations of embryonic cells have arisen largely through division and migration. They follow distinctly separate courses during later development.

Migrations, such as those described above, create new associations between cells, which, in turn, allow unique possibilities for subsequent development through interactions between the cell populations. Such interactions have been studied experimentally by isolating the different cell

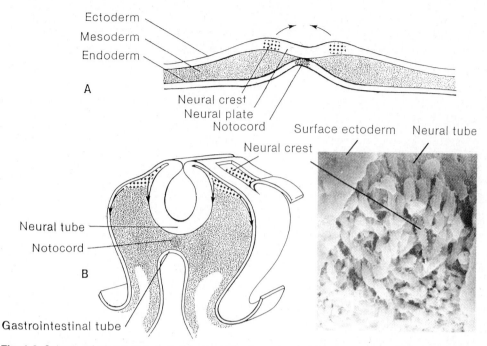

Fig. 1-3. Scheme of neural and gastrointestinal tube formation in higher vertebrate embryos (section planes illustrated in Fig. 1-1). **A,** Cross section through three-germ layer embryo. Similar structures are seen in both head and trunk regions. Neural crest cells (diamond pattern) are initially located between neural plate and surface ectoderm. Arrows indicate directions of folding processes. **B,** Neural tube, which later forms major components of brain and spinal cord, and gastrointestinal tube will separate from embryo surface after fusions are completed. Arrows indicate directions of migration of crest cells, which are initiated at about fourth week in human embryo. **C,** Scanning electron micrograph (SEM) of mouse embryo neural crest cells migrating over neural tube and under surface ectoderm near junction of brain and spinal cord following removal of piece of surface ectoderm as indicated in **B.** Such migrating cells are frequently bipolar (e.g., outlined cell at end of leader) and oriented in path of migration *(arrow).*

populations or tissues and recombining them in different ways in culture or in transplants. From these studies it is known, for example, that a median strip of mesoderm cells (the *chordamesoderm*) extending throughout the length of the embryo induces *neural plate* formation within the overlying ectoderm (Fig. 1-3). The prechordal plate is thought to have a similar role in the anterior neural plate region. The nature of such inductive stimuli is presently unknown. Sometimes cell-to-cell contact appears to be necessary, whereas in other cases (as in neural plate induction) the inductive influences appear to be able to act between cells separated by considerable distances and to consist of diffusible substances. It is known that inductive influences need only be present for a short time, after which the responding tissue is capable of independent development. For example, an induced neural plate isolated in culture will roll up into a tube, which then differentiates into the brain, spinal cord, and other structures.

In addition to inducing neural plate formation, the chordamesoderm appears to be responsible for developing the organizational plan of the head. As noted previously, the notochord and prechordal plates arise initially within the endoderm (Fig. 1-3, *A*), from which they eventually separate (Figs. 1-2, *G* and 1-3, *B*). The mesodermal portion differentiates into well-organized blocks of cells, called *somites*, caudal to the developing ear and less-organized *somitomeres* rostral to the ear (Figs. 1-2 and 1-6). Later these structures form myoblasts and some of the skeletal and connective tissues of the head. Besides inducing the neural plate from overlying ectoderm, the chordamesoderm organizes the positional relationships of various neural plate components, such as the initial primordium of the eye.

A unique population of cells develops from the ectoderm along the lateral margins of the neural plate. These are the neural crest cells. They undergo extensive migrations, usually beginning at about the time of tube closure (Fig. 1-3), and give rise to a variety of different cells that form components of many tissues. The crest cells that migrate in the trunk region form mostly neural, endocrine, and pigment cells, whereas those that migrate in the head and neck also contribute extensively to skeletal and connective tissues (i.e., cartilage, bone, dentin, dermis, etc.). In the trunk, all skeletal and connective tissues are formed by mesoderm. Of the skeletal or connective tissue of the facial region, it appears that tooth enamel (an acellular skeletal tissue) is the only one not formed by crest cells. The enamel-forming cells are derived from ectoderm lining the oral cavity.

The migration routes that cephalic (head) neural crest cells follow are illustrated in Fig. 1-4. They move around the sides of the head beneath the surface ectoderm, en masse, as a sheet of cells. They form all the mesenchyme* in the upper facial region, whereas in the lower facial region they surround mesodermal cores already present in the visceral arches. The pharyngeal region is then characterized by grooves (clefts and pouches) in the lateral pharyngeal wall endoderm and ectoderm that approach each other and appear to effectively segment the mesoderm into a number of bars that become surrounded by crest mesenchyme (Figs. 1-4, *C, D* and 1-7, *A*).

Toward the completion of migration, the trailing edge of the crest cell mass appears to attach itself to the neural tube at locations where sensory ganglia of the fifth, seventh, ninth, and tenth cranial nerves will form (Fig. 1-4, *C* and *D*). In the trunk sensory ganglia, supporting (e.g., Schwann) cells and all neurons are derived from neural crest cells. On the other hand, many of the sensory neurons of the cranial sensory ganglia originate from placodes in the surface ectoderm (Fig. 1-4, *C* and *F*).

Eventually, capillary endothelial cells derived from mesoderm cells invade the crest cell mesenchyme, and it is from this mesenchyme that the supporting cells of the developing blood vessels are derived. Initially, these supporting cells include only pericytes, which are closely apposed to the outer surfaces of endothelial cells. Later, additional crest cells differentiate into the fibroblasts and smooth muscle cells that will form the vessel wall. The developing blood vessels become interconnected to form vascular networks. These networks undergo a series of modifications, examples of which are illustrated in Fig. 1-5, before they eventually form the mature vascular system. The underlying mechanisms are not clearly understood.

---

*Mesenchyme is defined here as the loosely organized embryonic tissue, in contrast to epithelia, which are compactly arranged.

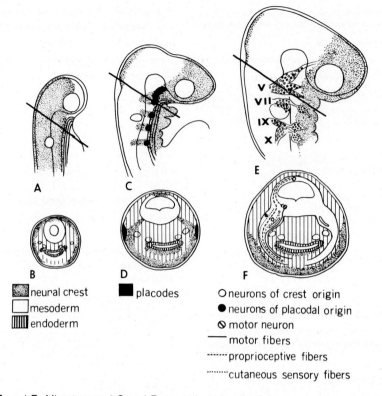

V
VII
IX
X

neural crest
mesoderm
endoderm

placodes

○ neurons of crest origin
● neurons of placodal origin
⊘ motor neuron
— motor fibers
------- proprioceptive fibers
········· cutaneous sensory fibers

Fig. 1-4. A and **B,** Migratory and **C** and **D,** postmigratory distributions of crest cells *(stipple)* and origins of cranial sensory ganglia. Initial ganglionic primordia **(C** and **D)** are formed by cords of neural crest cells that remain in contact with neural tube. Section planes in **C** and **E,** pass through primordium of trigeminal ganglion. Ectodermal "thickenings," termed placodes, form adjacent to distal ends of ganglionic primordia—for trigeminal (V) nerve as well as for cranial nerves VII, IX, and X. They contribute presumptive neuroblasts that migrate into previously purely crest cell ganglionic primordia. Distribution of crest and placodal neurons is illustrated in **E** and **F.** (Adapted from Johnston MC and Hazelton RD: Embryonic origins of facial structures related to oral sensory and motor functions. From Bosma JB, editor: Third symposium on oral sensation and perception, Springfield, IL, 1972, Charles C Thomas, Publisher.)

Almost all the myoblasts that subsequently fuse with each other to form the multinucleated striated muscle fibers are derived from mesoderm. The myoblasts that form the hypoglossal (tongue) muscles are derived from somites located beside the developing hindbrain. Somites are condensed masses of cells derived from mesoderm located adjacent to the neural tube. The myoblasts of the extrinsic ocular muscles originate from the prechordal plate (Fig. 1-2, *F*). They first migrate to poorly condensed blocks of mesoderm (somitomeres) located rostral to (in front of) the otocyst, from which they migrate to their final locations (Fig. 1-6). The supporting connective tissue found in facial muscles is derived from neural crest cells. Much of the development of the masticatory and other facial musculature is closely related to the final stages of visceral arch development and will be described later.

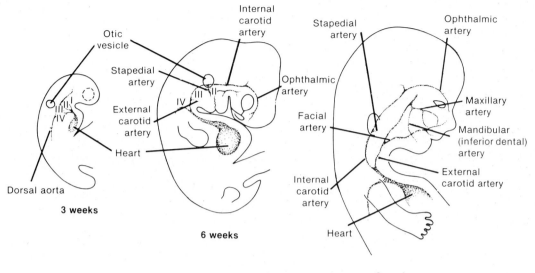

Fig. 1-5. Development of arterial system serving facial region with emphasis on its relation to visceral arches. In 3-week human embryo visceral arches are little more than conduits for blood traveling through aortic arch vessels (indicated by Roman numerals according to the visceral arch containing them) from heart to dorsal aorta. Other structures indicated are eye *(broken circle)* and ophthalmic artery. In 6-week embryo first two aortic arch vessels have regressed almost entirely, and distal portions of arches have separated from heart. Portion of third aortic arch vessel adjacent to dorsal aorta persists and eventually forms stem of external carotid artery by fusing with stapedial artery. Stapedial artery, which develops from second aortic arch vessel, temporarily (in humans) provides arterial supply for embryonic face. After fusion with external carotid artery, proximal portion of stapedial artery regresses. Aortic arch vessel of fourth visceral arch persists as arch of aorta. By 9 weeks primordium of definitive vascular system of face has been laid down. (From Ross RB, and Johnston MC: Cleft lip and palate, Baltimore, 1972, The Williams & Wilkins Co.)

A number of other structures in the facial region, such as the epithelial components or glands and the enamel organ of the tooth bud, are derived from epithelium that grows (invaginates) into underlying mesenchyme. Again, the connective tissue components in these structures (e.g., fibroblasts, odontoblasts, and the cells of tooth-supporting tissues) are derived from neural crest cells.

DEVELOPMENT OF FACIAL PROMINENCES

On the completion of the initial crest cell migration and the vascularization of the de-rived mesenchyme, a series of outgrowths or swellings termed "facial prominences" initiates the next stages of facial development (Figs. 1-7 and 1-8). The growth and fusion of upper facial prominences produce the primary and secondary palates. As will be described below, other prominences developing from the first two visceral arches considerably alter the nature of these arches.

Development of the frontonasal region: olfactory placode, primary palate, and nose. After the crest cells arrive in the future location of the upper face and midface, this area often is referred to as the frontonasal

Fig. 1-6. Migration paths followed by prospective skeletal muscle cells. Somites, or comparable structures from which muscle cells are derived, give rise to most skeletal (voluntary) myoblasts (differentiating muscle cells). Condensed somites tend not to form in head region of higher vertebrates, and their position in lower forms is indicated by broken lines. It is from these locations that extrinsic ocular and "tongue" (hypoglossal cord) muscle contractile cells are derived from postoptic somites. Recent studies indicate that myoblasts which contribute to visceral arch musculature have similar origins and originate as indicated by Roman numerals according to their nerves of innervation. At this stage of development (approximately day 34) they are still migrating *(arrowheads)* into cores of each visceral arch. Information about fourth visceral arch is still inadequate, as indicated by question mark *(?)*. Origin of extrinsic ocular myoblasts is complex (see text).

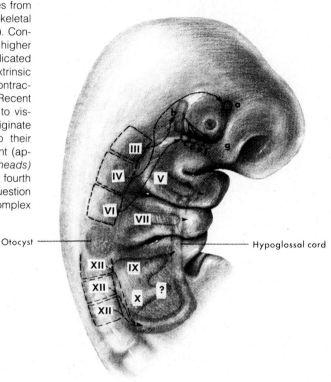

Otocyst

Hypoglossal cord

region. The first structures to become evident are the olfactory placodes. These are thickenings of the ectoderm that appear to be derived at least partly from the anterior rim of the neural plate (Fig. 1-2, *F*). Experimental evidence indicates that the lateral edges of the placodes actively curl forward, which enhance the initial development of the lateral nasal prominence (LNP, sometimes called the nasal wing—see Fig. 1-7, *A*). This morphogenetic movement combined with persisting high rates of cell proliferation rapidly brings the LNP forward so that it catches up with the medial nasal prominence (MNP), which was situated in a more forward position at the beginning of its development (Fig. 1-7, *A* and *C*). How-

Fig. 1-7. Scheme of development of facial prominences. After completion of crest cell migration. **A,** Facial prominence development begins, with curling forward, lateral portion of nasal placode **(B)** and is completed after fusion of prominences with each other or with other structures, **C.** (Details are given in text). Heart and adjacent portions of visceral arches have been removed in **A,** and most of heart has been removed in **B,** and **C.** Arrows indicate direction of growth and/or movement. Mesenchymal cell process meshwork *(CPM)* is exposed after removal of epithelium **(C)** and is illustrated to right side of **C.** Single mesenchymal cell body is outlined by broken line.

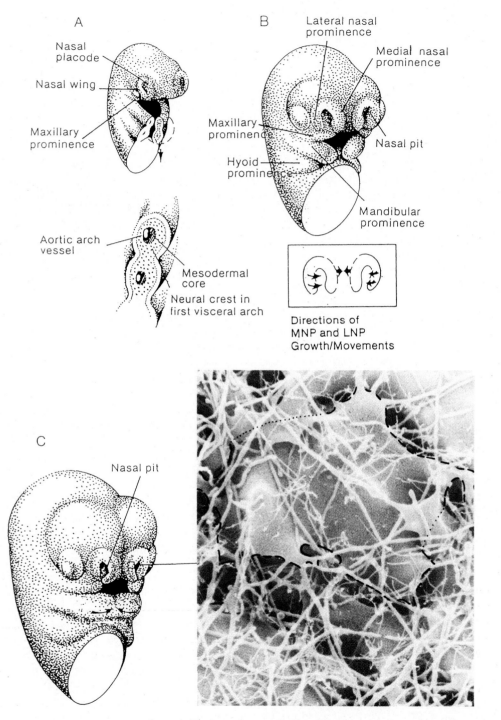

A

Nasal
placode

Nasal wing

Maxillary
prominence

Aortic arch
vessel

Mesodermal
core

Neural crest in
first visceral arch

B

Lateral nasal
prominence

Medial nasal
prominence

Maxillary
prominence

Nasal pit

Hyoid
prominence

Mandibular
prominence

Directions of
MNP and LNP
Growth/Movements

C

Nasal pit

Fig. 1-7. For legend see opposite page.

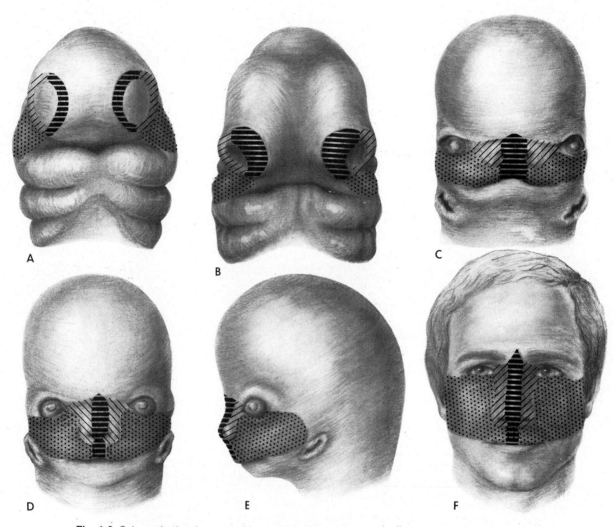

Fig. 1-8. Schematic development of human face: maxillary prominence *(stipple),* lateral nasal prominence *(oblique hatching),* and medial nasal prominence *(dark).* **A,** Embryo 4 to 6 mm in length, approximately 28 days. Prospective nasal and lateral nasal prominences are just beginning to form from mesenchyme surrounding olfactory placode. Maxillary prominence forming at proximal end of first (mandibular) arch under eye (compare to Fig. 1-3). **B,** Embryo 8 to 11 mm in length, approximately 37 days. Medial nasal prominence is beginning to make contact with lateral nasal and maxillary prominences. **C,** Embryo 16 to 18 mm in length, approximately 47 days. **D** and **E,** Embryo 23 to 28 mm in length, approximately 54 days. **F,** Adult face. Approximate derivatives of medial nasal prominence, lateral nasal prominence, and maxillary prominence are indicated.

[handwritten: initial for sep. of oral cavity 1) LNP 2) MNP 3) max.]

ever, before that contact is made, the maxillary prominence (MxP) has already grown forward from its origin at the proximal end of the first visceral arch (Figs. 1-7, *A* and 1-13) to merge with the LNP and make early contact with the MNP (Fig. 1-7, *G*). With development of the lateral nasal prominence—medial nasal prominence contact, all three prominences contribute to the initial separation of the developing oral cavity and nasal pit (Fig. 1-7, *C*). This separation is usually called the *primary palate* (Fig. 1-9, *A* to *C*). The combined right and left maxillary prominences are sometimes called the intermaxillary segment.

The contacting epithelia form the epithelial seam. Before contact many of the surface epithelial (peridermal) cells are lost, and the underlying basal epithelial cells appear to actively participate in the contact phenomenon by forming processes that span the space between the contacting epithelia. During the fifth week of human embryonic development, a portion of the epithelial seam breaks down and the mesenchyme of the three prominences becomes

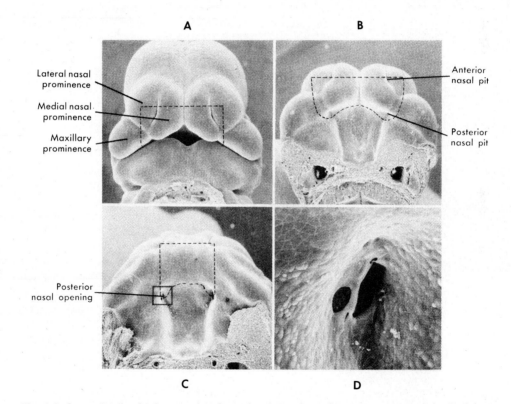

A

B

Lateral nasal prominence

Medial nasal prominence

Maxillary prominence

Anterior nasal pit

Posterior nasal pit

Posterior nasal opening

C

D

Fig. 1-9. Some details of primary palate formation, here shown in mouse, are conveniently demonstrated by scanning electron micrographs (SEMs). Area encompassed by developing primary palate is outlined by broken lines. **A** and **B,** Frontal and palatal views showing moderately advanced stage of primary palate formation. **C** and **D,** In this more advanced stage, elimination of epithelial connection between anterior and posterior nasal pits is nearing completion. Area outlined by solid lines in **C** is given in **D,** showing that last epithelial elements are regressing as nasal passage is now almost completely opened. *[handwritten: to oral cavity.]*

Oral (Nasal) Pharyngeal membrane

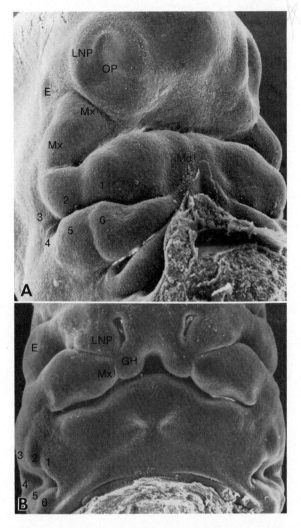

Fig. 1-10. Human embryos of approximately 29 and 35 days' gestational age. **A,** In younger embryo, lateral edge of olfactory placode *(OP)* is beginning to curl forward, initiating formation of lateral nasal prominence *(LNP)*. Groove between anterior extension *(Mx')* of maxillary prominences *(MP)* and olfactory placode will form lacrimal duct. Auricular hillocks of mandibular arch *(1, 2, and 3)* and hyoid arch *(4, 5, and 6)* will form external ear. Location of eye *(E)* is indicated. **B,** Globular process of His *(GH)* of medial nasal prominence of medial side and lateral nasal prominence and maxillary prominence *(Mx')* on lateral side fuse together to separate olfactory pit from oral cavity. Rapid growth of ventral midline portions of mandibular and hyoid prominences separates auricular hillocks. Eye *(E)* is now of considerable size. (From collection of K. K. Sulik.)

confluent. Fluid accumulates between the cells of the persisting epithelium behind the point of epithelial breakdown. Eventually, these fluid-filled spaces coalesce to form the initial nasal passageway connecting the olfactory pit with the roof of the primitive oral cavity (Fig. 1-9). The tissue resulting from development and fusion of these prominences is termed the *primary palate* (outlined by broken lines in Fig. 1-9). It forms the roof of the anterior portion of the primitive oral cavity, as well as forming the initial separation between the oral and nasal cavities. In later development, derivatives of the primary palate form portions of the upper lip, anterior maxilla, and upper incisor teeth.

The outlines of the developing external nose can be seen in Fig. 1-12. Although the nose is disproportionately large, the basic form is easily recognizable. Subsequent alterations in form lead to progressively more mature structure (Fig. 1-1, day 50 specimen). Fig. 1-8 is a schematic illustration of the contribution of various facial prominences to the development of the external face.

Development of maxillary prominences and secondary palate. New outgrowths from the medial edges of the maxillary prominences form the shelves of the secondary palate. These palatal shelves grow downward beside the tongue (Figs. 1-11), at which time the tongue partially fills the nasal cavities. At about the ninth gestational week, the shelves elevate, make contact, and fuse with each other above the tongue (Fig. 1-12). In the anterior region, the shelves are brought to the horizontal position by a rotational (hingelike) movement. In the more posterior regions, the shelves appear to alter their position by changing shape (remodeling) as well as by rotation. Available evidence indicates that the shelves are incapable of elevation until the tongue is first withdrawn from between them. Although

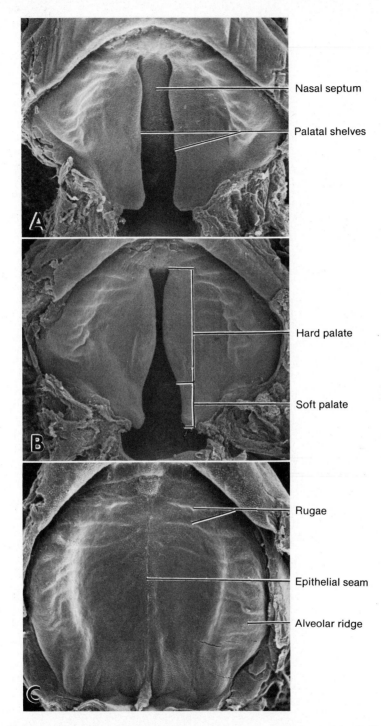

Fig. 1-11. Scanning electron micrographs of developing human secondary palate. **A,** Near completion of shelf elevation; **B,** palatal shelves almost in contact; **C,** contact between shelf edges has been made almost throughout entire length of hard and soft palate. Contacting epithelial seam rapidly disappears (see text). (From Russell MM: Comparative Morphogenesis of the Secondary Palate in Murine and Human Embryos, PhD thesis, University of North Carolina, 1986.)

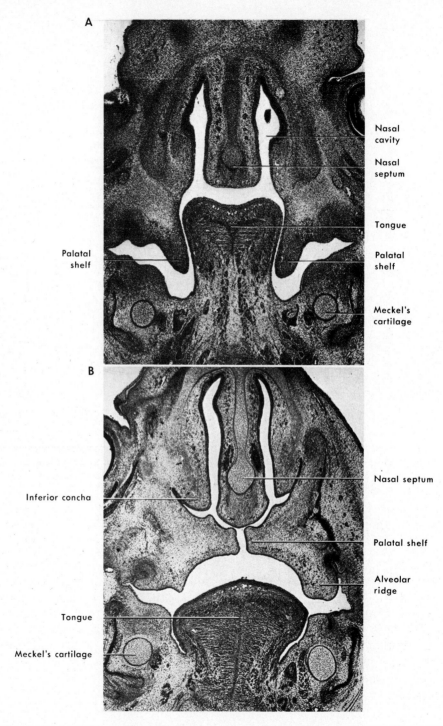

A

Nasal
cavity

Nasal
septum

Tongue

Palatal
shelf

Palatal
shelf

Meckel's
cartilage

B

Inferior concha

Nasal septum

Palatal shelf

Alveolar
ridge

Tongue

Meckel's cartilage

Fig. 1-12. For legend see opposite page.

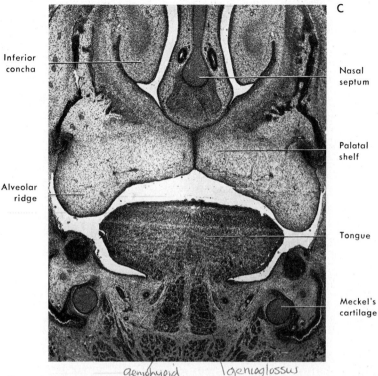

Inferior
concha

C

Nasal
septum

Palatal
shelf

Alveolar
ridge

Tongue

Meckel's
cartilage

geniohyoid   genioglossus

Fig. 1-12. Coronal sections through secondary palates of human embryos showing progressive stages of development. **A,** Frontal section through head of 7-week embryo. Tongue is high and narrow between vertical palatal shelves. Meckel's cartilage is first visceral arch cartilage. **B,** Frontal section through head of slightly more advanced embryo. Tongue has left space between palatal shelves and lies flat and wide within mandibular arch. Palatal shelves have assumed horizontal positon. **C,** Frontal section through head of embryo slightly older than that in **B.** Horizontal palatal shelves are fusing with each other and with nasal septum. Secondary palate separates nasal cavities from oral cavity. (**A** and **B** courtesy P. Gruenwald, Richmond, Va.)

the motivating force for shelf elevation is not clearly defined, contractile elements may be involved.

Fusion of palatal shelves requires alterations in the epithelium of the medial edges that begin prior to elevation. These alterations consist of cessation of cell division, which appears to be mediated through distinct underlying biochemical pathways, including a rise in cyclic AMP levels. There is also loss of some surface epithelial (peridermal) cells (Fig. 1-13) and production of extracellular surface sub-

stances, particularly glycoproteins, that appear to enhance adhesion between the shelf edges as well as between the shelves and inferior margin of the nasal septum (Fig. 1-12).

The ultimate fate of these remaining epithelial cells is controversial. Some of them appear to undergo cell death and eventually are phagocytized, but recent studies indicate that many undergo direct transformation in mesenchymal cells. The fate of cells in the epithelial seam of the primary palate described previously also is ques-

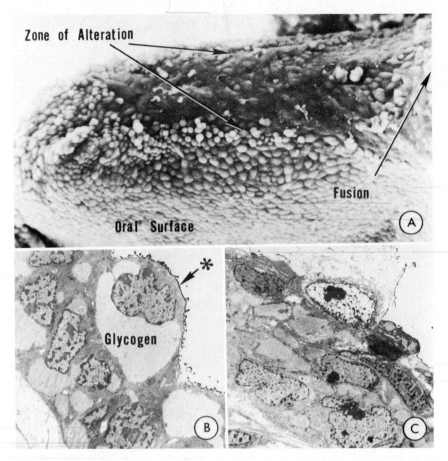

Fig. 1-13. Scanning and transmission electron micrographs of palatal shelf of human embryo at same stage of development as reconstruction in Fig. 1-9, *B.* **A,** Posterior region of palatal shelf viewed from below and from opposite side. Fusion will occur in "zone of alteration," where surface epithelial (peridermal) cells have been lost (see text). Transmission electron micrographs of specimen in **A.** Surface cells of oral epithelium in **B** contain large amounts of glycogen, whereas those of zone of alteration in **C** are undergoing degenerative changes and many of them are presumably desquamated into oral cavity fluids. Asterisk in **B** indicates heavy metal deposited on embryo surfaces for scanning electron microscopy. (**A** to **C** from Waterman RE and Meller SM: Anat Rec 180:11, 1974.)

tionable. Some of the epithelial cells remain indefinitely in clusters (cell rests) along the fusion line. Eventually, most of the hard palate and all of the soft palate form from the secondary palate (see Chapter 8).

Development of visceral arches and tongue. The pituitary gland develops as a result of inductive interactions between the ventral forebrain and oral ectoderm and is derived in part from both tissues (Figs. 1-14 and 1-15). Following initial crest cell migration (Fig. 1-7, A), these cells invade the area of the developing pituitary gland and are continuous with cells that will later form the maxillary prominence. Eventually, crest cells form the connective tissue components of the gland.

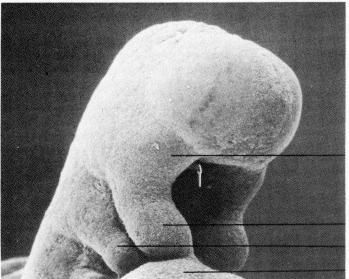

Maxillary
prominence

Mandibular
visceral arch

Hyoid viscera
arch

Heart

Fig. 1-14. Scanning electron micrograph of ferret embryo showing intermediate stage of visceral arch development. Eventually both mandibular and hyoid visceral arches come together in ventral midline as heart recedes caudally. *Arrow,* Opening to Rathke's pouch is located at medial edge of maxillary prominence, which is just beginning to form recognizable structure. (Courtesy A.J. Steffek and D. Mujwid, Chicago.)

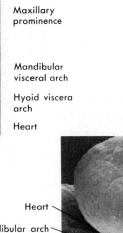

Heart

Mandibular arch

Hyoid arch

B

Forebrain

Oral fossa

Buccopharyngeal
membrane

A Mandibular arch

Foregut

Heart

Notochord

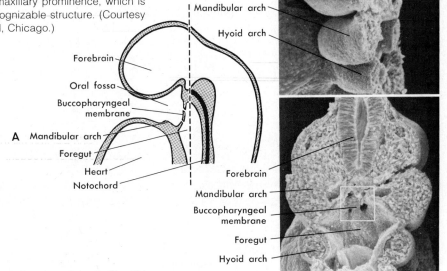

Forebrain

Mandibular arch

Buccopharyngeal
membrane

Foregut

Hyoid arch

C

Fig. 1-15. Oropharyngeal development. **A,** Diagram of sagittal section through head of 3½- to 4-week-old human embryo. Oral fossa is separated from foregut by double layer of epithelium (buccopharyngeal membrane), which is in its early stages of breakdown. **B** and **C,** Scanning electron micrographs (SEMs) of mouse head sectioned in plane indicated by broken line in **A. B,** More lateral view of specimen while in **C** it is viewed from its posterior aspect. Rupturing buccopharyngeal membrane is outlined by rectangle in this figure.

In humans there is a total of six visceral arches, of which the fifth is rudimentary. The proximal portion of the first (mandibular) arch becomes the maxillary prominence (Figs. 1-1 and 1-14). As the heart recedes caudally, the mandibular and hyoid arches develop further at their distal portions to become consolidated in the ventral midline (Figs. 1-7, 1-14, and 1-15). As noted previously, the mesodermal core of each visceral arch (Fig. 1-7, A) is concerned primarily with the formation of vascular endothelial cells. As noted below, these cells appear to be later replaced by cells that eventually form visceral arch myoblasts.

The first (mandibular) and second (hyoid) visceral arches undergo further developmental changes. As the heart recedes caudally, both arches send out bilateral processes that merge with their opposite members in the ventral midline (Figs. 1-7 and 1-14).

Nerve fibers from the fifth, seventh, ninth, and tenth cranial nerves extend into the mesoderm of the first four visceral arches. The mesoderm of the definitive mandibular and hyoid arches gives rise to the fifth and seventh nerve musculature, while mesoderm associated with the less well developed third and fourth arches forms the ninth and tenth nerve musculature. Recent studies show that myoblast cells in the visceral arches actually originate from mesoderm more closely associated with the neural tube (as do the cells that form the hypoglossal and extrinsic eye musculature; Fig. 1-6). They would then migrate into the visceral arches and replace the mesodermal cells that initiated blood vessel formation earlier (see p. 5). It therefore appears that myoblasts forming voluntary striated muscle fibers of the facial region would then originate from mesoderm *adjacent to the neural tube.*

Groups of visceral arch myoblasts that are destined to form individual muscles each take a branch of the appropriate visceral arch nerve. Myoblasts from the second visceral arch, for example, take branches of the seventh cranial nerve and migrate very extensively throughout the head and neck to form the contractile components of the "muscles of facial expression." Myoblasts from the first arch contribute mostly to the muscles of mastication, while those from the third and fourth arches contribute to the pharyngeal and soft palate musculature. As noted earlier, connective tissue components of each muscle in the facial region are provided by mesenchymal cells of crest origin.

The crest mesenchymal cells of the visceral arches give rise to skeletal components such as the temporary visceral arch cartilages (e.g., Meckel's cartilage; Fig. 1-12), middle ear cartilages, and mandibular bones. Also visceral arch crest cells form connective tissues such as dermis and the connective tissue components of the tongue.

The tongue forms in the ventral floor of the pharynx after arrival of the hypoglossal muscle cells. The significance of the lateral lingual tubercles (Fig. 1-16) and other swellings in the forming tongue has not been carefully documented. It is known that the anterior two thirds of the tongue is covered by ectoderm whereas endoderm covers the posterior one third. The thyroid gland forms by invagination of the most anterior endoderm (thyroglossal duct). A residual pit (the foramen cecum; Fig. 1-16, C) left in the epithelium at the site of invagination marks the junction between the anterior two thirds and posterior one third of the tongue, which are, respectively, covered by epithelia of ectodermal and endodermal origin. It is also known that the connective tissue components of the anterior two thirds of the tongue are derived

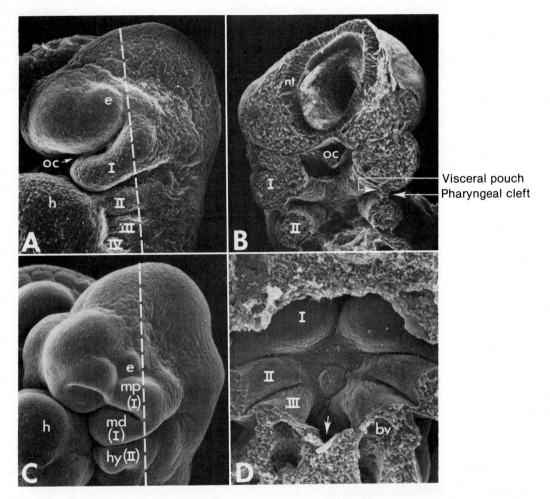

Fig. 1-16. Scanning electron micrographs of developing visceral arches and tongue of mouse embryos. Planes of section illustrated in **B** and **D** (dorsal views of floor of pharynx) are shown in **A** and **C. A** and **B,** Embryos whose developmental age is approximately equivalent to that of human 30-day-old embryos. (See Fig. 1-1.) Development of medial and lateral nasal prominences has yet to be initiated. Visceral arches are indicated by Roman numerals. First (mandibular) arch is almost separated from heart *(h).* Other structures indicated are eye *(e),* oral cavity *(oc;* compare to buccopharyngeal membrane in Fig. 1-14, *C),* and neural tube *(nt).* **C** and **D,** These are comparable to 35-day-old human embryos. The mandibular arch now has two distinct prominences, maxillary prominence *(mp),* and mandibular prominence *(md).* Second arch is called hyoid arch *(hy).* In **D** blood vessel exiting from third arch is labeled *bv.* Arrow indicates entry into lower pharynx.

Continued.

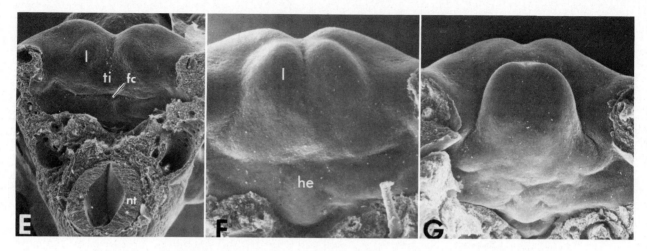

Fig. 1-16 cont'd. E to **G,** Older specimens, prepared in a manner similar to **B** and **D,** illustrate development of tongue. Lingual swellings *(l)* presumably represent accumulations of myoblasts derived from hypoglossal cord. Tuberculum impar *(ti)* also contributes to anterior two thirds of tongue. Foramen cecum *(fc)* is site of endodormal invagination that gives rise to epithelial components of thyroid gland. It lies at junction between anterior two thirds and posterior one third of tongue. Hypobranchial eminence *(he)* is primordium of epiglottis. (From Johnston MC and Sulik KK: Embryology of the head and neck. In Serafin D, and Georgiade NG, editors: Pediatric plastic surgery, vol I, St Louis, 1984, The CV Mosby Co.)

from first-arch mesenchyme, whereas those of the posterior one third appear to be primarily derived from the third-arch mesenchyme.

The epithelial components of a number of glands are derived from the endodermal lining of the pharynx. In addition to the thyroid, these include the parathyroid and thymus. The epithelial components of the salivary and anterior pituitary glands are derived from oral ectoderm.

Finally, a lateral extension from the inner groove between the first and second arch gives rise to the eustachian tube, which connects the pharynx with the ear. The external ear, or pinna, is formed at least partially from tissues of the first and second arches (Fig. 1-1, day 44).

FINAL DIFFERENTIATION OF FACIAL TISSUES

The extensive cell migrations referred to above bring cell populations into new relationships and lead to further inductive interactions, which, in turn, lead to progressively more differentiated cell types. For example, some of the crest cells coming into contact with pharyngeal endoderm are induced by the endoderm to form visceral arch cartilages (see Chapter 8). Recent studies indicate the early epithelial interactions are also involved in bone formation. The exact interactions involved in tooth formation are somewhat controversial. Mesenchymal cells of crest origin must be involved, and these cells form the dental papilla and the mesenchyme surrounding the epithelial enamel organ. Whether the epithelium or mesenchyme is initially responsible for determining which tooth (e.g., incisor or molar) forms from a tooth germ is controversial. Interestingly, epithelia from species that ceased forming teeth many centuries ago (e.g., the chick) can still form enamel under experimental conditions.

In many instances, such as those cited above, only crest mesenchymal cells and not mesodermal mesenchymal cells will respond to inducing tissues such as pharyngeal endoderm. In other cases, as in the differentiation of dermis and meninges, it appears that the origin of the mesenchyme is of no consequence. In any case it is clear that one function the formation of skeletal and connective tissues, ordinarily performed by mesodermal cells in other regions, has been usurped by neural crest cells in the facial region. The crest cells therefore play a very dominant role in facial development, since they form all nonepithelial components except endothelial cells and the contractile elements of skeletal (voluntary) muscle.

The onset of bone formation or the establishment of all the organ systems (about the eighth week of development) is considered the termination of the embryonic period. Bone formation and other aspects of the final differentiation of facial tissues will be considered in detail elsewhere in this text.

CLINICAL CONSIDERATIONS

Aberrations in embryonic facial development lead to a wide variety of defects. Although any step may be impaired, defects of primary and secondary palate development are most common. There is evidence that other developmental defects may be even more common but they are not compatible with completion of intrauterine life and are therefore not as well documented.

Facial clefts

Most cases of clefts of the lip with or without associated cleft palate (Fig. 1-17) appear to form a group etiologically different from clefts involving only the secondary palate. For example, when more than one child in a family has facial clefts, the clefts are almost always found to belong only to one group.

Some evidence now indicates that there are two major etiologically and developmentally distinct types of cleft lips and palate. In the larger group, deficient medial nasal prominences appear to be the major developmental alteration, whereas in the smaller group the major developmental alteration appears to be underdevelopment of the maxillary prominence. Increases in clefting rates have been associated with children born to epileptic mothers undergoing phenytoin (Dilantin) therapy and to mothers who smoke cigarettes; in the latter case the embryonic effects are thought to result from hypoxia. When pregnant mice are exposed to hypoxia, the portion of the olfactory placode undergoing morphogenetic movements (Fig. 1-1) breaks down, and this is associated with underdevelopment of the lateral nasal prominence. Reduction in the size of the lateral nasal prominence that is more severe than that of other facial prominences also has been observed in an animal model of phenytoin-induced cleft lip and palate. Combinations of developmental alterations (e.g., placodal breakdown associated with medial nasal prominence deficiency) may relate to the multifactorial etiology thought to be responsible for many human cleft cases.

About two thirds of patients with clefts of the primary palate also have clefts of the secondary palate. Studies of experimental animals suggest that excessive separation of jaw segments as a result of the primary palate cleft prevents the palatal shelves

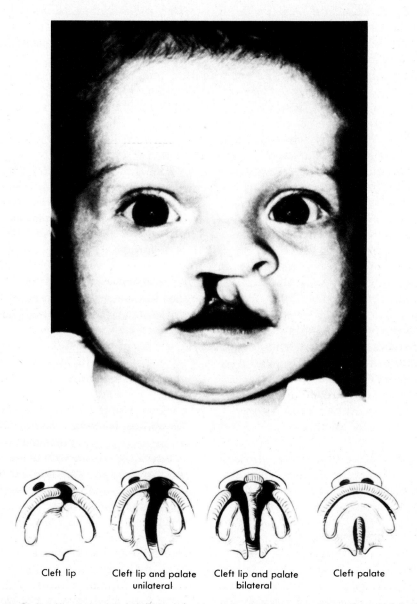

Fig. 1-17. Clefts of lip and palate in infants. Infant in photograph has complete unilateral cleft of lip and palate. (From Ross RB, and Johnston MC: Cleft lip and palate, Baltimore, 1972, The Williams & Wilkins Co.)

from contacting after elevation. The degree of clefting is highly variable. Clefts may be either bilateral or unilateral (Fig. 1-17) and complete or incomplete. Most of this variation results from differing degrees of fusion and may be explained by variable degrees of mesenchyme in the facial prominences. Some of the variation may represent different initiating events.

Clefts involving only the secondary palate (cleft palate, Fig. 1-17) constitute, after clefts involving the primary palate, the second most frequent facial malformation in humans. Cleft palate can also be produced in experimental animals with a wide variety of chemical agents or other manipulations affecting the embryo. Usually, such agents retard or prevent shelf elevation. In other cases, however, it is shelf growth that is retarded so that, although elevation occurs, the shelves are too small to make contact. There is also some evidence that indicates that failure of the epithelial seam or failure of it to be replaced by mesenchyme occurs after the application of some environmental agents. Cleft formation could then result from rupture of the persisting seam, which would not have sufficient strength to prevent such rupture indefinitely.

Less frequently, other types of facial clefting are observed. In most instances they can be explained by failure of fusion or merging between facial prominences of reduced size, and similar clefts can be produced experimentally. Examples include failure of merging and fusion between the maxillary prominence and the lateral nasal prominence, leading to oblique facial clefts, or failure of merging of the maxillary prominence and mandibular arch, leading to lateral facial clefts (macrostomia). Many of the variations in the position or degree of these rare facial clefts may depend on the timing or position of arrest of growth of

the maxillary prominence that normally merges and fuses with adjacent structures (Fig. 1-8). Other rare facial malformations (including oblique facial clefts) may also result from abnormal pressures or fusions with folds in the fetal (e.g., amniotic) membranes.

Also new evidence regarding the apparent role of epithelial-mesenchymal interactions via the mesenchymal cell process meshwork (CPM) may help to explain the frequent association between facial abnormalities, especially clefts, and limb defects. Genetic and/or environmental influences on this interaction might well affect both areas in the same individual.

Hemifacial microsomia

The term "hemifacial microsomia" is used to describe malformations involving underdevelopment and other abnormalities of the temporomandibular joint, the external and middle ear, and other structures in this region, such as the parotid gland and muscles of mastication. Substantial numbers of cases have associated malformations of the vertebrae and clefts of the lip and/or palate. The combination with vertebral anomalies is often considered to denote a distinct etiologic syndrome (oculo-auriculo-vertebral syndrome, etc.). As a group these malformations constitute the third most common group of major craniofacial malformations, after the two major groups of facial clefts.

Somewhat similar malformations have resulted from inadvertent use of the acne drug retinoic acid (Accutane) in pregnant women. Animal models using this drug have produced very similar malformations, many of which appear to result from major effects on neural crest cells. This has resulted in reevaluation of an earlier animal model that indicated that the malformation resulted from hemorrhage at the point where the external carotid artery fuses with the stapedial artery (Fig. 1-5). It now appears probable that at least some aspects of many hemifacial microsomia cases result from primary effects on crest cells. Malformations similar to hemifacial microsomia occurred in the fetuses of women who had taken the drug thalidomide.

Treacher Collins' syndrome

Treacher Collins' syndrome (mandibulofacial dysostosis) is an inherited disorder that results from the action of a dominant gene and may be almost as common as hemifacial microsomia. The syndrome consists of underdevelopment of the tissues derived from the maxillary, mandibular, and hyoid prominences. The external, middle, and inner ear are often defective, and clefts of the secondary palate are found in about one third of the cases. Defects of a similar nature result from the action of an abnormal gene in mice and can also be produced experimentally with excessive doses of retinoic acid (Accutane) administered at a later stage in development. Here, the primary effect appears to be on ganglionic placodal cells (Fig. 1-4). Although not limited to placodal cells of the massive trigeminal ganglion, most of the characteristic alterations in development appear to result from secondary effects on crest cells in this area.

Labial pits

Small pits may persist on either side of the midline of the lower lip. They are caused by the failure of the embryonic labial pits to disappear.

Lingual anomalies

Median rhomboid glossitis, an innocuous, red, rhomboidal smooth zone of the tongue in the midline in front of the foramen cecum, is considered the result of persistance of the tuberculum impar. Lack of fusion between the two lateral lingual prominences may produce a bifid tongue. Thyroid tissue may be present in the base of the tongue.

Developmental cysts

Epithelial rests in lines of union, of facial or oral prominences or from epithelial organs, (e.g., *vestigial nasopalatine ducts*) may give rise to cysts lined with epithelium.

Branchial cleft (cervical) cysts or fistulas may arise from the rests of epithelium in the visceral arch area. They usually are laterally disposed on the neck. Thyroglossal duct cysts may occur at any place along the course of the duct, usually at or near the midline.

Cysts may arise from epithelial rests after the fusion of medial, maxillary, and lateral nasal prominences. They are called globulomaxillary cysts and are lined with pseudostratified columnar epithelium and squamous epithelium. They may, however, develop as primordial cysts from a supernumerary tooth germ.

Anterior palatine cysts are situated in the midline of the maxillary alveolar prominence. Once believed to be from remnants of the fusion of two prominences, they may be primordial cysts of odontogenic origin; their true nature is a subject of discussion.

Nasolabial cysts, originating in the base of the wing of the nose and bulging into the nasal and oral vestibule and the root of the upper lip, sometimes causing a flat depression on the anterior surface of the alveolar prominence, are also explained as originating from epithelial remnants in the cleft-lip line. It is, however, more probable that they derive from excessive epithelial proliferations that normally, for some time in embryonic life, plug the nostrils. It is also possible that they are retention cysts of vestibular nasal glands or that they develop from the epithelium of the nasolacrimal duct.

REFERENCES

Adelmann HB: The problem of cyclopia, Q Rev Biophys 11:61, 284, 1937.

Ardinger HH, Buetow KH, Bell GI et al: Association of genetic variation of the transforming growth factor-alpha gene with cleft lip and palate, Am J Hum Genet 45:348, 1989.

Bronsky PT, Johnston MC, and Sulik KK: Morphogenesis of hypoxia-induced cleft lip in CL/Fr mice, J Craniofac Genet Dev Biol (suppl)2:113, 1986.

Chung CS, Bixler D, Watanabe T et al: Segregation analysis of cleft lip with or without cleft palate: a comparison of Danish and Japanese data, Am J Hum Genet 39:603, 1986.

Couly GF and Le Douarin NM: The fate map of the cephalic neural primordium at the presomitic to the 3-somite stage in the avian embryo, Development 103 Supplement 101-113, 1988.

Eichele G and Thaller C: Characterization of concentration gradients of a morphogenetically active retinoid in the chick limb bud, J Cell Biol 105:1917, 1987.

Erickson CA: Morphogenesis of the neural crest. In Browder LW, editor: Developmental biology: a comprehensive synthesis, vol 2, New York, 1986, Plenum Press.

Fitchett JE and Hay ED: Medial edge epithelium transforms to mesenchyme after embryonic palatal shelves fuse, Dev Biol 131:455, 1989.

Gasser RF: The development of the facial muscles in man, Am J Anat 120:357, 1967.

Goulding EH and Pratt RM: Isotretinoin teratogenicity in mouse whole embryo culture, J Craniofac Genet Dev Biol 6:99, 1986.

Hall BK: The embryonic development of bone, Amer Scientist 76(2):174, 1988.

Hamilton WJ and Mossman H: Human embryology, ed 4, Cambridge, 1972, W Heffer & Sons, Ltd.

Hay ED and Meier S: Tissue interactions in development. In Shaw JH et al, editors: Textbook of oral biology, Philadelphia, 1978, WB Saunders Co.

Hazelton RB: A radioautographic analysis of the migration and fate of cells derived from the occipital somites of the chick embryo with specific reference to the hypoglossal musculature, J Embryol Exp Morphol 24:455, 1971.

Hinrichsen K: The early development of morphology and patterns of the face in the human embryo, Adv Anat Embryol Cell Biol 98:1, 1985.

Holtfreter JE: A new look at Spemann's organizer. In Browder LW, editor: Developmental biology: a comprehensive synthesis, vol 5, New York, 1988, Plenum Publishing Corp.

Jirásek JE: Atlas of human prenatal morphogenesis, Hingham, Mass, 1983, Martinus Nijhoff Publishers.

Johnston MC: Embryology of the head and neck. In McCarthy J, editor: Plastic surgery, Philadelphia, WB Saunders Co (in press).

Johnston MC, Bhakdinaronk A, and Reid YC: An expanded role for the neural crest in oral and pharyngeal development. In Bosma JF editor: Oral sensation and preception: development in the fetus and infant, Washington, DC, 1974, US Government Printing Office.

Johnston MC, Bronsky PT, and Millicovsky G: Embryogenesis of cleft lip. In McCarthy J, editor: Plastic surgery, Philadelphia, WB Saunders Co (in press).

Johnston MC and Hunter WS: Cleft lip and/or palate in twins: evidence for two major cleft lip groups, Teratology 39:461, 1989.

Johnston MC and Listgarten MA: The migration interaction and early differentiation of oral-facial tissues. In Slavkin HS and Bavetta LA, editors: Developmental aspects of oral biology, New York, 1972, Academic Press, Inc.

Johnston MC, Noden DM, Hazelton RD et al: Origins of avian ocular and periocular tissues, Exp Eye Res 29:27, 1979.

Johnston MC and Sulik KK: Embryology of the head and neck. In Serafin D and Georgiade NG, editors: Pediatric plastic surgery, vol 1, St Louis, 1984, The CV Mosby Co.

Johnston MC, Vig K, and Ambrose L: Neurocristopathy as a unifying concept: clinical correlations, Adv Neurol 29:97, 1981.

Keels MA: The role of maternal cigarette smoking in the etiology of cleft lip with or without cleft palate, doctoral dissertation, University of North Carolina, Chapel Hill (in preparation).

Kraus BS, Kitamura H, and Latham RA: Atlas of the developmental anatomy of the face, New York, 1966, Harper & Row, Publishers.

LeLievre C and LeDouarin NM: Mesenchymal derivatives of the neural crest: analysis of chimeric quail and chick embryos, J Embryol Exp Morphol 34:125, 1975.

Millicovsky G and Johnston MC: Hyperoxia and hypoxia in pregnancy: simple experimental manipulation alters the incidence of cleft lip and palate in CL/Fr mice, Proc Natl Acad Sci USA 9:4723, 1981.

Minkoff R and Kuntz AJ: Cell proliferation during morphogenetic changes: analysis of frontonasal morphogenesis in the chick embryo employing DNA labelling indices, J Embryol Exp Morphol 40:101, 1977.

Minkoff R and Kuntz AJ: Cell proliferation and cell density of mesenchyme in the maxillary process on adjacent regions during facial development in the chick embryo, J Embryol Exp Morphol 46:65, 1978.

Moore KL: The developing human, ed 4, Philadelphia, 1989, WB Saunders Co.

Nicolet G: Analyse autoradiographique de la localisation des différentes ébauches présomptives dans la ligne primitive de l'embryon de poulet, J Embryol Exp Morphol 23:79, 1970.

Nishimura H: Incidence of malformations in abortions. In Fraser FC and McKusick VA, editors: Congenital malformations, Amsterdam, 1969, Excerpta Medica Press.

Nishimura H, Semba R, Tanimura P, and Tanaka O.: Prenatal development of humans with special reference to craniofacial structures: an atlas, Washington, DC, 1977, US Government Printing Office.

Noden DM: Interactions directing the migration and cytodifferentiation of avian neural crest cells. In Garrod DR, editor: Specificity of embryological interactions, vol 5, London, 1978, Chapman & Hall Ltd.

Noden DM: Embryonic origins of avain cephalic and cervial muscles and associated connective tissue, Am J Anat 168:257, 1983.

Noden DM: Interactions and fates of avian craniofacial mesenchyme, Development 103(Supplement): 121-140, 1988.

Patterson S, Minkoff R, and Johnston MC: Autoradiographic studies of cell migration during primary palate formation, J Dent Res 58:113, 1979 (abstract).

Poswillo D: The pathogenesis of the first and second branchial arch syndrome, Oral Surg 35:302, 1973.

Pourtois M: Morphogenesis of the primary and secondary palate. In Slavkin HS and Bavetta LA, editors: Developmental aspects of oral biology, New York, 1972, Academic Press.

Pratt RM and Martin GR: Epithelial cell death and elevated cyclic AMP during palatal development, Proc Natl Acad Sci USA 72:814, 1975.

Ross RB and Johnston MC: Cleft lip and palate, Baltimore, 1972, The Williams & Wilkins Co.

Sadler TW: Langman's medical embryology, ed 6, Baltimore, 1990, Williams & Wilkins.

Sicher H and Tandler J: Anatomie fur Zahnarzte (Anatomy for dentists), Berlin, 1928, Springer Verlag.

Smuts MK: Rapid nasal pit formation in mouse stimulated by ATP-containing medium, J Exp Zool 216:409, 1981.

Sperberg GH: Craniofacial embryology, Bristol, England, 1976, John Wright & Sons, Ltd.

Streeter GL: Developmental horizons in human embryos, Contrib Embryol 32:133, 1948.

Sulik KK, Cook CS, and Webster WS: Teratogens and craniofacial malformations: relationships to cell death, Development 103 (Supplement): 213-232, 1988.

Sulik KK and Johnston MC: Sequence of developmental changes following ethanol exposure in mice: craniofacial features in the fetal alcohol syndrome (FAS), Am J Anat 166:257, 1983.

Sulik KK, Johnston MC, Ambrose JLH, and Dorgan DR: Phenytoin (Dilantin)-induced cleft lip, a scanning and transmission electron microscopic study, Anat Rec 195:243, 1979.

Sulik KK, Johnston MC, Smiley SJ et al: Mandibulofacial dysostosis (Treacher Collins' syndrome): a new proposal for its pathogenesis, Am J Med Genet 27:359, 1987.

Tam PPL and Beddington RSP: The formation of mesodermal tissues in the mouse embryo during gastrulation and early organogenesis, Development 99:109, 1987.

Tam PPL and Meier S: The establishment of a somitomeric pattern in the mesoderm of the gastrulating mouse embryo, J Anat 164:209, 1982.

Tamarin A and Boyde A: Facial and visceral arch development in the mouse embryo: a study by scanning electron microscopy, J Anat 124:563, 1977.

Tan SS and Morriss-Kay G: The development and distribution of cranial neural crest in the ray embryo, Cell Tissue Res 240:403, 1985.

Tan SS and Morriss-Kay GM: Analysis of cranial neural crest cell migration and early fates in postimplantation rat, Morphology 98:21, 1986.

Tessier R: Anatomical classification of facial, craniofacial and latero-facial clefts, J Maxillofac Surg 4:69, 1976.

Tolarova M: Orofacial clefts in Czechoslovakia, Scand J Plast Reconstr Surg 21:19, 1987.

Tosney KW: The segregation and early migration of cranial neural crest cells in the avian embryo, Dev Biol 89:13, 1982.

Trasler DG: Pathogenesis of cleft lip and its relation to embryonic face shape in A/Jax and C57BL mice, Teratology 1:33, 1968.

Trasler DG and Fraser FC: Time-position relationships with particular references to cleft lip and cleft palate. In Wilson JC and Fraser FC, editors: Handbook of teratology, vol 2, New York, 1977, Plenum Press.

Wachtler F and Jacob M: Origin and development of the cranial skeletal muscles, Bibl Anat 29:24, 1986.

Waterman RE and Meller SM: A scanning electron microscope study of secondary palate formation in the human, Anat Rec 175:464, 1973.

Waterman RE and Meller SM: Normal facial development in the human embryo. In Shaw JH et al., editors: Textbook of oral biology, Philadelphia, 1978, WB Saunders Co.

Webster WS, Johnston MC, Lammer EJ, and Sulik KK: Isotretinoin embryopathy and the cranial neural crest: an in vivo and in vitro study, J Craniofac Genet Dev Biol 6:211, 1986.

Weston JA: The migration and differentiation of neural crest cells, Adv Morphol 8:41, 1970.

2

DEVELOPMENT AND GROWTH OF TEETH

The primitive oral cavity, or stomodeum, is lined by stratified squamous epithelium called the oral ectoderm. The oral ectoderm contacts the endoderm of the foregut to form the buccopharyngeal membrane (Fig. 1-9). At about the twenty-seventh day of gestation this membrane ruptures and the primitive oral cavity establishes a connection with the foregut. Most of the connective tissue cells underlying the oral ectoderm are neural crest or ectomesenchyme in origin. These cells are thought to instruct or induce the overlying ectoderm to start tooth development, which begins in the anterior portion of what will be the future maxilla and mandible and proceeds posteriorly. (See Chapter 1 for more details on embryonic induction.)

DENTAL LAMINA

Two or 3 weeks after the rupture of the buccopharyngeal membrane, when the embryo is about 6 weeks old, certain areas of basal cells of the oral ectoderm proliferate more rapidly than do the cells of the adjacent areas. This leads to the formation of the dental lamina, which is a band of epithelium that has invaded the underlying ectomesenchyme along each of the horseshoe-shaped future dental arches (Figs. 2-1, A, and 2-3). The dental laminae serve as the primordium for the ectodermal portion of the deciduous teeth. Later, during the development of the jaws, the permanent molars arise directly from a distal extension of the dental lamina.

The development of the first permanent

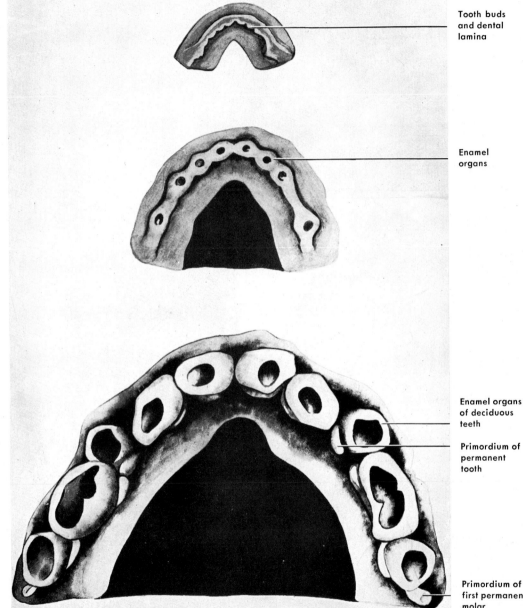

A

Tooth buds
and dental
lamina

B

Enamel
organs

C

Enamel organs
of deciduous
teeth

Primordium of
permanent
tooth

Primordium of
first permanent
molar

Fig. 2-1. Diagrammatic reconstruction of dental lamina and enamel organs of mandible. **A,** 22 mm embryo, bud stage (eighth week). **B,** 43 mm embryo, cap stage (tenth week). **C,** 163 mm embryo, bell stage (about 4 months). Primordia of permanent teeth are seen as thickenings of dental lamina on lingual side of each tooth germ. Distal extension of dental lamina with primordium of first molar.

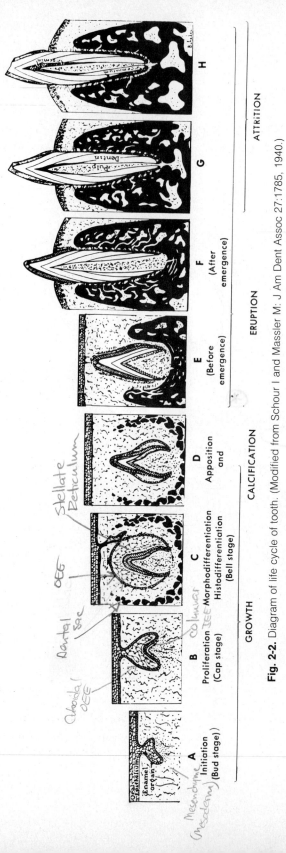

Fig. 2-2. Diagram of life cycle of tooth. (Modified from Schour I and Massler M: J Am Dent Assoc 27:1785, 1940.)

molar is initiated at the fourth month in utero. The second molar is initiated at about the first year after birth, the third molar at the fourth or fifth years. The distal proliferation of the dental lamina is responsible for the location of the germs of the permanent molars in the ramus of the mandible and the tuberosity of the maxilla. The successors of the deciduous teeth develop from a lingual extension of the free end of the dental lamina opposite to the enamel organ of each deciduous tooth (Fig. 2-2, *C*). The lingual extension of the dental lamina is named the successional lamina and develops from the fifth month in utero (permanent central incisor) to the tenth month of age (second premolar).

Fate of dental lamina. It is evident that the total activity of the dental lamina extends over a period of at least 5 years. Any particular portion of the dental lamina functions for a much briefer period since only a relatively short time elapses after initiation of tooth development before the dental lamina begins to degenerate at that particular location. However, the dental lamina may still be active in the third molar region after it has disappeared elsewhere, except for occasional epithelial remnants. As the teeth continue to develop, they lose their connection with the dental lamina. They later break up by mesenchymal invasion, which is at first incomplete and does not perforate the total thickness of the lamina (Fig. 2-8). Remnants of the dental lamina persist as epithelial pearls or islands within the jaw as well as in the gingiva.

Vestibular lamina. Labial and buccal to the dental lamina in each dental arch, another epithelial thickening develops independently and somewhat later. It is the vestibular lamina, also termed the lip furrow band (Figs. 2-6 and 2-7). It subsequently hollows and forms the oral vestibule be-

tween the alveolar portion of the jaws and the lips and cheeks (Figs. 2-10 and 2-11).

TOOTH DEVELOPMENT

At certain points along the dental lamina, each representing the location of one of the 10 mandibular and 10 maxillary deciduous teeth, the ectodermal cells multiply still more rapidly and form little knobs that grow into the underlying mesenchyme (Figs. 2-2 and 2-4). Each of these little downgrowths from the dental lamina represents the beginning of the *enamel organ* of the tooth bud of a deciduous tooth. Not all of these enamel organs start to develop at the same time, and the first to appear are those of the anterior mandibular region.

As cell proliferation continues, each enamel organ increases in size and changes in shape. As it develops, it takes on a shape that resembles a cap, with the outside of the cap directed toward the oral surface (Figs. 2-5 and 2-7).

On the inside of the cap (i.e., inside the depression of the enamel organ), the ectomesenchymal cells increase in number. The tissue appears more dense than the surrounding mesenchyme and represents the beginning of the *dental papilla*. Surrounding the combined enamel organ and dental papilla, the third part of the tooth bud forms. It is the *dental sac,* and it consists of ectomesenchymal cells and fibers that surround the dental papilla and the enamel organ (Fig. 2-8).

During and after these developments the shape of the enamel organ continues to change. The depression occupied by the dental papilla deepens until the enamel organ assumes a shape resembling a bell. As this development takes place, the dental lamina, which had thus far connected the enamel organ to the oral epithelium, breaks up and the tooth bud loses its connection with the epithelium of the primitive oral cavity.

DEVELOPMENTAL STAGES

Although tooth development is a continuous process, the developmental history of a tooth is divided into several morphologic "stages" for descriptive purposes. While the size and shape of individual teeth are different, they pass through similar stages of development. They are named after the shape of the epithelial part of the tooth germ and are called the bud, cap, and bell stages (Fig. 2-2, A to C).

Bud stage

The epithelium of the dental laminae is separated from the underlying ectomesenchyme by a basement membrane (Fig. 2-3). Simultaneous with the differentiation of each dental lamina, round or ovoid swellings arise from the basement membrane at 10 different points, corresponding to the future positions of the deciduous teeth. These are the primordia of the enamel organs, the tooth buds (Fig. 2-4). Thus the development of tooth germs is initiated, and the cells continue to proliferate faster than adjacent cells. The dental lamina is

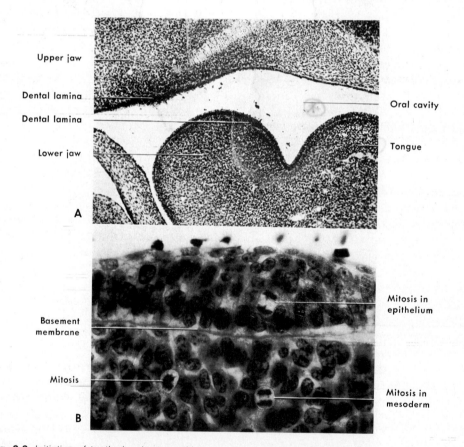

Upper jaw

Dental lamina

Dental lamina

Lower jaw

Oral cavity

Tongue

A

Basement membrane

Mitosis

Mitosis in epithelium

Mitosis in mesoderm

B

Fig. 2-3. Initiation of tooth development. Human embryo 13.5 mm in length, fifth week. **A,** Sagittal section through upper and lower jaws. **B,** High magnification of thickened oral epithelium. (From Orban B: Dental histology and embryology, Philadelphia, 1929, P Blakiston's Son & Co.)

shallow, and microscopic sections often show tooth buds close to the oral epithelium. Since the main function of certain epithelial cells of the tooth bud is to form the tooth enamel, these cells constitute the enamel organ, which is critical to normal tooth development. In the bud stage, the enamel organ consists of peripherally located low columnar cells and centrally located polygonal cells (Fig. 2-4). Many cells of the tooth bud and the surrounding mesenchyme undergo mitosis (Fig. 2-4). As a

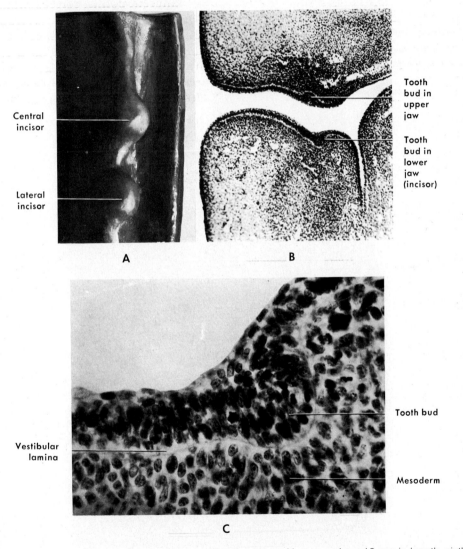

Central incisor

Lateral incisor

A

Tooth bud in upper jaw

Tooth bud in lower jaw (incisor)

B

Vestibular lamina

Tooth bud

Mesoderm

C

Fig. 2-4. Bud stage of tooth development, proliferation stage. Human embryo 16 mm in length, sixth week. **A,** Wax reconstruction of germs of lower central and lateral incisors. **B,** Sagittal section through upper and lower jaws. **C,** High magnification of tooth germ of lower incisor in bud stage. (From Orban B: Dental histology and embryology, Philadelphia, 1929, P Blakiston's Son & Co.)

result of the increased mitotic activity and the migration of neural crest cells into the area the ectomesenchymal cells surrounding the tooth bud condense. The area of ectomesenchymal condensation immediately subjacent to the enamel organ is the dental papilla. The condensed ectomesenchyme that surrounds the tooth bud and the dental papilla is the dental sac (Figs. 2-6, to 2-8). Both the dental papilla and the dental sac become more well defined as the enamel organ grows into the cap and bell shapes (Fig. 2-8). The cells of the dental papilla will form tooth pulp and dentin. The cells in the dental sac will form cementum and the periodontal ligament.

Cap stage

As the tooth bud continues to proliferate, it does not expand uniformly into a larger sphere. Instead, unequal growth in different parts of the tooth bud leads to the cap stage, which is characterized by a shallow invagination on the deep surface of the bud (Figs. 2-2, *B*, and 2-5).

Outer and inner enamel epithelium. The peripheral cells of the cap stage are cuboidal, cover the convexity of the "cap," and are

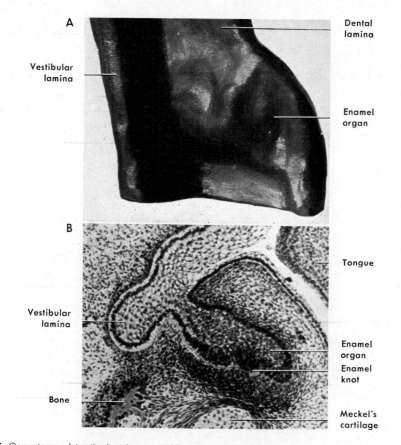

Fig. 2-5. Cap stage of tooth development. Human embryo 31.5 mm in length, ninth week. **A,** Wax reconstruction of enamel organ of lower lateral incisor. **B,** Labiolingual section through same tooth. (From Orban B: Dental histology and embryology, Philadelphia, 1929, P Blakiston's Son & Co.)

called the outer enamel (dental) epithelium. The cells in the concavity of the "cap" become tall, columnar cells and represent the inner enamel (dental) epithelium (Figs. 2-6 and 2-7). The outer enamel epithelium is separated from the dental sac, and the inner enamel epithelium from the dental papilla, by a delicate basement membrane. Hemidesmosomes anchor the cells to the basal lamina.

Stellate reticulum (enamel pulp). Polygonal cells located in the center of the epithelial enamel organ, between the outer and inner enamel epithelia, begin to separate as more intercellular fluid is produced and form a cellular network called the stellate reticu-

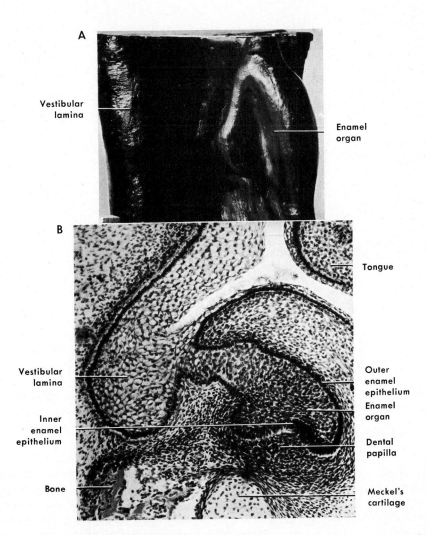

Fig. 2-6. Cap stage of tooth development. Human embryo 41.5 mm in length, tenth week. **A,** Wax reconstruction of enamel organ of lower central incisor. **B,** Labiolingual section through same tooth. (From Orban B: Dental histology and embryology, Philadelphia, 1929, P Blakiston's Son & Co.)

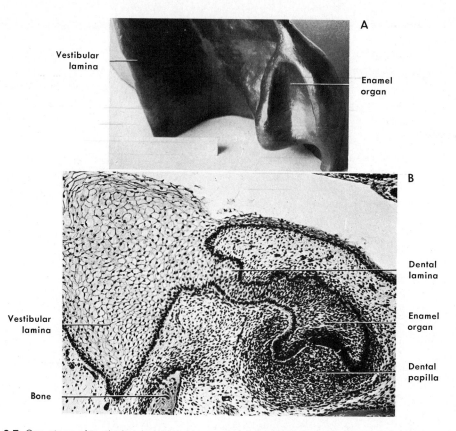

Vestibular
lamina

A

Enamel
organ

B

Dental
lamina

Enamel
organ

Dental
papilla

Vestibular
lamina

Bone

Fig 2-7. Cap stage of tooth development. Human embryo 60 mm in length, eleventh week. **A,** Wax reconstruction of enamel organ of lower lateral incisor. **B,** Labiolingual section through same tooth. (From Orban B: Dental histology and embryology, Philadelphia, 1929, P Blakiston's Son & Co.)

lum (Figs. 2-8 and 2-9). The cells assume a branched reticular form. The spaces in this reticular network are filled with a mucoid fluid that is rich in albumin, which gives the stellate reticulum a cushionlike consistency that may support and protect the delicate enamel-forming cells.

The cells in the center of the enamel organ are densely packed and form the *enamel knot* (Fig. 2-5). This knot projects in part toward the underlying dental papilla, so that the center of the epithelial in-

vagination shows a slightly knoblike enlargement that is bordered by the labial and lingual enamel grooves (Fig. 2-5). At the same time there arises in the increasingly high enamel organ a vertical extension of the enamel knot, called the *enamel cord* (Fig. 2-8). Both are temporary structures that disappear before enamel formation begins. The function of the enamel knot and cord may be to act as a reservoir of dividing cells for the growing enamel organ.

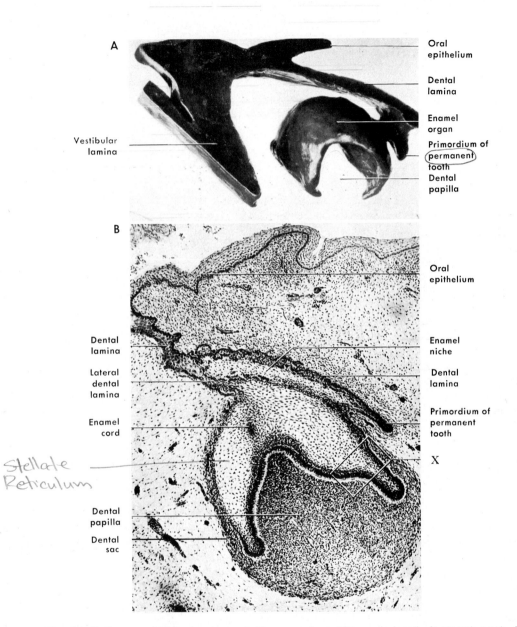

A

Oral
epithelium

Dental
lamina

Enamel
organ

Primordium of
permanent
tooth

Dental
papilla

Vestibular
lamina

B

Oral
epithelium

Dental
lamina

Lateral
dental
lamina

Enamel
cord

Stellate
Reticulum

Dental
papilla

Dental
sac

Enamel
niche

Dental
lamina

Primordium of
permanent
tooth

X

Fig. 2-8. Bell stage of tooth development. Human embryo 105 mm in length, fourteenth week. **A,** Wax reconstruction of lower central incisor. **B,** Labiolingual section of the same tooth. X, See Fig. 2-9. (From Orban B: Dental histology and embryology, Philadelphia, 1929, P Blakiston's Son & Co.)

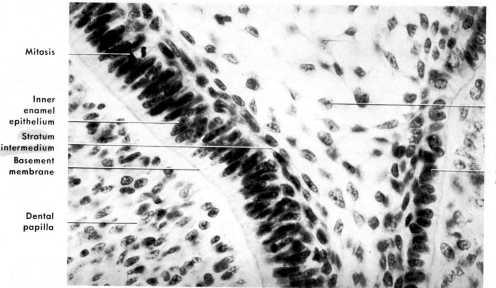

Mitosis

Inner enamel epithelium

Stratum intermedium

Basement membrane

Dental papilla

Stellate reticulum

Outer enamel epithelium

Fig. 2-9. Layers of epithelial enamel organ at high magnification. Area X of Fig. 2-8.

Dental papilla. Under the organizing influence of the proliferating epithelium of the enamel organ, the ectomesenchyme (neural crest cells) that is partially enclosed by the invaginated portion of the inner enamel epithelium proliferates. It condenses to form the dental papilla, which is the formative organ of the dentin and the primordium of the pulp (Figs. 2-5 and 2-6). The changes in the dental papilla occur concomitantly with the development of the epithelial enamel organ. Although the epithelium exerts a dominating influence over the adjacent connective tissue, the condensation of the latter is not a passive crowding by the proliferating epithelium. The dental papilla shows active budding of capillaries and mitotic figures, and its peripheral cells adjacent to the inner enamel epithelium enlarge and later differentiate into the odontoblasts. → Dentin

Dental sac. Concomitant with the devel-opment of the enamel organ and the dental papilla, there is a marginal condensation in the ectomesenchyme surrounding the enamel organ and dental papilla. Gradually, in this zone, a denser and more fibrous layer develops, which is the primitive dental sac. The cells of the dental sac are important for the formation of cementum and the periodontal ligament.

The epithelial enamel organ, the dental papilla, and the dental sac are the formative tissues for an entire tooth and its supporting structures.

Bell stage

As the invagination of the epithelium deepens and its margins continue to grow, the enamel organ assumes a bell shape (Figs. 2-2, *C*, and 2-8). Four different types of epithelial cells can be distinguished on light microscopic examination of the bell stage of the enamel organ. The cells form the inner enamel epithelium, the stratum intermedium, the stellate reticulum, and the outer enamel epithelium.

Inner enamel epithelium. The inner enamel epithelium consists of a single layer of cells that differentiate prior to amelogenesis into tall columnar cells called ameloblasts (Figs. 2-8 and 2-9). These cells are 4 to 5 micrometers (μm) in diameter and about 40 μm high. These elongated cells are attached to one another by junctional complexes laterally and to cells in the stratum intermedium by desmosomes (Fig. 2-9). The fine structure of inner enamel epithelium and ameloblasts is described in Chapter 3.

The cells of the inner enamel epithelium exert an organizing influence on the underlying mesenchymal cells in the dental papilla, which later differentiate into odontoblasts.

Stratum intermedium. A few layers of squamous cells form the stratum intermedium, between the inner enamel epithelium and the stellate reticulum (Fig. 2-9). These cells are closely attached by desmosomes and gap junctions. The well-developed cytoplasmic organelles, acid mucopolysaccharides, and glycogen deposits indicate a high degree of metabolic activity. This layer seems to be essential to enamel formation. It is absent in the part of the tooth germ that outlines the root portions of the tooth but does not form enamel.

Stellate reticulum. The stellate reticulum expands further, mainly by an increase in the amount of intercellular fluid. The cells are star shaped, with long processes that anastomose with those of adjacent cells (Fig. 2-9). Before enamel formation begins, the stellate reticulum collapses, reducing the distance between the centrally situated ameloblasts and the nutrient capillaries near the outer enamel epithelium. Its cells then are hardly distinguishable from those

of the stratum intermedium. This change begins at the height of the cusp or the incisal edge and progresses cervically (see Fig. 3-37).

Outer enamel epithelium. The cells of the outer enamel epithelium flatten to a low cuboidal form. At the end of the bell stage, preparatory to and during the formation of enamel, the formerly smooth surface of the outer enamel epithelium is laid in folds. Between the folds the adjacent mesenchyme of the dental sac forms papillae that contain capillary loops and thus provide a rich nutritional supply for the intense metabolic activity of the avascular enamel organ.

Dental lamina. In all of the teeth, except the permanent molars, the dental lamina proliferates at its deep end to give rise to the enamel organs of the permanent teeth (Figs. 2-10 and 2-11).

Dental papilla. The dental papilla is enclosed in the invaginated portion of the enamel organ. Before the inner enamel epithelium begins to produce enamel, the peripheral cells of the mesenchymal dental papilla differentiate into odontoblasts under the organizing influence of the epithelium. First, they assume a cuboidal form; later they assume a columnar form and acquire the specific potential to produce dentin.

The basement membrane that separates the enamel organ and the dental papilla just prior to dentin formation is called the *membrana preformativa*.

Dental sac. Before formation of dental tissues begins, the dental sac shows a circular arrangement of its fibers and resembles a capsular structure. With the development of the root, the fibers of the dental sac differentiate into the periodontal fibers that become embedded in the developing cementum and alveolar bone.

Advanced bell stage. During the advanced

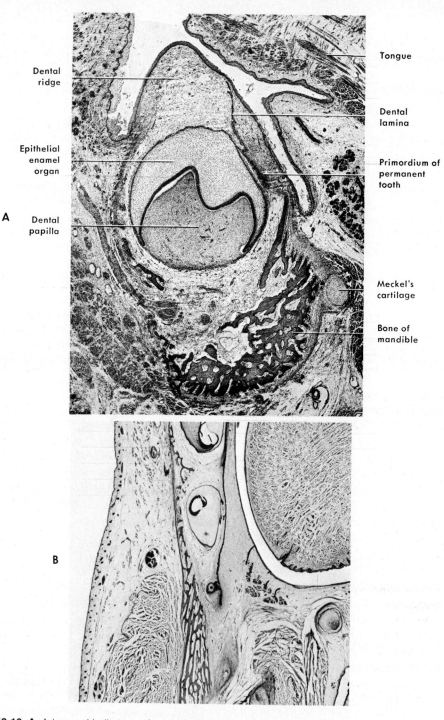

Dental ridge

Tongue

Dental lamina

Epithelial enamel organ

Primordium of permanent tooth

A

Dental papilla

Meckel's cartilage

Bone of mandible

B

Fig. 2-10. A, Advanced bell stage of tooth development. Human embryo 200 mm in length, about 18 weeks. Labiolingual section through deciduous lower first molar. **B,** Horizontal section through human embryo about 20 mm in length showing extension of dental lamina distal to second deciduous molar and formation of permanent first molar tooth germ. (**B** from Bhaskar SN: Synopsis of oral histology, ed 5, St Louis, 1977, The CV Mosby Co.)

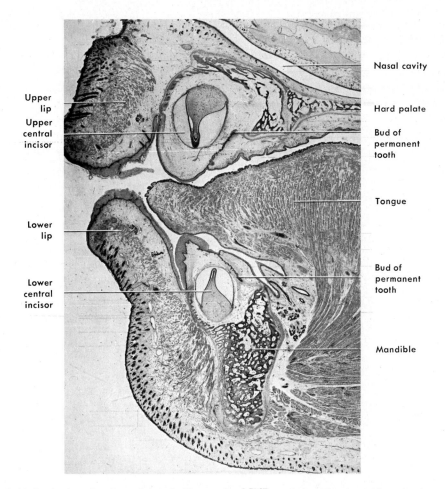

Fig. 2-11. Sagittal section through head of human fetus 200 mm in length, about 18 weeks, in region of central incisors.

bell stage, the boundary between inner enamel epithelium and odontoblasts outlines the future dentinoenamel junction (Figs. 2-8 and 2-10). In addition, the cervical portion of the enamel organ gives rise to the epithelial root sheath of Hertwig.

Hertwig's epithelial root sheath and root formation

The development of the roots begins after enamel and dentin formation has reached the future cementoenamel junction. The enamel organ plays an important part in root development by forming Hertwig's epithelial root sheath, which molds the shape of the roots and initiates radicular dentin formation. Hertwig's root sheath consists of the outer and inner enamel epithelia only, and therefore it does not include the stratum intermedium and stellate reticulum. The cells of the inner layer remain short and normally do not produce enamel. When these cells have induced the differentiation of radicular cells into odontoblasts and the first layer of dentin has been laid down, the epithelial root sheath loses its structural continuity and its close relation to the surface of the root. Its remnants persist as an epithelial network of strands or tubules near the external surface of the root. These epithelial remnants are found in the periodontal ligament of erupted teeth and are called *rests of Malassez* (see Chapter 7).

There is a pronounced difference in the development of Hertwig's epithelial root sheath in teeth with one root and in those with two or more roots. Prior to the beginning of root formation, the root sheath forms the epithelial diaphragm (Fig. 2-12). The outer and inner enamel epithelia bend at the future cementoenamel junction into

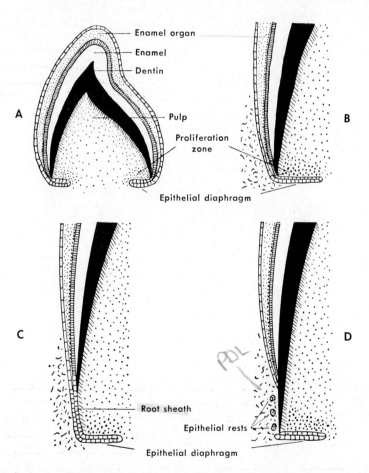

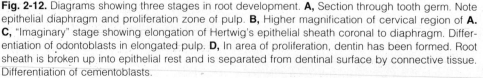

Fig. 2-12. Diagrams showing three stages in root development. **A,** Section through tooth germ. Note epithelial diaphragm and proliferation zone of pulp. **B,** Higher magnification of cervical region of **A.** **C,** "Imaginary" stage showing elongation of Hertwig's epithelial sheath coronal to diaphragm. Differentiation of odontoblasts in elongated pulp. **D,** In area of proliferation, dentin has been formed. Root sheath is broken up into epithelial rest and is separated from dentinal surface by connective tissue. Differentiation of cementoblasts.

a horizontal plane, narrowing the wide cervical opening of the tooth germ. The plane of the diaphragm remains relatively fixed during the development and growth of the root (see Chapter 11). The proliferation of the cells of the epithelial diaphragm is accompanied by proliferation of the cells of the connective tissue of the pulp, which occurs in the area adjacent to the diaphragm. The free end of the diaphragm does not grow into the connective tissue, but the epithelium proliferates coronal to the epithelial diaphragm (Fig. 2-12, B). The differentiation of odontoblasts and the formation of dentin follow the lengthening of the root sheath. At the same time the connective tissue of the dental sac surrounding the root

sheath proliferates and invades the continuous double epithelial layer (Fig. 2-12, C) dividing it into a network of epithelial strands (Fig. 2-12, D). The epithelium is moved away from the surface of the dentin so that connective tissue cells come into contact with the outer surface of the dentin and differentiate into cementoblasts that deposit a layer of cementum onto the surface of the dentin. The rapid sequence of proliferation and destruction of Hertwig's root sheath explains the fact that it cannot be seen as a continuous layer on the surface of the developing root (Figs. 2-12, D, and 2-14). In the last stages of root development, the proliferation of the epithelium in the diaphragm lags behind that of the

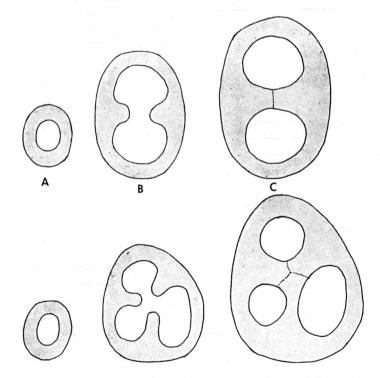

Fig. 2-13. Three stages in development of tooth with two roots and one with three roots. Surface view of epithelial diaphragm. During growth of tooth germ, simple diaphragm, **A,** expands eccentrically so that horizontal epithelial flaps are formed. **B,** Later these flaps proliferate and unite (dotted lines in **C**) and divide single cervical opening into two or three openings.

pulpal connective tissue. The wide apical foramen is reduced first to the width of the diaphragmatic opening itself and later is further narrowed by apposition of dentin and cementum to the apex of the root.

Differential growth of the epithelial diaphragm in multirooted teeth causes the division of the root trunk into two or three roots. During the general growth of the enamel organ the expansion of its cervical opening occurs in such a way that long tonguelike extensions of the horizontal diaphragm develop (Fig. 2-13). Two such extensions are found in the germs of lower molars and three in the germs of upper molars. Before division of the root trunk occurs, the free ends of these horizontal epithelial flaps grow toward each other and

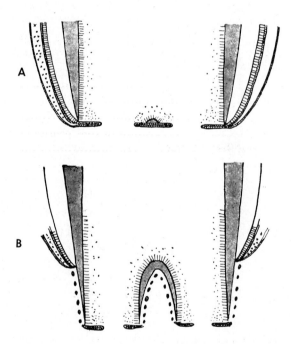

Fig. 2-14. Two stages in development of two-rooted tooth. Diagrammatic mesiodistal sections of lower molar. **A,** Beginning of dentin formation at bifurcation. **B,** Formation of two roots in progress. (Details as shown in Fig. 2-12.)

fuse. The single cervical opening of the coronal enamel organ is then divided into two or three openings. On the pulpal surface of the dividing epithelial bridges, dentin formation starts (Fig. 2-14, *A*), and on the periphery of each opening, root development follows in the same way as described for single-rooted teeth (Fig. 2-14, *B*).

If cells of the epithelial root sheath remain adherent to the dentin surface, they may differentiate into fully functioning ameloblasts and produce enamel. Such droplets of enamel, called *enamel pearls*, are sometimes found in the area of furcation of the roots of permanent molars. If the continuity of Hertwig's root sheath is broken or is not established prior to dentin formation, a defect in the dentinal wall of the pulp ensues. Such defects are found in the pulpal floor corresponding to the furcation or on any point of the root itself if the fusion of the horizontal extensions of the diaphragm remains incomplete. This accounts for the development of accessory root canals opening on the periodontal surface of the root (see Chapter 5).

HISTOPHYSIOLOGY AND CLINICAL CONSIDERATIONS

A number of physiologic growth processes participate in the progressive development of the teeth (Table 1). Except for their initiation, which is a momentary event, these processes overlap considerably, and many are continuous throughout the various morphologic stages of odontogenesis. Nevertheless, each physiologic process tends to predominate in one stage more than in another.

For example, the process of histodifferentiation characterizes the bell stage, in which the cells of the inner enamel epithelium differentiate into functional ameloblasts. However, proliferation still pro-

Table 1. Stages in tooth growth

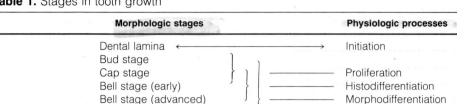

Morphologic stages	Physiologic processes
Dental lamina ⟷	Initiation
Bud stage	
Cap stage	Proliferation
Bell stage (early)	Histodifferentiation
Bell stage (advanced)	Morphodifferentiation
Formation of enamel and dentin matrix	Apposition

gresses at the deeper portion of the enamel organ.

Initiation. The dental laminae and associated tooth buds represent those parts of the oral epithelium that have the potential for tooth formation. Specific cells within the horseshoe-shaped dental laminae have the potential to form the enamel organ of certain teeth by responding to those factors that initiate or induce tooth development. Different teeth are initiated at definite times. Initiation induction requires ectomesenchymal-epithelial interaction. The mechanism of such interaction is not clearly understood. However, it has been demonstrated that dental papilla mesenchyme can induce or instruct tooth epithelium and even nontooth epithelium to form enamel.

Teeth may develop in abnormal locations, for example, in the ovary (dermoid tumors or cysts) or in the hypophysis. In such instances the tooth undergoes stages of development similar to those in the jaws.

A lack of initiation results in the absence of either a single tooth or multiple teeth (partial anodontia), most frequently the permanent upper lateral incisors, third molars, and lower second premolars. There also may be a complete lack of teeth (anodontia). On the other hand, abnormal initiation may result in the development of single or multiple supernumerary teeth.

Proliferation. Enhanced proliferative activity ensues at the points of initiation and results successively in the bud, cap, and bell stages of the odontogenic organ. Proliferative growth causes regular changes in the size and proportions of the growing tooth germ (Figs. 2-3 and 2-7).

Even during the stage of proliferation, the tooth germ already has the potential to become more highly developed. This is illustrated by the fact that explants of these early stages continue to develop in tissue culture through the subsequent stages of histodifferentiation and appositional growth. A disturbance or experimental interference has entirely different effects, according to the time of occurrence and the stage of development that it affects.

Histodifferentiation. Histodifferentiation succeeds the proliferative stage. The formative cells of the tooth germs developing during the proliferative stage undergo definite morphologic as well as functional changes and acquire their functional assignment (the appositional growth potential). The cells become restricted in their functions. They differentiate and give up their capacity to multiply as they assume their new function; this law governs all differentiating cells. This phase reaches its highest development in the bell stage of the enamel organ, just preceding the beginning of formation and apposition of dentin and enamel (Fig. 2-8).

The organizing influence of the inner

enamel epithelium on the mesenchyme is evident in the bell stage and causes the differentiation of the adjacent cells of the dental papilla into odontoblasts. With the formation of dentin, the cells of the inner enamel epithelium differentiate into ameloblasts and enamel matrix is formed opposite the dentin. Enamel does not form in the absence of dentin, as demonstrated by the failure of transplanted ameloblasts to form enamel when dentin is not present. Dentin formation therefore precedes and is essential to enamel formation. The differentiation of the epithelial cells precedes and is essential to the differentiation of the odontoblasts and the initiation of dentin formation.

In vitro studies on tooth development

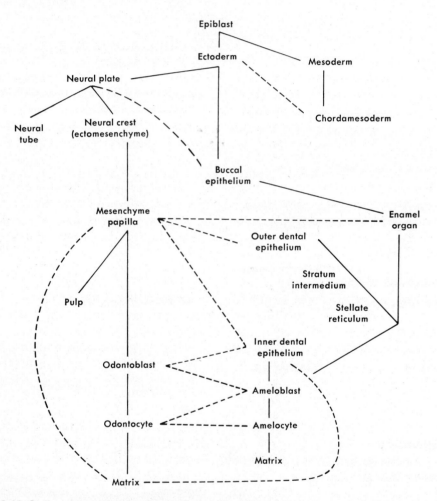

Fig. 2-15. Outline of development of tooth. *Broken lines,* Known or suspected interactions that occur between tissues. Data suggesting placement of these lines derive from transplantations and in vitro studies. Words "amelocyte" and "odontocyte" are employed only to indicate that these cells may possess different capabilities for interaction with other tissues after their overt differentiation. (Courtesy Dr. William E. Koch., Chapel Hill, NC.)

have provided vital information concerning the interaction of dermal-epidermal components of tooth tissues on differentiation of odontoblasts and ameloblasts. The importance of the basement membrane of this interface has been recognized. However, the criteria for the development of this complex organ system will have to await the delineation of the precise roles of the stellate reticulum, the stratum intermedium, and the outer dental epithelial components. One of the models that has been suggested for the interactions that may occur between tissues during the development of a tooth is presented in Fig. 2-15.

In vitamin A deficiency the ameloblasts fail to differentiate properly. Consequently, their organizing influence on the adjacent mesenchymal cells is disturbed, and atypical dentin, known as osteodentin, is formed.

Morphodifferentiation. The morphologic pattern, or basic form and relative size of the future tooth, is established by morphodifferentiation, that is, by differential growth. Morphodifferentiation therefore is impossible without proliferation. The advanced bell stage marks not only active histodifferentiation but also an important stage of morphodifferentiation in the crown, outlining the future dentinoenamel junction (Figs. 2-8 and 2-10).

The dentinoenamel and dentinocemental junctions, which are different and characteristic for each type of tooth, act as a blueprint pattern. In conformity with this pattern the ameloblasts, odontoblasts, and cementoblasts deposit enamel, dentin, and cementum, respectively, and thus give the completed tooth its characteristic form and size. For example, the size and form of the cuspal portion of the crown of the first permanent molar are established at birth long before the formation of hard tissues begin.

The frequent statement in the literature that endocrine disturbances affect the size or form of the crown of teeth is not tenable unless such effects occur during morphodifferentiation, that is, in utero or in the first year of life. Size and shape of the root, however, may be altered by disturbances in later periods. Clinical examinations show that the retarded eruption that occurs in persons with hypopituitarism and hypothyroidism results in a small clinical crown that is often mistaken for a small anatomic crown.

Disturbances in morphodifferentiation may affect the form and size of the tooth without impairing the function of the ameloblasts or odontoblasts. New parts may be differentiated (supernumerary cusps or roots), twinning may result, a suppression of parts may occur (loss of cusps or roots), or the result may be a peg or malformed tooth with enamel and dentin that may be normal in structure (e.g., the upper central incisor may become notched at the edge, or "screw driver" shaped, in individuals born with congenital syphilis; this condition is known as Hutchinson's incisor).

Apposition. Apposition is the deposition of the matrix of the hard dental structures. It will be described in separate chapters on enamel, dentin, and cementum. This chapter deals with certain aspects of apposition in order to complete the discussion of the physiologic processes concerned in the growth of teeth.

Appositional growth of enamel and dentin is a layerlike deposition of an extracellular matrix. This type of growth is therefore additive. It is the fulfillment of the plans outlined at the stages of histodifferentiation and morphodifferentiation. Appositional growth is characterized by regular and rhythmic deposition of the extracellular matrix, which is of itself incapable of further growth. Periods of activity and rest alternate at definite intervals during tooth formation.

Genetic and environmental factors may disturb the normal synthesis and secretion of the organic matrix of enamel leading to a condition called *enamel hypoplasia.*

If the organic matrix is normal but its mineralization is defective, then the enamel or dentin is said to be hypocalcified or hypomineralized. Both hypoplasia and hypocalcification can occur as a result of an insult to the cells responsible for the apposition stage of tooth development (see Chapter 3, Clinical Considerations).

REFERENCES

Avery JK: Embryology of the teeth, J Dent Res 30:490, 1951.

Avery JK: Primary induction of tooth formation, J Dent Res 33:702, 1954 (abstract).

Bhaskar SN: Synopsis of oral pathology, ed 7, St Louis, 1986, The CV Mosby Co.

Diamond M and Applebaum E: The epithelial sheath, J Dent Res 21:403, 1942.

Fisher AR: The differentiation of the molar tooth germ of the mouse in vivo and in vitro with special reference to cusp development, doctoral thesis, 1957, University of Bristol.

Fleming HS: Homologous and heterologous intraocular growth of transplanted tooth germs, J Dent Res 31:166, 1952.

Gaunt WA: The vascular supply to the dental lamina during early development, Acta Anat (Basel) 37:232, 1959.

Glasstone S: Regulative changes in tooth germs grown in tissue culture, J Dent Res 42:1364, 1963.

Hoffman R and Gillete R: Mitotic patterns in pulpal and periodontal tissue in developing teeth, Fortieth General Meeting of the International Association of Dental Research, St Louis, 1962.

Johnson PL and Bevelander G: The role of the stratum intermedium in tooth development, Oral Surg 10:437, 1957.

Koch WE: Tissue interaction during in vitro odontogenesis. In Slavkin HS and Bavetta LA, editors: Developmental aspects of oral biology, New York, 1972, Academic Press, Inc.

Kollar EJ: Histogenetics of dermal-epidermal interactions. In Slavkin HS and Bavetta LA, editors: Developmental aspects of oral biology, New York, 1972, Academic Press, Inc.

Kraus BS: Calcification of the human deciduous teeth, J Am Dent Assoc 59:1128, 1959.

Lefkowitz W and Swayne P: Normal development of tooth buds cultured in vitro, J Dent Res 37:1100, 1958.

Marsland EA: Histological investigation of amelogenesis in rats, Br Dent J 91:251, 1951.

Marsland EA: Histological investigation of amelogenesis in rats, Br Dent J 92:109, 1952.

Orban B: Growth and movement of the tooth germs and teeth, J Am Dent Assoc 15:1004, 1928.

Orban B: Dental histology and embryology, Philadelphia, 1929, P Blakiston's Son & Co.

Orban B and Mueller E: The development of the bifurcation of multirooted teeth, J Am Dent Assoc 16:297, 1929.

Schour I and Massler M: Studies in tooth development: the growth pattern of human teeth, J Am Dent Assoc 27:1778, 1940.

Sicher H: Tooth eruption: axial movement of teeth with limited growth, J Dent Res 21:395, 1942.

Slavkin HC: Embryonic tooth formation. In Melcher AH and Zarb GA, editors: Oral sciences reviews 4, Copenhagen, 1974, Munksgaard, International Booksellers & Publishers, Ltd.

3
ENAMEL

HISTOLOGY
Physical characteristics

Enamel forms a protective covering of variable thickness over the entire surface of the crown. On the cusps of human molars and premolars the enamel attains a maximum thickness of about 2 to 2.5 mm, thinning down to almost a knife edge at the neck of the tooth. The shape and contour of the cusps receive their final modeling in the enamel.

Because of its high content of mineral salts and their crystalline arrangement, enamel is the hardest calcified tissue in the human body. The function of the enamel is to form a resistant covering of the teeth, rendering them suitable for mastication. The structure and hardness of the enamel render it brittle, which is particularly apparent when the enamel loses its foundation of sound dentin. The specific gravity of enamel is 2.8.

Another physical property of enamel is its permeability. It has been found with radioactive tracers that the enamel can act in a sense like a semipermeable membrane, permitting complete or partial passage of certain molecules: ^{14}C-labeled urea, I, etc. The same phenomenon has also been demonstrated by means of dyes.

The color of the enamel-covered crown ranges from yellowish white to grayish

49

white, It has been suggested that the color is determined by differences in the translucency of enamel, yellowish teeth having a thin, translucent enamel through which the yellow color of the dentin is visible and grayish teeth having a more opaque enamel. The translucency may be attributable to variations in the degree of calcification and homogeneity of the enamel. Grayish teeth frequently show a slightly yellowish color at the cervical areas, presumably because the thinness of the enamel permits the light to strike the underlying yellow dentin and be reflected. Incisal areas may have a bluish tinge where the thin edge consists only of a double layer of enamel.

Chemical properties

The enamel consists mainly of inorganic material (96%) and only a small amount of organic substance and water (4%). The inorganic material of the enamel is similar to apatite. The bar graph in Fig. 3-1 indicates the composition by volume of mineralized tissues in which odontoblast processes have been replaced with peritubular den-

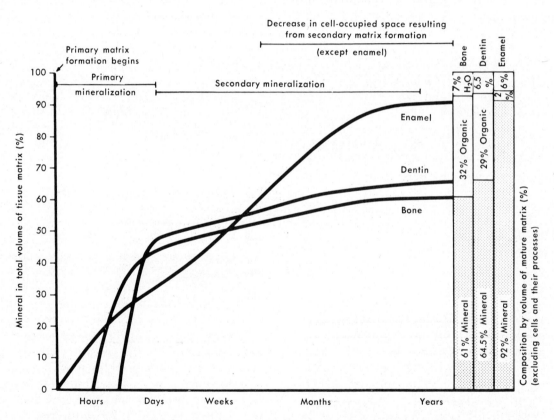

Fig. 3-1. Formation, mineralization, and maturation of some mineralized tissues. (Figures for bone from Robinson RA: In Rodahl K, Nicholson JT, and Brown EM, editors: Bone as a tissue, New York, 1960, The Blakiston Division, McGraw-Hill Book Co, pp 186-250. Figures for dentin and enamel from Brudevold F: In Sognnaes RF, editor: Chemistry and prevention of dental caries, Springfield, Ill, 1962, Charles C Thomas, Publisher, pp 32-88.)

tin (sclerotic dentin) and the equivalent situation in bone in which osteocyte lacunae are filled with mineral.

The origins shown at the left of Fig. 3-1 reflect the facts that enamel matrix mineralization begins immediately after it is secreted and that the lag in mineralization after matrix formation is greater in dentin than in bone. Enamel primary mineralization and secondary mineralization (maturation) increase mineral content in a relatively smooth curve. In both bone and dentin, well over one half of the mineral accumulates rapidly (primary mineralization). The curves then flatten as secondary mineralization occurs. The curves continue to rise slowly as cell-occupied space is filled with mineralized matrix (secondary matrix formation) in bone and dentin.

The relative *space occupied* by the organic framework and the entire enamel is almost equal. Fig. 3-2 illustrates this by comparing a stone and a sponge of approximately *equal size*. The stone represents the mineral content, and the sponge represents the organic framework of the enamel. Although their sizes are almost equal, their weights are vastly different. The stone is more than 100 times heavier than the sponge, or expressed in percentage, the weight of the sponge is less than 1% of that of the stone.

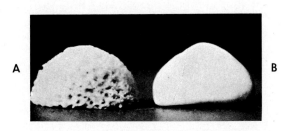

Fig. 3-2. A sponge, **A,** and a stone, **B,** are comparable to organic and mineral elements of enamel. Their sizes are approximately equal, but their weights differ greatly. (From Bodecker CF: Dent Rev 20:317, 1906.)

The nature of the organic elements of enamel is incompletely understood. During development the histologic staining reactions of the enamel matrix resemble keratinizing epidermis. More specific methods have revealed sulfhydryl groups and other reactions suggestive of keratin. However, chemical analyses of the matrix of mature enamel indicate that the amino acid composition is not closely related to keratin and is distinctly different from collagen. Proteins can be isolated in several different fractions, and they generally contain high percentages of serine, glutamic acid, and glycine. Roentgen-ray diffraction studies reveal that the molecular structure is typical of the group of proteins called cross-β-proteins. In addition, histochemical reactions have suggested that the enamel-forming cells of developing teeth also contain a polysaccharide-protein complex and that an acid mucopolysaccharide enters the enamel itself at the time when calcification becomes a prominent feature. Tracer studies have indicated that the enamel of erupted teeth of rhesus monkeys can transmit and exchange radioactive isotopes originating from the saliva and the pulp. Considerable investigation is still required to determine the normal physiologic characteristics and the age changes that occur in the enamel.

Structure

Rods. The enamel is composed of enamel rods or prisms, rod sheaths, and in some regions a cementing interprismatic substance. The number of enamel rods has been estimated as ranging from 5 million in the lower lateral incisors to 12 million in the upper first molars. From the dentinoenamel junction the rods run somewhat tortuous courses outward to the surface of the tooth. The length of most rods is greater than the thickness of the enamel because of

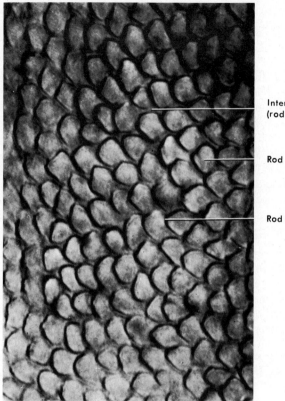

Interrod substance
(rod "tail")

Rod

Rod sheath

Fig. 3-3. Decalcified section of enamel of human tooth germ. Rods cut transversely have appearance of fish scales.

the oblique direction and the wavy course of the rods. The rods located in the cusps, the thickest part of the enamel, are longer than those at the cervical areas of the teeth. It is stated generally that, as observed with the light microscope, the diameter of the rods averages 4 μm, but this measurement necessarily varies, since the outer surface of the enamel is greater than the dentinal surface where the rods originate. It is claimed that the diameter of the rods increases from the dentinoenamel junction toward the surface of the enamel at a ratio of about 1:2.

The enamel rods normally have a clear crystalline appearance, permitting light to pass through them. In cross section under the light microscope they occasionally appear hexagonal. Sometimes they appear round or oval. In cross sections of human enamel, many rods resemble fish scales (Fig. 3-3).

Submicroscopic structure. Since many features of enamel rods are below the limit of resolution of the light microscope, many questions concerning their morphology can only be answered by electron microscopy. Although many areas of human enamel seem to contain rods surrounded by rod sheaths and separated by interrod sub-

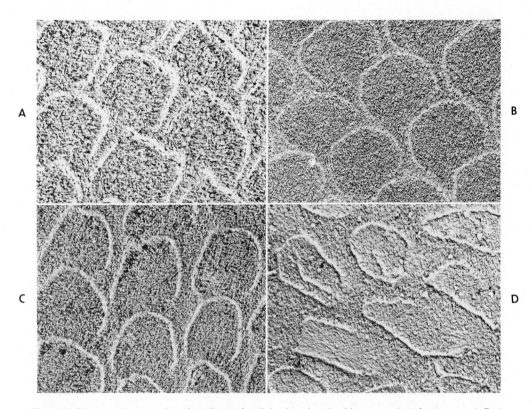

Fig. 3-4. Electron micrographs of replicas of polished and etched human subsurface enamel. Rods are cut in cross section. Various patterns are apparent. **A,** "Keyholes." **B,** "Staggered arches." **C,** "Stacked arches." **D,** Irregular rods near dentinoenamel junction. (Approximately ×3000.) (From Swancar VR, Scott DB, and Njemirovskij Z: J Dent Res 49:1025, 1970. Copyright by the American Dental Association. Reprinted by permission.)

stance (Fig. 3-4), a more common pattern is a keyhole- or paddle-shaped prism in human enamel (Fig. 3-5). When cut longitudinally (Fig. 3-6), sections pass through the "heads" or "bodies" of one row of rods and the "tails" of an adjacent row. This produces an appearance of rods separated by interrod substance. These rods measure about 5 μm in breadth and 9 μm in length. Rods of this shape can be packed tightly together (Fig. 3-7), and enamel with this structure explains many bizarre patterns seen with the electron microscope. The

"bodies" of the rods are nearer occlusal and incisal surfaces, whereas the "tails" point cervically.

Studies with polarized light and roentgen-ray diffraction have indicated that the apatite crystals are arranged approximately parallel to the long axis of the prisms, although deviations of up to 40 degrees have been reported. Careful electron microscope studies have made it possible to describe more precisely the orientation of these crystals. They are approximately parallel to the long axes of the rods in their "bodies"

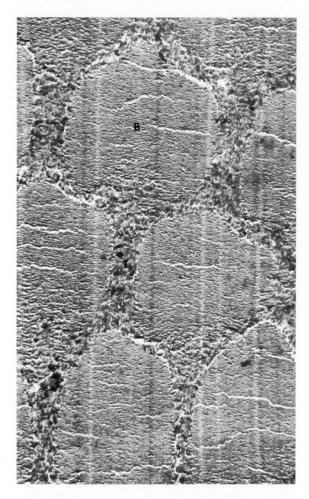

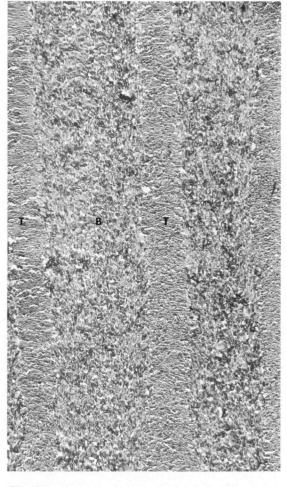

Fig. 3-5. Electron micrograph of cross sections of rods in mature human enamel. Rods are keyhole shaped, and crystal orientation is different in "bodies," *B*, than in "tails," *T*. (Approximately ×5000.) (From Meckel AH, Griebstein WJ, and Neal RJ: Arch Oral Biol 10:775, 1965.)

Fig. 3-6. Electron micrograph of longitudinal section through mature human enamel. Alternating "tails," *T*, and "bodies," *B*, of rods are defined by abrupt changes in crystal direction where they meet. (Approximately ×5000.) (From Meckel AH, Griebstein WJ, and Neal RJ: Arch Oral Biol 10:775, 1965.)

or "heads" and deviate about 65 degrees from this axis as they fan out into the "tails" of the prisms (Fig. 3-8). Since it is extremely difficult to prepare a section that is exactly parallel to the long axes of the crystals, there is some question about their length, but they are estimated to vary be-

tween 0.05 and 1 μm. When cut in cross section, the crystals of human enamel are somewhat irregular in shape (Fig. 3-9) and have an average thickness of about 30 nanometers* (nm; 300 angstrom units [Å])

---

*1 nanometer (new terminology) = 10 Å.

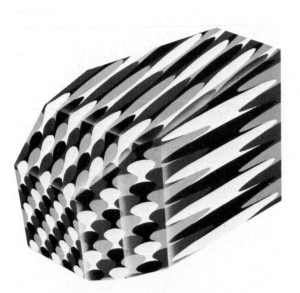

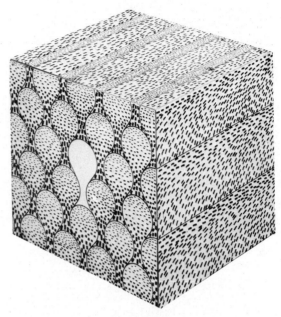

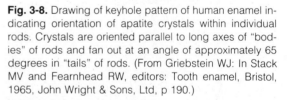

Fig. 3-7. Model indicating packing of keyhole-shaped rods in human enamel. Various patterns can be produced by changing plane of sectioning. (From Meckel AH, Griebstein WJ, and Neal RJ: Arch Oral Biol 10:775, 1965.)

Fig. 3-8. Drawing of keyhole pattern of human enamel indicating orientation of apatite crystals within individual rods. Crystals are oriented parallel to long axes of "bodies" of rods and fan out at an angle of approximately 65 degrees in "tails" of rods. (From Griebstein WJ: In Stack MV and Fearnhead RW, editors: Tooth enamel, Bristol, 1965, John Wright & Sons, Ltd, p 190.)

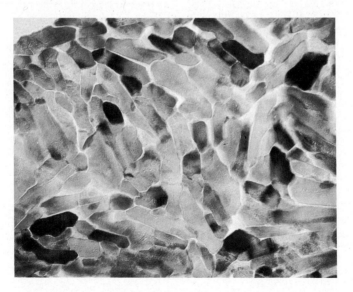

Fig. 3-9. Cross section of apatite crystals within enamel rod in human enamel. Crystals are tightly packed and irregular in shape. (Approximately ×168,000.) (From Frazier PD: J Ultrastruct Res 22:1, 1968.)

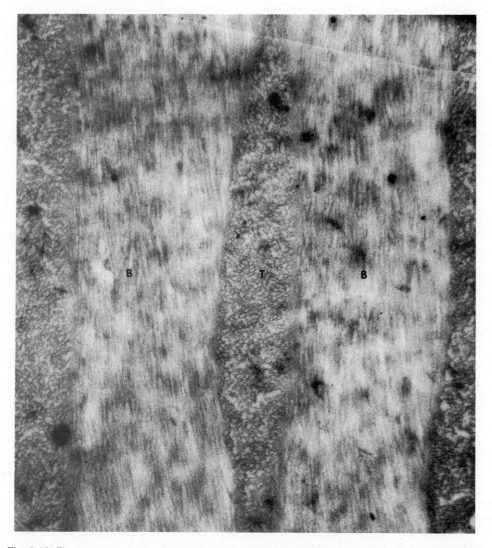

Fig. 3-10. Electron micrograph of decalcified section of immature bovine enamel. Although shape of rods in bovine enamel is not clearly established, this electron micrograph reproduces pattern one would expect in longitudinal sections through human enamel. Organic sheaths around individual apatite crystals are oriented parallel to long axes of rods in their "bodies," *B,* and more nearly perpendicular to long axes in their "tails," *T.* (Approximately ×38,000.) (From Travis DF and Glimcher MJ: J Cell Biol 23:447, 1964.)

and an average width of about 90 μm (900 Å).

Early investigators using electron microscopy described a network of fine organic fibrils running throughout the rods and interrod substance. Recent improvements in preparative methods have disclosed that the organic matrix probably forms an envelope surrounding each apatite crystal (Fig. 3-10). In electron micrographs the surfaces of rods are visible because of abrupt changes in crystal orientation from one rod to another. For this reason the crystals are not as tightly packed and there may be more space for organic matrix at these surfaces. This accounts for the rod sheath visible in the light microscope (Fig. 3-3).

Striations. Each enamel rod is built up of segments separated by dark lines that give it a striated appearance (Fig. 3-11). These transverse striations demarcate rod segments and become more visible by the action of mild acids. The striations are more pronounced in enamel that is insufficiently calcified. The rods are segmented because the enamel matrix is formed in a rhythmic manner. In humans these segments seem to be a uniform length of about 4 μm.

Direction of rods. Generally the rods are oriented at right angles to the dentin surface. In the cervical and central parts of the crown of a deciduous tooth they are approximately horizontal (Fig. 3-12, A). Near the incisal edge or tip of the cusps they change gradually to an increasingly oblique direction until they are almost vertical in the region of the edge or tip of the cusps. The arrangement of the rods in permanent teeth is similar in the occlusal two thirds of the crown. In the cervical region, however, the rods deviate from the horizontal in an apical direction (Fig. 3-12, B).

The rods are rarely, if ever, straight throughout. They follow a wavy course

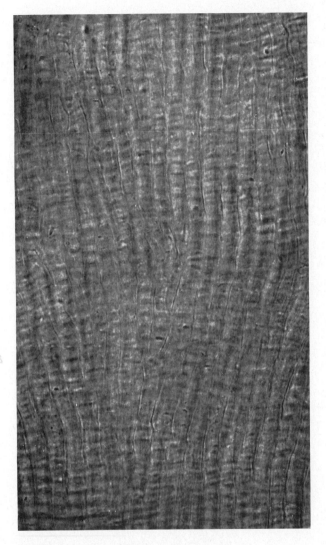

Fig. 3-11. Ground section through enamel. Rods cut longitudinally. Cross-striation of rods.

from the dentin to the enamel surface. The most significant deviations from a straight radial course can be described as follows. If the middle part of the crown is divided into thin horizontal discs, the rods in the adjacent discs bend in opposite directions. For instance, in one disc the rods start from

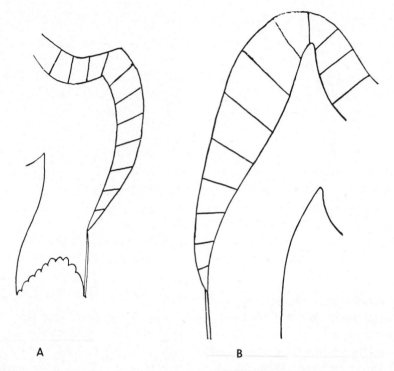

Fig. 3-12. Diagrams indicating general direction of enamel rods. **A,** Deciduous tooth. **B,** Permanent tooth.

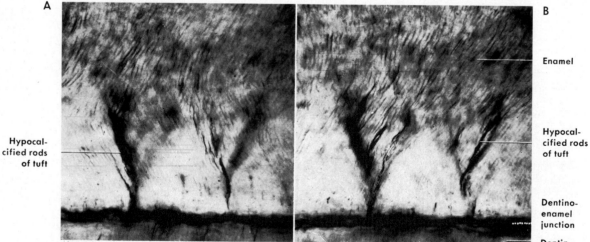

Fig. 3-13. Horizontal ground section through enamel near dentinoenamel junction. **A** and **B** show change in direction of rods in two adjacent layers of enamel, which is made visible by change in focus of microscope.

the dentin in an oblique direction and bend more or less sharply to the left side (Fig. 3-13, *A*), whereas in the adjacent disc the rods bend toward the right (Fig. 3-13, *B*). This alternating clockwise and counterclockwise deviation of the rods from the radial direction can be observed at all levels of the crown if the discs are cut in the planes of the general rod direction.

If the discs are cut in an oblique plane, especially near the dentin in the region of the cusps or incisal edges, the rod arrangement appears to be further complicated—the bundles of rods seem to intertwine more irregularly. This optical appearance of enamel is called *gnarled enamel*.

The enamel rods forming the developmental fissures and pits, as on the occlusal surface of molar and premolars, converge in their outward course.

Hunter-Schreger bands. The more or less regular change in the direction of rods may be regarded as a functional adaptation, minimizing the risk of cleavage in the axial direction under the influence of occlusal masticatory forces. The change in the direction of rods is responsible for the appearance of the Hunter-Schreger bands. These are alternating dark and light strips of varying widths (Fig. 3-14, *A*) that can best be seen in a longitudinal ground section under oblique reflected light. They

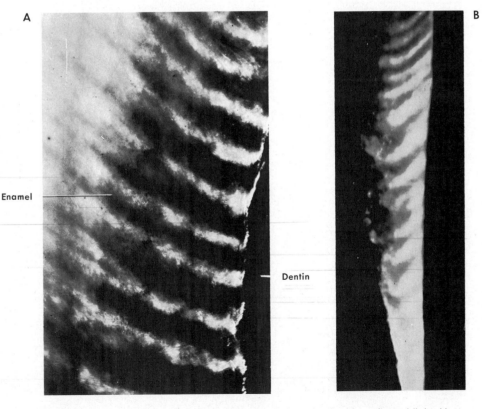

Fig. 3-14. A, Longitudinal ground section through enamel photographed by reflected light. Hunter-Schreger bands. **B,** Decalcified enamel, photographed by reflected light, showing Hunter-Schreger bands.

originate at the dentinoenamel border and pass outward, ending at some distance from the outer enamel surface. Some investigators claim that there are variations in calcification of the enamel that coincide with the distribution of the bands of Hunter-Schreger. Careful decalcification and staining of the enamel have provided further evidence that these structures may not be the result solely of an optical phenomenon but that they are composed of alternate zones having a slightly different permeability and a different content of organic material (Fig. 3-14, *B*).

Incremental lines of Retzius. The incremental lines of Retzius appear as <u>brownish bands in ground sections of the enamel</u>. They illustrate the incremental pattern of the enamel, that is, the successive apposition of layers of enamel during formation of the crown. In longitudinal sections they surround the tip of the dentin (Fig. 3-15, *A*). In the cervical parts of the crown they run obliquely. From the dentinoenamel junction to the surface they deviate occlusally (Fig. 3-15, *B*). In transverse sections of a tooth the incremental lines of Retzius appear as <u>concentric circles</u> (Fig. 3-16). They

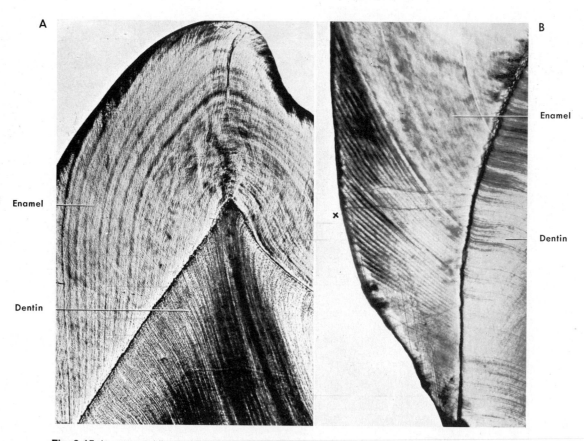

Fig. 3-15. Incremental lines of Retzius in longitudinal ground sections. **A,** Cuspal region. **B,** Cervical region, X.

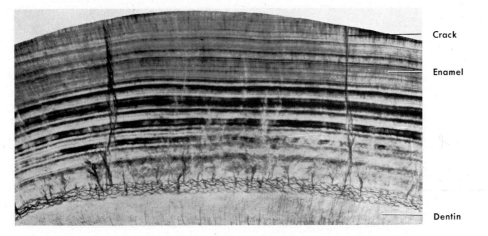

Crack

Enamel

Dentin

Fig. 3-16. Incremental lines of Retzius in transverse ground section, arranged concentrically.

may be compared to the growth rings in the cross section of a tree. The term "incremental lines" designates these structures appropriately, for they do, in fact, reflect variations in structure and mineralization, either hypomineralization or hypermineralization, that occur during growth of the enamel. The exact nature of these developmental changes is not known. The incremental lines have been attributed to periodic bending of the enamel rods, to variations in the basic organic structure (Fig. 3-17), or to a physiologic calcification rhythm.

The incremental lines of Retzius, if

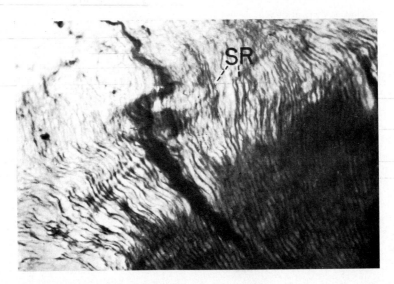

SR

Fig. 3-17. Carefully decalcified section through enamel. Thickening of sheath substance, *SR,* in Retzius lines. (From Bodecker CF: Dent Rev 20:317, 1906.)

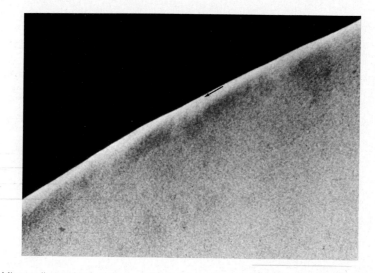

Fig. 3-18. Microradiograph of ground section of sound human enamel. Relatively structureless surface layer *(arrow)* is more radiopaque than bulk of enamel below it. (Approximately ×200.) (Courtesy Dr. A.J. Gwinnett, Stony Brook, NY)

present in moderate intensity, are considered normal. However, the rhythmic alteration of periods of enamel matrix formation and of rest can be upset by metabolic disturbances, causing the rest periods to be unduly prolonged and close together. Such an abnormal condition is responsible for the broadening of the incremental lines of Retzius, rendering them more prominent.

Surface structures. A relatively structureless layer of enamel, approximately 30 μm thick, has been described in 70% of permanent teeth and all deciduous teeth. This structureless enamel is found least often over the cusp tips and most commonly toward the cervical areas of the enamel surface. In this surface layer no prism outlines are visible, and all of the apatite crystals are parallel to one another and perpendicular to the striae of Retzius. It is also somewhat more heavily mineralized than the bulk of enamel beneath it (Fig. 3-18). Other microscopic details that have been observed on outer enamel surfaces of newly

erupted teeth are perikymata, rod ends, and cracks (lamellae).

Perikymata are transverse, wavelike grooves, believed to be the external manifestations of the striae of Retzius. They are continuous around a tooth and usually lie parallel to each other and to the cementoenamel junction (Figs. 3-19 and 3-20). Ordinarily there are about 30 perikymata per millimeter in the region of the cementoenamel junction, and their concentration gradually decreases to about 10 per millimeter near the occlusal or incisal edge of a surface. Their course usually is fairly regular, but in the cervical region it may be quite irregular.

The enamel rod ends are concave and vary in depth and shape. They are shallowest in the cervical regions of surfaces and deepest near the incisal or occlusal edges (Fig. 3-19, *B*).

The term "cracks" originally was used to describe the narrow, fissurelike structures that are seen on almost all surfaces (Fig. 3-

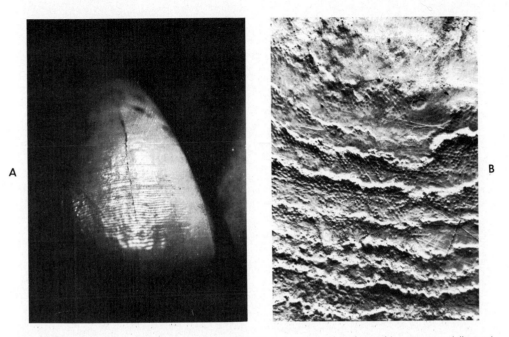

Fig. 3-19. A, Perikymata on lateral incisor. **B,** Shadowed replica of surface of intact enamel (buccal surface of upper left second molar showing perikymata). (×1500.) (**B** from Scott DB and Wyckoff RWG: Public Health Rep 61:1397, 1946.)

20, *D*). It has since been demonstrated that they are actually the outer edges of lamellae (see discussion of enamel lamellae). They extend for varying distances along the surface, at right angles to the dentinoenamel junction, from which they originate. Most of them are less than a millimeter in length, but some are longer, and a few reach the occlusal or incisal edge of a surface. They are fairly evenly spaced, but long lamellae appear thicker than short ones.

The enamel of the deciduous teeth develops partly before and partly after birth. The boundary between the two portions of enamel in the deciduous teeth is marked by an accentuated incremental line of Retzius, the *neonatal line* or *neonatal ring* (Fig. 3-21). It appears to be the result of the abrupt change in the environment and nutrition of the newborn infant. The prenatal enamel usually is better developed than the postnatal enamel. This is explained by the fact that the fetus develops in a well-protected environment with an adequate supply of all the essential materials, even at the expense of the mother. Because of the undisturbed and even development of the enamel prior to birth, perikymata are absent in the occlusal parts of the deciduous teeth, whereas they are present in the postnatal cervical parts.

Enamel cuticle. A delicate membrane called *Nasmyth's membrane*, after its first investigator, or the *primary enamel cuticle* covers the entire crown of the newly erupted tooth but is probably soon removed by mastication. Electron microscope studies have indicated that this membrane is a typical basal lamina found

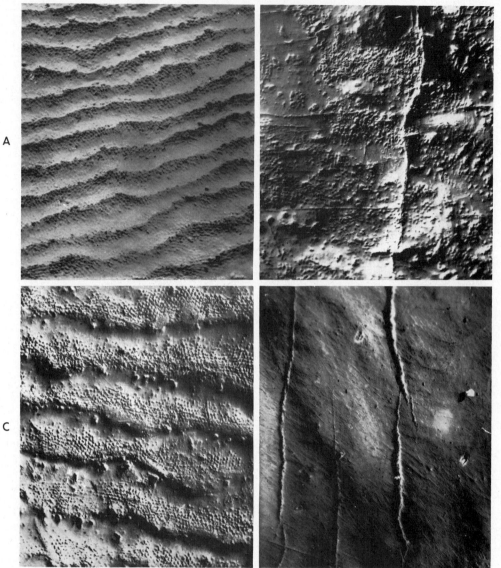

Fig. 3-20. Progressive loss of surface structure with advancing age. **A,** Surface of recently erupted tooth showing pronounced enamel prism ends and perikymata. Patient is 12 years of age. **B,** Early stage of structural loss that occurs during first few years (wear is more rapid on anterior teeth than on posterior teeth and more rapid on facial or lingual surfaces than on proximal surfaces). Note small regions where prism ends are worn away. Patient is 25 years of age. **C,** Later stage. Here elevated parts between perikymata are worn smooth, while structural detail in depths of grooves is still more or less intact. Eventually wearing proceeds to point where all prism ends and perikymata disappear. Patient is 52 years of age. (Since these are negative replicas, surface details appear inverted. Raised structures represent depressions in actual surface.) **D,** Surface worn completely smooth and showing only "cracks," which actually represent outer edges of lamellae. Patient is 50 years of age. (All magnifications ×105.) (From Scott DB and Wyckoff RWG: J Am Dent Assoc 39:275, 1949.)

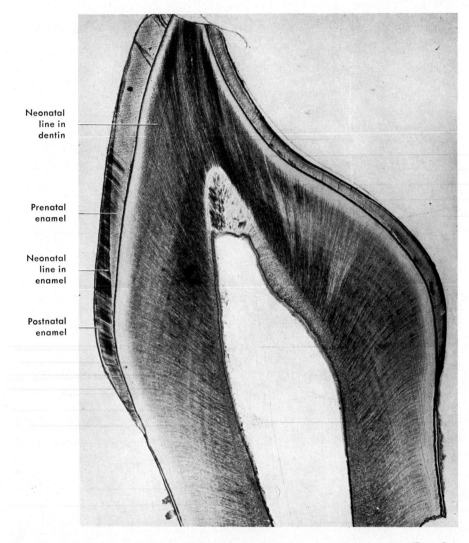

Neonatal
line in
dentin

Prenatal
enamel

Neonatal
line in
enamel

Postnatal
enamel

Fig. 3-21. Neonatal line in enamel. Longitudinal ground section of deciduous canine. (From Schour I: J Am Dent Assoc 23:1946, 1936.)

beneath most epithelia (Fig. 3-22). It is probably visible with the light microscope because of its wavy course. This basal lamina is apparently secreted by the ameloblasts when enamel formation is completed. It has also been reported that the cervical area of the enamel is covered by afibrillar cementum, continuous with the cementum and probably of mesodermal origin (Fig. 3-23). This cuticle is apparently secreted after the epithelial enamel organ retracts from the cervical region during tooth development.

Finally, erupted enamel is normally covered by a *pellicle*, which is apparently a precipitate of salivary proteins (Fig. 3-24).

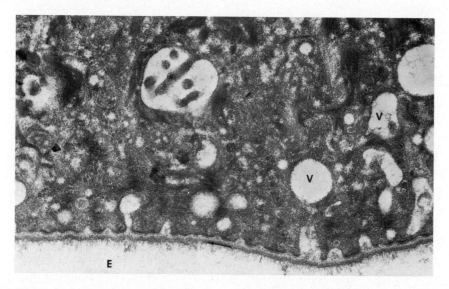

Fig. 3-22. Electron micrograph of reduced enamel epithelium covering surface of unerupted human tooth. Enamel has been removed by demineralization, *E.* Typical basal lamina separates enamel space from epithelium *(arrow).* Epithelial cells contain a number of intracytoplasmic vacuoles, *V.* (Approximately ×24,000.) (From Listgarten MA: Arch Oral Biol 11:999, 1966.)

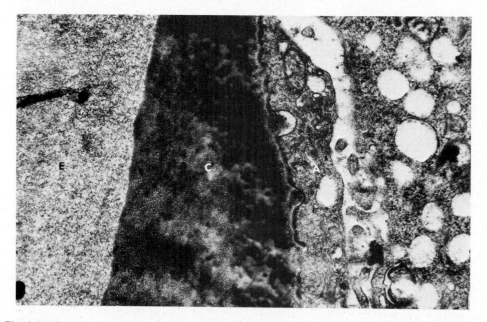

Fig. 3-23. Electron micrograph of gingival area of erupted human tooth. Remnants of enamel matrix appear at left, *E.* Cuticle, *C,* separates enamel matrix from epithelial cells of attached epithelial cuff, *A.* Inner layers of cuticle (afibrillar cementum) are deposited before eruption; origin of outer layers is not known. (Approximately ×37,000.) (From Listgarten MA: Am J Anat 119:147, 1966.)

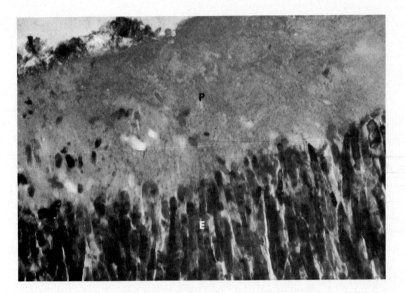

Fig. 3-24. Electron micrograph of surface of undemineralized human enamel. Enamel surface, *E,* is covered by pellicle, *P.* Individual crystals can be seen in enamel. (Approximately ×58,000.) (From Houver G and Frank RM: Arch Oral Biol 12:1209, 1967.)

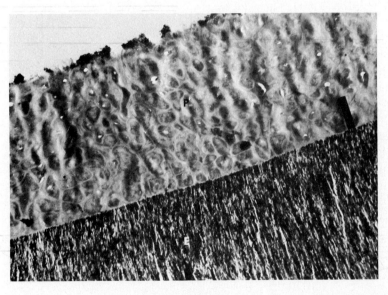

Fig. 3-25. Electron micrograph of undemineralized human enamel surface. Enamel, *E,* is covered by a bacterial plaque, *P. Black bar at right,* Thickness of pellicle seen in Fig. 3-24. (Approximately ×12,000.) (From Frank RM and Brendel A: Arch Oral Biol 11:883, 1966.)

This pellicle re-forms within hours after an enamel surface is mechanically cleaned. Within a day or two after the pellicle has formed, it becomes colonized by microorganisms to form a bacterial plaque (Fig. 3-25).

Enamel lamellae. Enamel lamellae are thin, leaflike structures that extend from the enamel surface toward the dentinoenamel junction (Fig. 3-26). They may extend to, and sometimes penetrate into, the dentin. They consist of organic material, with but little mineral content. In ground sections these structures may be confused with cracks caused by grinding of the specimen (Fig. 3-16). Careful decalcification of ground sections of enamel makes possible the distinction between cracks and enamel lamellae. The former disappear, whereas the latter persist (Figs. 3-26, *A*, and 3-27).

Lamellae may develop in planes of tension. Where rods cross such a plane, a short segment of the rod may not fully calcify. If the disturbance is more severe, a crack may develop that is filled either by surrounding cells, if the crack occurred in the unerupted tooth, or by organic substances from the oral cavity, if the crack developed after eruption. Three types of lamellae can thus be differentiated: type A, lamellae composed of poorly calcified rod segments (Fig. 3-27, *B*); type B, lamellae consisting of degenerated cells; and type C, lamellae arising in erupted teeth where the cracks are filled with organic matter, presumably originating from saliva. The last type may be more common than formerly believed. Although lamellae of type A are restricted to the enamel, those of types B and C may reach into the dentin (Fig. 3-28). If cells from the enamel organ fill a crack in the enamel, those in the depth degenerate, whereas those close to the surface may remain vital for a time and produce a hornified cuticle in the cleft. In such cases the inner parts of the lamella consist of an organic cell detritus, the outer parts of a double layer of the cuticle. If connective tissue

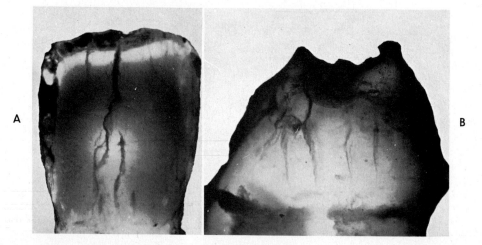

A

B

Fig. 3-26. A, Decalcified incisor with moderately severe mottled enamel. Numerous lamellae can be observed. (×8.) **B,** Maxillary first permanent molar of caries-free 2-year-old rhesus monkey. Numerous bands of organic matter, lamellae, can be seen after decalcification. (×8.) (**B** from Sognnaes RF: J Dent Res 29:260, 1950.)

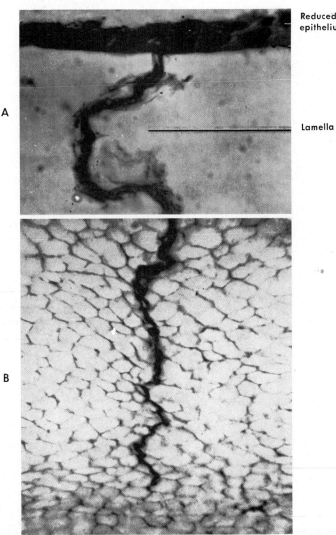

A   Reduced enamel
               epithelium

               Lamella

B

Fig. 3-27. A, Paraffin section through reduced enamel epithelium, enamel cuticle, and lamella, isolated together by acid flotation from surface of unerupted human tooth. Note intimate relationship between three elements. (Hematoxylin and eosin; ×1300.) **B,** Paraffin section of decalcified enamel of human molar showing relation between lamella and surrounding organic sheath substance. (Hematoxylin and eosin; ×1000.) (**A** from Ussing MJ: Acta Odontal Scand 13:23, 1955; reprinted in J West Soc Periodont 3:71, 1955; **B** courtesy Dr. R.F. Sognnaes, Los Angeles.)

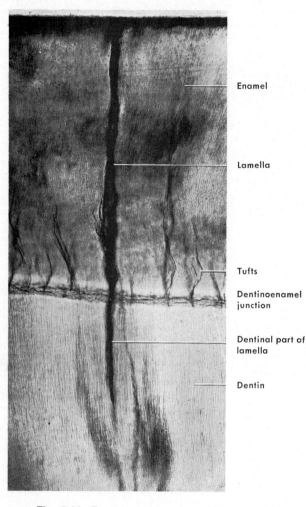

Enamel

Lamella

Tufts

Dentinoenamel
junction

Dentinal part of
lamella

Dentin

Fig. 3-28. Transverse ground section through lamella reaching from surface into dentin.

invades a crack in the enamel, cementum may be formed. In such cases lamellae consist entirely or partly of cementum.

Lamellae extend in the longitudinal and radial direction of the tooth, from the tip of the crown toward the cervical region (Fig. 3-26). This arrangement explains why they can be observed better in horizontal sections. It has been suggested that enamel

lamellae may be a site of weakness in a tooth and may form a road of entry for bacteria that initiate caries.

Enamel tufts. Enamel tufts (Fig. 3-29) arise at the (dentinoenamel junction) and reach into the enamel to about one fifth to one third of its thickness. They were so termed because they resemble tufts of grass when viewed in ground sections. This picture is erroneous. An enamel tuft does not spring from a single small area but is a narrow, ribbonlike structure, the inner end of which arises at the dentin. The impression of a tuft of grass is created by examining such structures in thick sections under low magnification. Under these circumstances the imperfections, lying in different planes and curving in different directions (Fig. 3-13), are projected into one plane (Fig. 3-29).

Tufts consist of hypocalcified enamel rods and interprismatic substance. Like the lamellae, they extend in the direction of the long axis of the crown. Therefore they are seen abundantly in horizontal, and rarely in longitudinal, sections. Their presence and their development are a consequence of, or an adaptation to, the spatial conditions in the enamel.

Dentinoenamel junction. The surface of the dentin at the dentinoenamel junctions is pitted. Into the shallow depressions of the dentin fit rounded projections of the enamel. This relation assures the firm hold of the enamel cap on the dentin. In sections, therefore, the dentinoenamel junction appears not as a straight but as a scalloped line (Figs. 3-29 and 3-30). The convexities of the scallops are directed toward the dentin. The pitted dentinoenamel junction is preformed even before the development of hard tissues and is evident in the arrangement of the ameloblasts and the basement membrane of the dental papilla (Fig. 3-43).

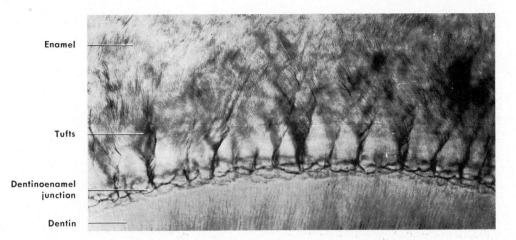

Fig. 3-29. Transverse ground section through tooth under low magnification. Numerous tufts extend from dentinoenamel junction into enamel.

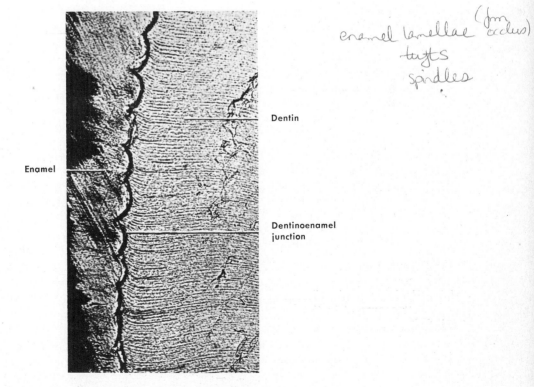

enamel lamellae (from occlus)
tufts
spindles

Fig. 3-30. Longitudinal ground section. Scalloped dentinoenamel junction.

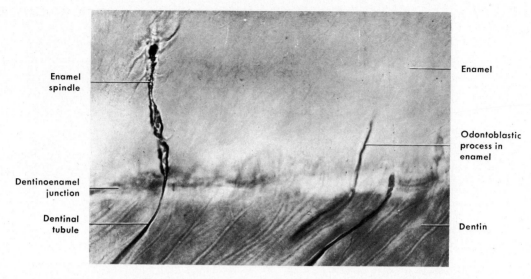

Enamel spindle

Enamel

Odontoblastic process in enamel

Dentinoenamel junction

Dentinal tubule

Dentin

Fig. 3-31. Ground section. Odontoblast processes extend into enamel as enamel spindles.

In microradiographs of ground sections a hypermineralized zone about 30 μm thick can sometimes be demonstrated at the dentinoenamel junction. It is most prominent before mineralization is complete.

Odontoblast processes and enamel spindles. Occasionally odontoblast processes pass across the dentinoenamel junction into the enamel. Since many are thickened at their end (Fig. 3-31), they have been termed *enamel spindles.* They seem to originate from processes of odontoblasts that extended into the enamel epithelium before hard substances were formed. The direction of the odontoblast processes and spindles in the enamel corresponds to the original direction of the ameloblasts—at right angles to the surface of the dentin. Since the enamel rods are formed at an angle to the axis of the ameloblasts, the direction of spindles and rods is divergent. In ground sections of dried teeth the organic content of the spindles disintegrates and is replaced by air, and the spaces appear dark in transmitted light.

Age changes

The most apparent age change in enamel is attrition or wear of the occlusal surfaces and proximal contact points as a result of mastication. This is evidenced by a loss of vertical dimension of the crown and by a flattening of the proximal contour. In addition to these gross changes, the outer enamel surfaces themselves undergo posteruptive alterations in structure at the microscopic level. These result from environmental influences and occur with a regularity that can be related to age (Fig. 3-20).

The surfaces of unerupted and recently erupted teeth are covered completely with pronounced rod ends and perikymata. At the points of highest contour of the surfaces these structures soon begin to disappear. This is followed by a generalized loss of the rod ends and a much slower flattening of the perikymata. Finally, the perikymata disappear completely. The rate at which structure is lost depends on the location of the surface of the tooth and on the location of the tooth in the mouth. Facial and lingual surfaces lose their structure much more rapidly than do proximal surfaces, and anterior teeth lose their structure more rapidly than do posterior teeth.

Age changes within the enamel proper have been difficult to discern microscopically. The fact that alterations do occur has been demonstrated by chemical analysis, but the changes are not well understood. For example, the total amount of organic matrix is said by some to increase, by others to remain unchanged, and by still others to decrease. Localized increases of certain elements such as nitrogen and fluorine, however, have been found in the superficial enamel layers of older teeth. This suggests a continuous uptake, probably from the oral environment, during aging. As a result of age changes in the organic portion of enamel, presumably near the surface, the teeth may become darker, and their resistance to decay may be increased. Suggestive of an aging change is the greatly reduced permeability of older teeth to fluids. There is insufficient evidence to show that enamel becomes harder with age.

Clinical considerations

The course of the enamel rods is of importance in cavity preparations. The choice of instruments depends on the location of the cavity in the tooth. Generally the rods run at a right angle to the underlying dentin or tooth surface. Close to the cementoenamel junction the rods run in a more horizontal direction (Fig. 3-12, *B*). In preparing cavities, it is important that unsupported enamel rods are not left at the cavity margins because they would soon break and produce leakage. Bacteria would lodge in these spaces, inducing secondary dental caries. Enamel is brittle and does not withstand forces in thin layers or in areas where it is not supported by the underlying dentin (Fig. 3-32, *A*).

Deep enamel fissures predispose teeth to caries. Although these deep clefts between adjoining cusps cannot be regarded as pathologic, they afford areas for retention of caries-producing agents. Caries penetrate the floor of fissures rapidly because the enamel in these areas is very thin (Fig. 3-32, *B*). As the destructive process reaches the dentin, it spreads along the dentinoenamel junction, undermining the enamel. An extensive area of dentin becomes carious without giving any warning to the patient because the entrance to the cavity is minute. Careful examination is necessary to discover such cavities because most enamel fissures are more minute than a single toothbrush bristle and cannot be detected with the dental probe.

Dental lamellae may also be predisposing locations for caries because they contain much organic material. Primarily from the standpoint of protection against caries, the structure and reactions of the outer enamel surface are subject to much current research. In vitro tests have shown that the acid solubility of enamel can be greatly reduced by treatment with fluoride compounds. Clinical trials based on these studies have demonstrated reductions of 40% or more in the incidence of caries in children after topical applications of sodium or stannous fluoride. Incorporation of fluorides in dentifrices is now a well-accepted means of caries prevention. Fluoride-containing mixtures such as stannous fluoride pastes, sodium fluoride rinses, and acidulated phosphate fluoride are also used by the dentist to alter the outer surface of the enamel in such a manner that it becomes more resistant to decay.

The most effective means for mass control of dental caries to date has been adjustment of the fluoride level in communal wa-

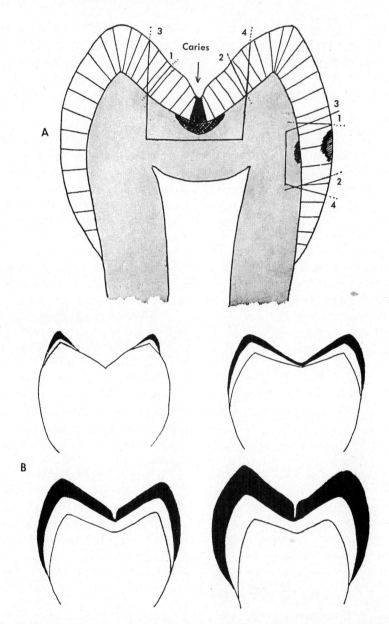

Fig. 3-32. A, Diagram of course of enamel rods in molar in relation to cavity preparation. *1* and *2* indicate wrong preparation of cavity margins. *3* and *4* indicate correct preparation. **B,** Diagram of development of deep enamel fissure. Note thin enamel layer forming floor of fissure. (**B** from Kronfeld R: J Am Dent Assoc 22:1131, 1935.)

ter supplies to 1 part per million. Epidemiologic studies in areas in which the drinking water contained natural fluoride revealed that the caries prevalence in both children and adults was about 65% lower than in nonfluoride areas, and long-term studies have demonstrated that the same order of protection is afforded through water fluoridation programs. The mechanisms of action are believed to be primarily a combination of changes in enamel resistance, brought about by incorporation of fluoride during calcification, and alterations in the environment of the teeth, particularly with respect to the oral bacterial flora.

The surface of the enamel in the cervical region should be kept smooth and well polished by proper home care and by regular cleansing by the dentist. If the surface of the cervical enamel becomes decalcified or otherwise roughened, food debris, bacterial plaques, and so on accumulate on this surface. The gingiva in contact with this roughened, debriscovered enamel surface undergoes inflammatory changes. The ensuing gingivitis, unless promptly treated, may lead to more serious periodontal disease.

One of the more recently developed techniques in operative dentistry consists of the use of composite resins. These materials can be mechanically "bonded" directly to the enamel surface. In this procedure the enamel surface is first etched with an acid (phosphoric acid 37%) to remove the smear layer on the enamel that was created during cavity preparation. Smear layers are about 1 μm thick and are made up of burnished cutting debris. Because the particles that constitute the smear layer are very small, the layer is very acid labile. Acid etching of enamel removes this smear layer. This produces an uneven dissolution of the enamel rods and their "sheaths" or enamel "heads" and their "tails" so that a relatively smooth enamel surface becomes pitted and irregular. When a composite resin is put on this irregular surface, it can achieve mechanical bonding with the enamel. The same principle is used in coating the susceptible areas of the enamel with the so-called pit fissure sealants.

DEVELOPMENT
Epithelial enamel organ

The early development of the enamel organ and its differentiation have been discussed in Chapter 2. At the stage preceding the formation of hard structures (dentin and enamel) the enamel organ, originating from the stratified epithelium of the primitive oral cavity, consists of four distinct layers: outer enamel epithelium, stellate reticulum, stratum intermedium, and inner enamel epithelium (ameloblastic layer) (Fig. 3-33). The borderline between the inner enamel epithelium and the connective tissue of the dental papilla is the subsequent dentinoenamel junction. Thus its outline determines the pattern of the occlusal or incisal part of the crown. At the border of the wide basal opening of the enamel organ, the inner enamel epithelium reflects onto the outer enamel epithelium. This is the *cervical loop*. The inner and outer enamel epithelia are elsewhere separated from each other by a large mass of cells differentiated into two distinct layers. The layer that is close to the inner enamel epithelium consists of two or three rows of flat polyhedral cells—the stratum intermedium. The other layer, which is more loosely arranged, constitutes the stellate reticulum.

The different layers of epithelial cells of the enamel organ are named according to their morphology, function, or location. The stellate reticulum derives its name from the morphology of its cells. The outer enamel epithelium and the stratum inter-

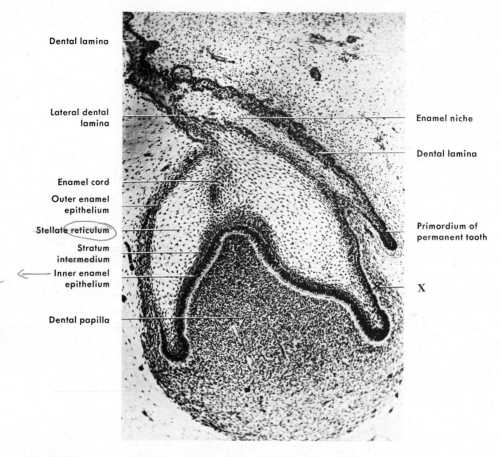

Dental lamina

Lateral dental lamina

Enamel cord

Outer enamel epithelium

Stellate reticulum

Stratum intermedium

Inner enamel epithelium

Dental papilla

ameloblastic layer ⟵

Enamel niche

Dental lamina

Primordium of permanent tooth

X

Fig. 3-33. Tooth germ (deciduous lower incisor) of human embryo 105 mm, fourth month. Four layers of enamel organ. Area at X is shown at a higher magnification in Fig. 3-35.

medium are so named because of their location. The inner enamel epithelium is so named on the basis of its position. On the basis of function it is called the ameloblastic layer.

Outer enamel epithelium. In the early stages of development of the enamel organ the outer enamel epithelium consists of a single layer of cuboid cells, separated from the surrounding connective tissue of the dental sac by a delicate basement membrane (Fig. 3-34). Prior to the formation of hard structures, this regular arrangement of

the outer enamel epithelium is maintained only in the cervical parts of the enamel organ. At the highest convexity of the organ (Fig. 3-33) the cells of the outer enamel epithelium become irregular in shape and cannot be distinguished easily from the outer portion of the stellate reticulum. The capillaries in the connective tissue surrounding the epithelial enamel organ proliferate and protrude toward it (Fig. 3-34). Immediately before enamel formation commences, capillaries may even indent the stellate reticulum. This increased vascular-

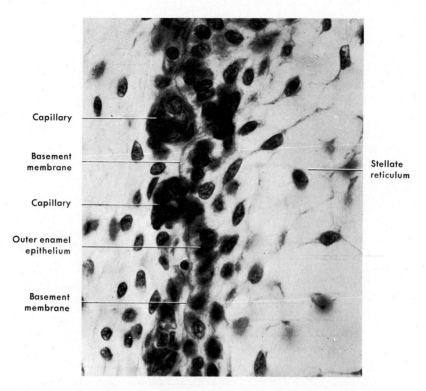

Capillary

Basement
membrane

Capillary

Outer enamel
epithelium

Basement
membrane

Stellate
reticulum

Fig. 3-34. Capillaries in contact with outer enamel epithelium. Basement membrane separates outer enamel epithelium from connective tissue.

ity ensures a rich metabolism when a plentiful supply of substances from the bloodstream to the inner enamel epithelium is required (Fig. 3-35).

During enamel formation, cells of the outer enamel epithelium develop villi and cytoplasmic vesicles and large numbers of mitochondria, all indicating cell specialization for the active transport of materials. The capillaries in contact with the outer enamel epithelium show areas with very thin walls, a structural modification also commonly found in areas of active transport.

Stellate reticulum. In the stellate reticulum, which forms the middle part of the enamel organ, the neighboring cells are separated by wide intercellular spaces filled by a large amount of intercellular substance. The cells are star shaped, with long processes reaching in all directions from a central body (Figs. 3-34 and 3-36). They are connected with each other and with the cells of the outer enamel epithelium and the stratum intermedium by desmosomes.

The structure of the stellate reticulum renders it resistant and elastic. Therefore it seems probable that it acts as a buffer against physical forces that might distort the conformation of the developing dentinoenamel junction, giving rise to gross morphologic changes. It seems to permit only a limited flow of nutritional elements

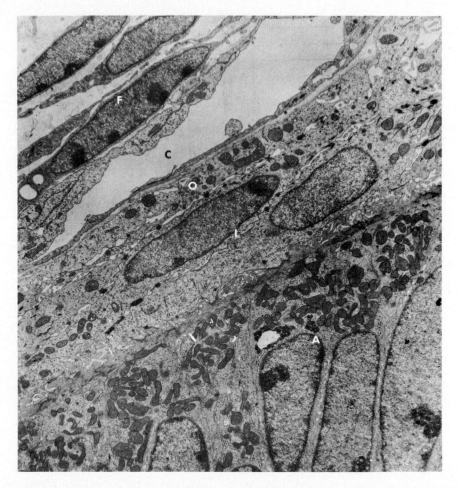

Fig. 3-35. Electron micrograph of epithelial enamel organ over area of rodent incisor in which enamel secretion is underway. From above downward are fibroblasts of dental sac, *F;* capillary, *C;* cells of outer enamel epithelium, *O;* cells of stratum intermedium, *I;* and proximal ends of ameloblasts, *A.* (Approximately ×7000.) (Courtesy Dr. P.R. Garant, Stony Brook, NY)

from the outlying blood vessels to the formative cells. Indicative of this is the fact that the stellate reticulum is noticeably reduced in thickness when the first layers of dentin are laid down, and the inner enamel epithelium is thereby cut off from the dental papilla, its original source of supply (Fig. 3-37).

Stratum intermedium. The cells of the stratum intermedium are situated between the stellate reticulum and the inner enamel epithelium. They are flat to cuboid in shape and are arranged in one to three layers. They are connected with each other and with the neighboring cells of the stellate reticulum and the inner enamel epithelium

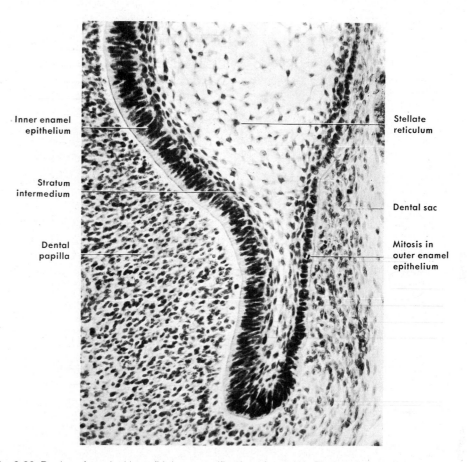

Inner enamel
epithelium

Stratum
intermedium

Dental
papilla

Stellate
reticulum

Dental sac

Mitosis in
outer enamel
epithelium

Fig. 3-36. Region of cervical loop (higher magnification of area X in Fig. 3-33). Transition of outer into inner enamel epithelium.

by desmosomes. Tonofibrils, with an orientation parallel to the surface of the developing enamel, are found in the cytoplasm. The function of the stratum intermedium is not understood, but it is believed to play a role in production of the enamel itself, either through control of fluid diffusion into and out of the ameloblasts or by the actual contribution of necessary formative elements or enzymes. The cells of the stratum intermedium show mitotic division even after the cells of the inner enamel epithelium cease to divide.

Inner enamel epithelium. The cells of the inner enamel epithelium are derived from the basal cell layer of the oral epithelium. Before enamel formation begins, these cells assume a columnar form and differentiate into ameloblasts that produce the enamel matrix. The changes in shape and structure that the cells of the inner enamel epithelium undergo will be described in detail in the discussion of the life cycle of the ameloblasts. It should be mentioned, however, that cell differentiation occurs earlier in the region of the incisal edge or

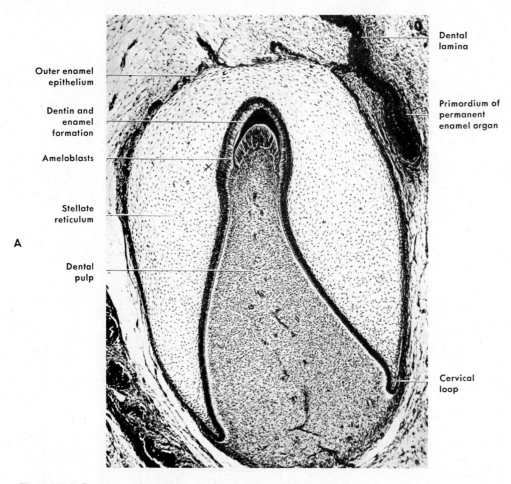

Outer enamel
epithelium

Dentin and
enamel
formation

Ameloblasts

Stellate
reticulum

A

Dental
pulp

Dental
lamina

Primordium of
permanent
enamel organ

Cervical
loop

Fig. 3-37. A, Tooth germ (lower incisor) of human fetus (fifth month). Beginning of dentin and enamel formation. Stellate reticulum at tip of crown is reduced in thickness.

cusps than in the area of the cervical loop.

Cervical loop. At the free border of the enamel organ the outer and inner enamel epithelial layers are continuous and reflected into one another as the cervical loop (Figs. 3-33 and 3-35). In this zone of transition between the outer enamel epithelium and the inner enamel epithelium the cuboid cells gradually gain in length. When the crown has been formed, the cells

of this portion give rise to Hertwig's epithelial root sheath (see Chapter 2).

Life cycle of the ameloblasts

According to their function, the life span of the cells of the inner enamel epithelium can be divided into six stages: (1) morphogenic, (2) organizing, (3) formative, (4) maturative, (5) protective, and (6) desmolytic. Since the differentiation of ameloblasts is

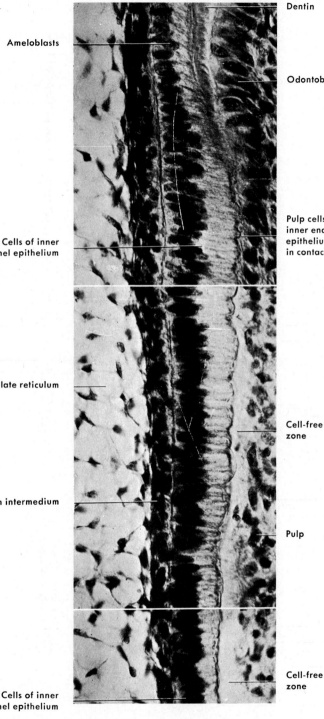

Dentin

Ameloblasts

Odontoblasts

Pulp cells and
inner enamel
epithelium
in contact

Cells of inner
enamel epithelium

B

Stellate reticulum

Cell-free
zone

Stratum intermedium

Pulp

Cell-free
zone

Cells of inner
enamel epithelium

Fig. 3-37, cont'd. B, High magnification of inner enamel epithelium from area X in **A.** In cervical region, cells are short, and outermost layer of pulp is cell free. Occlusally cells are long, and cell-free zone of pulp has disappeared. Ameloblasts are again shorter where dentin formation has begun and enamel formation is imminent. (**B** from Diamond M and Weinmann JP: J Dent Res 21:403, 1942.)

most advanced in the region of the incisal edge or tips of the cusps and least advanced in the region of the cervical loop, all or some stages of the developing ameloblasts can be observed in one tooth germ.

Morphogenic stage. Before the ameloblasts are fully differentiated and produce enamel, they interact with the adjacent mesenchymal cells, determining the shape of the dentinoenamel junction and the crown (Fig. 3-37, *A*). During this morphogenic stage the cells are short and columnar, with large oval nuclei that almost fill the cell body.

The Golgi apparatus and the centrioles are located in the proximal end of the cell,* whereas the mitochondria are evenly dispersed throughout the cytoplasm. During

---

*In modern usage, to conform with the terminology applied to other secretory cells, the dentinal end of the ameloblast, at which enamel is formed, is called *distal*, and the end facing the stratum intermedium is called *basal* or *proximal*.

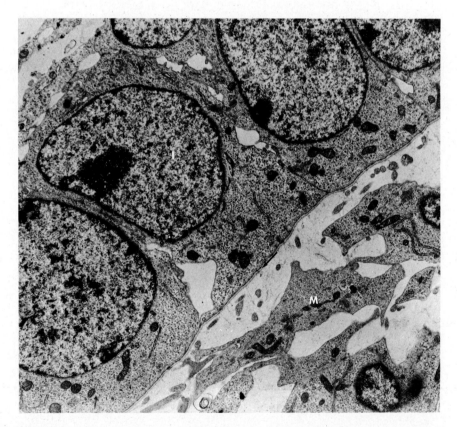

Fig. 3-38. Electron micrograph of inner enamel epithelium, *I,* and adjacent mesenchymal cells of dental papilla, *M,* at early stage of tooth formation. Cytoplasm of cells of inner enamel epithelium is filled with mitochondria and free ribosomes. Typical basement membrane separates epithelium from mesenchyme *(arrow).* Reticular fibers and cytoplasmic processes of mesenchymal cells appear between inner enamel epithelium and cells of dental papilla. (Approximately ×9000.) (Courtesy Dr. P.R. Garant, Stony Brook, NY)

ameloblast differentiation, terminal bars appear concomitantly with the migration of the mitochondria to the basal region of the cell (Fig. 3-44). The terminal bars represent points of close contact between cells. They were previously believed to consist of dense intercellular substance, but under the electron microscope it has been found that they comprise thickening of the opposing cell membranes, associated with condensations of the underlying cytoplasm.

The inner enamel epithelium is separated from the connective tissue of the dental papilla by a delicate basal lamina. The adjacent pulpal layer is a cell-free, narrow, light zone containing fine argyrophil fibers and the cytoplasmic processes of the superficial cells of the pulp (Figs. 3-37, B, and 3-38).

Organizing stage. In the organizing stage of development the inner enamel epithelium interacts with the adjacent connective tissue cells, which differentiate into odontoblasts. This stage is characterized by a change in the appearance of the cells of the inner enamel epithelium. They become longer, and the nucleus-free zones at the distal ends of the cells become almost as long as the proximal parts containing the nuclei (Fig. 3-37, B). In preparation for this development a reversal of the functional polarity of these cells takes place by the migration of the centrioles and Golgi regions from the proximal ends of the cells into their distal ends (Fig. 3-39).

Special staining methods reveal the presence of fine acidophil granules in the proximal part of the cell. Electron miscroscope studies have shown that these granules are actually the mitochondria, which have become concentrated in this part of the cell. At the same time the clear cell-free zone between the inner enamel epithelium and the dental papilla disappears (Fig. 3-37, B), probably because of elongation of the epi-

thelial cells toward the papilla. Thus the epithelial cells come into close contact with the connective tissue cells of the pulp, which differentiate into odontoblasts. During the terminal phase of the organizing stage the formation of the dentin by the odontoblasts begins (Fig. 3-37, B).

The first appearance of dentin seems to be a critical phase in the life cycle of the inner enamel epithelium. As long as it is in contact with the connective tissue of the dental papilla, it receives nutrient material from the blood vessels of this tissue. When dentin forms, however, it cuts off the ameloblasts from their original source of nourishment, and from then on they are supplied by the capillaries that surround and may even penetrate the outer enamel epithelium. This reversal of nutritional source is characterized by proliferation of capillaries of the dental sac and by reduction and gradual disappearance of the stellate reticulum (Figs. 3-35 and 3-37, A). Thus the distance between the capillaries and the stratum intermedium and the ameloblast layer is shortened. Experiments with vital stains demonstrate this reversal of the nutritional stream.

Formative stage. The ameloblasts enter their formative stage (Fig. 3-39) after the first layer of dentin has been formed. The presence of dentin seems to be necessary for the beginning of enamel matrix formation just as it was necessary for the epithelial cells to come into close contact with the connective tissue of the pulp during differentiation of the odontoblasts and the beginning of dentin formation. This mutual interaction between one group of cells and another is one of the fundamental laws of organogenesis and histodifferentiation.

During formation of the enamel matrix the ameloblasts retain approximately the same length and arrangement. Changes in the organization and number of cytoplas-

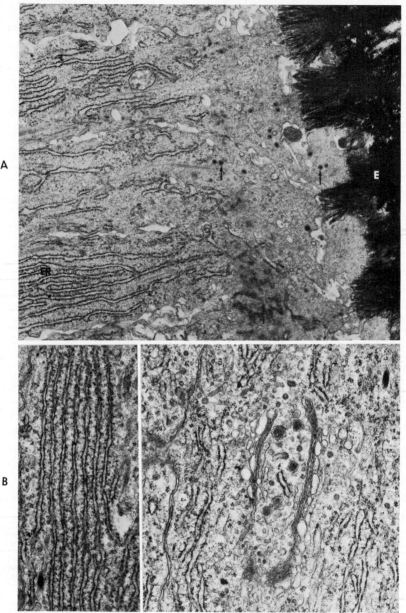

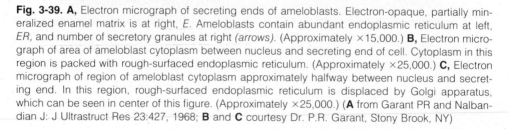

Fig. 3-39. A, Electron micrograph of secreting ends of ameloblasts. Electron-opaque, partially mineralized enamel matrix is at right, *E*. Ameloblasts contain abundant endoplasmic reticulum at left, *ER,* and number of secretory granules at right *(arrows).* (Approximately ×15,000.) **B,** Electron micrograph of area of ameloblast cytoplasm between nucleus and secreting end of cell. Cytoplasm in this region is packed with rough-surfaced endoplasmic reticulum. (Approximately ×25,000.) **C,** Electron micrograph of region of ameloblast cytoplasm approximately halfway between nucleus and secreting end. In this region, rough-surfaced endoplasmic reticulum is displaced by Golgi apparatus, which can be seen in center of this figure. (Approximately ×25,000.) (**A** from Garant PR and Nalbandian J: J Ultrastruct Res 23:427, 1968; **B** and **C** courtesy Dr. P.R. Garant, Stony Brook, NY)

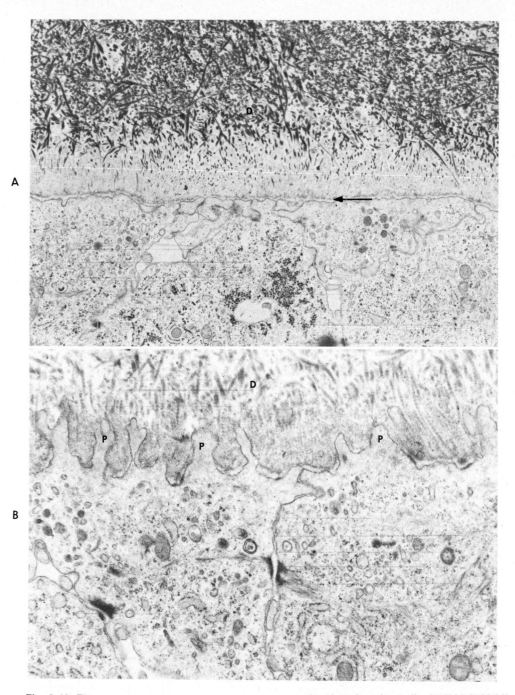

Fig. 3-40. Electron micrographs of distal (secretory) ends of ameloblasts in stage of differentiation shortly before enamel formation begins. **A,** Relatively smooth ameloblast surfaces are separated from predentin *(D)* by basal lamina *(arrow)*. (Approximately ×11,000.) **B,** At slightly later stage, ameloblast cell processes *(P)* have penetrated basal lamina and protrude into predentin *(D)*. (Approximately ×16,000.) (From Kallenbach E: Am J Anat 145:283, 1976.)

mic organelles and inclusions are related to the initiation of secretion of enamel matrix.

The earliest apparent change is the development of blunt cell processes on the ameloblast surfaces, which penetrate the basal lamina and enter the predentin (Fig. 3-40).

Maturative stage. Enamel maturation (full mineralization) occurs after most of the thickness of the enamel matrix has been formed in the occlusal or incisal area. In the cervical parts of the crown, enamel matrix formation is still progressing at this time. During enamel maturation the ameloblasts are slightly reduced in length and are closely attached to enamel matrix. The cells of the stratum intermedium lose their cuboidal shape and regular arrangement and assume a spindle shape. It is certain that the ameloblasts also play a part in the maturation of the enamel. During maturation, ameloblasts display microvilli at their distal extremities, and cytoplasmic vacuoles containing material resembling enamel matrix are present (Figs. 3-50 and 3-52). These structures indicate an absorptive function of these cells.

Protective stage. When the enamel has completely developed and has fully calcified, the ameloblasts cease to be arranged in a well-defined layer and can no longer be differentiated from the cells of the stratum intermedium and outer enamel epithelium (Fig. 3-50). These cell layers then form a stratified epithelial covering of the enamel, the so-called reduced enamel epithelium. The function of the reduced enamel epithelium is that of protecting the mature enamel by separating it from the connective tissue until the tooth erupts. If connective tissue comes in contact with the enamel, anomalies may develop. Under such conditions the enamel may be either resorbed or covered by a layer of cementum.

During this phase of the life cycle of ameloblasts the epithelial enamel organ may retract from the cervical edge of the enamel. The adjacent mesenchymal cells may then deposit afibrillar cementum on the enamel surface (Fig. 3-41).

Desmolytic stage. The reduced enamel epithelium proliferates and seems to induce atrophy of the connective tissue separating it from the oral epithelium, so that fusion of the two epithelia can occur (see Chapter 9). It is probable that the epithelial cells elaborate enzymes that are able to destroy connective tissue fibers by desmolysis. Premature degeneration of the reduced enamel epithelium may prevent the eruption of a tooth.

Amelogenesis

On the basis of ultrastructure and composition, two processes are involved in the development of enamel: organic matrix formation and mineralization. Although the inception of mineralization does not await the completion of matrix formation, the two processes will be treated separately.

Formation of the enamel matrix

The ameloblasts begin their secretory activity when a small amount of dentin has been laid down. The ameloblasts lose the projections that had penetrated the basal lamina separating them from the predentin (compare Figs. 3-40, B, and 3-42, A), and islands of enamel matrix are deposited along the predentin (Fig. 3-42, B,). As enamel deposition proceeds, a thin, continuous layer of enamel is formed along the dentin (Figs. 3-37, B, and 3-43). This has been termed the dentinoenamel membrane. Its presence accounts for the fact that the distal ends of the enamel rods are not in direct contact with the dentin.

Development of Tomes' processes. The surfaces of the ameloblasts facing the develop-

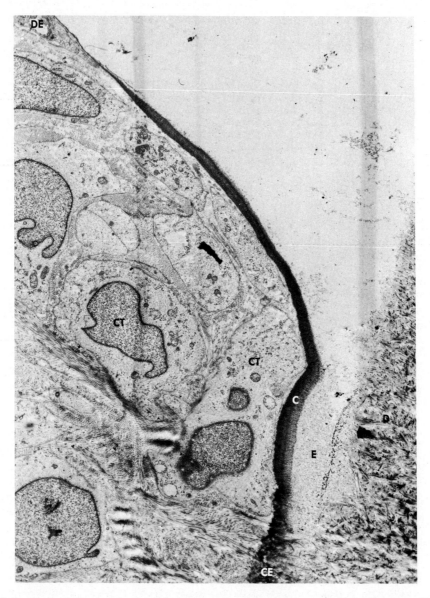

Fig. 3-41. Electron micrograph of cervical region of unerupted human tooth. Dentin matrix, *D,* and remnants of demineralized enamel matrix, *E,* are at right. Afibrillar cementum, apparently of meso-dermal origin, runs through center of figure, *C,* and is continuous with cementum, *CE.* Cells of adja-cent connective tissue, *CT,* and retracted end of enamel organ, *DE,* are at left. (Approximately ×6500.) (From Listgarten MA: Arch Oral Biol 11:999, 1966.)

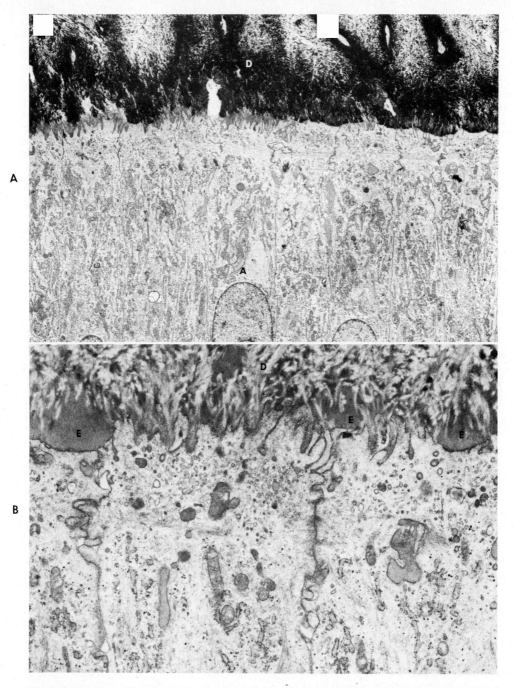

Fig. 3-42. Electron micrographs of ameloblasts in later stage of differentiation than those in Fig. 3-40. **A,** Ameloblasts (A) at left still retain their processes, while those at right, at a slightly later stage of differentiation, have smooth surfaces facing dentin (D). (Approximately ×2700.) **B,** Higher magnification of region similar to that in **A.** In this decalcified section, dentin (D) is pale and islands of enamel matrix (E) are more darkly stained. (Approximately ×12,000.) (From Kallenbach E: Am J Anat 145:283, 1976.)

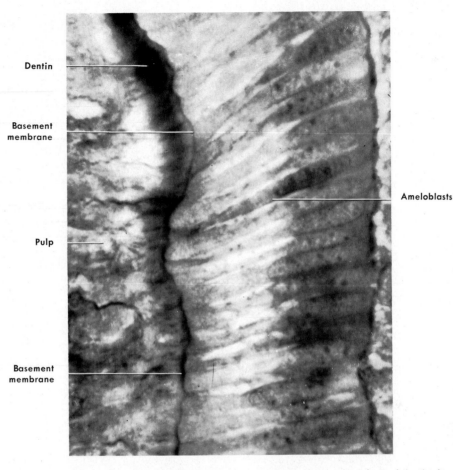

Dentin

Basement
membrane

Pulp

Basement
membrane

Ameloblasts

Fig. 3-43. Basement membrane of dental papilla can be followed on outer surface of dentin, forming dentinoenamel membrane. (From Orban B, Sicher H, and Weinmann JP: J Am Coll Dent 10:13, 1943.)

ing enamel are not smooth. There is an interdigitation of the cells and the enamel rods that they produce (Fig. 3-44). This interdigitation is partly a result of the fact that the long axes of the ameloblasts are not parallel to the long axes of the rods (Figs. 3-45 and 3-46). The projections of the ameloblasts into the enamel matrix have been named Tomes' processes. It was once believed that these processes were transformed into enamel matrix, but more recent

electron microscope studies have demonstrated that matrix synthesis and secretion by ameloblasts are very similar to the same processes occurring in other protein-secreting cells. Although Tomes' processes are partly delineated by incomplete septa (Fig. 3-45), they also contain typical secretion granules as well as rough endoplasmic reticulum and mitochondria (Figs. 3-39, 3-47, *B*, and 3-53, *B*).

Fig. 3-46 is a drawing derived from the

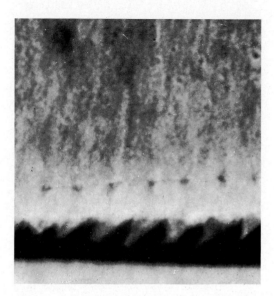

Fig. 3-44. "Picket fence" arrangement of Tomes' processes. Rods are at angle to ameloblasts and Tomes' processes. (From Orban B, Sicher H, and Weinmann JP: J Am Coll Dent 10:13, 1943.)

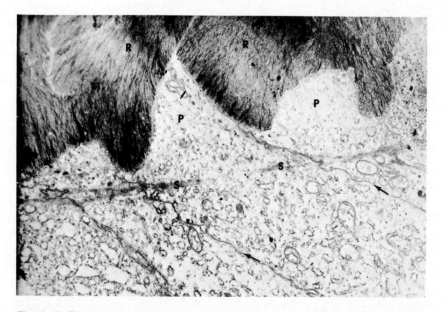

Fig. 3-45. Electron micrograph of ends of ameloblasts and adjacent enamel in developing human deciduous tooth. Positions of ameloblast cell membranes *(arrows)* indicate that cells are nearly perpendicular to long axes of rods, *R*. An incomplete septum, *S,* can be seen, indicating approximate position of Tomes' processes, *P.* (Approximately ×16,000.) (From Rönnholm E: J Ultrastruct Res 6:249, 1962.)

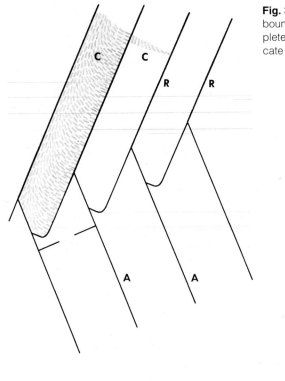

Fig. 3-46. Drawing derived from Fig. 3-45. Dark lines indicate rod boundaries, *R,* and ameloblast cell surfaces, *A,* as well as incomplete septum near distal end of ameloblast at left. Gray lines indicate approximate orientation of apatite crystals, *C.*

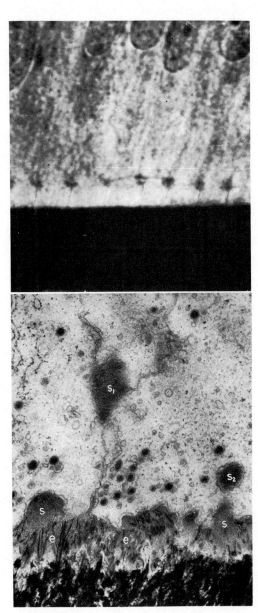

Fig. 3-47. A, Formation of Tomes' processes and terminal bars as first step in enamel rod formation. Rat incisor. **B,** Electron photomicrograph showing an early stage in formation of enamel in lower incisor of rat. At this stage, dentin (at bottom of photomicrograph) is well developed. Enamel, *e,* appears as a less dense layer on surface of dentin and consists of thin, ribbon-shaped elements running more or less perpendicular to dentinoenamel junction and masses of a less dense stippled material, *s.* Separating enamel from cytoplasm of ameloblasts, which occupies most of upper part of photomicrograph, is ameloblast plasma membrane. Parts of three ameloblasts are shown. In middle of photomicrograph in region bounded by membranes of three ameloblasts lies another mass of stippled material, s_1, while a second mass, s_2, lies at right, surrounded by membrane, but within bounds of ameloblast. Numerous small, membrane-bound granules lie within cytoplasm. Contents of these have same general consistency as stippled material, but rather higher density. It is possible that these represent unsecreted granules of stippled material, which in turn is a precursor of enamel matrix. (×24,000.) (**A** from Orban B, Sicher H, and Weinmann JP: J Am Coll Dent 10:13, 1943; **B** from Watson ML: J Biophys Biochem Cytol 7:489, 1960.)

electron micrograph in Fig. 3-45. It is clear from this sketch that at least two amelo-blasts are involved in the synthesis of each enamel rod. If the surface of developing enamel is examined in the scanning elec-tron microscope, which permits a three-di-mensional visualization of the surface, the depressions resulting from the presence of Tomes' processes are quite obvious (Fig. 3-48). One interpretation of the relationships between the keyhole-shaped enamel rods and the roughly hexagonal ameloblasts is indicated in Fig. 3-49. The bulk of the "head" of each rod is formed by one amelo-blast, whereas three others contribute com-ponents to the "tail" of each rod. According to this interpretation, each rod is formed by four ameloblasts, and each ameloblast con-tributes to four different rods.

Distal terminal bars. At the time Tomes' processes begin to form, terminal bars ap-pear at the distal ends of the ameloblasts, separating the Tomes' processes from the

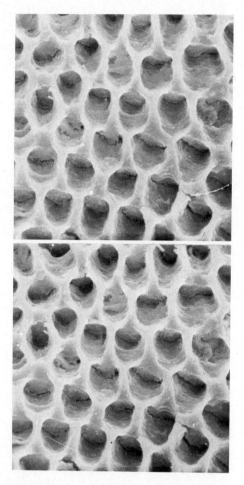

Fig. 3-48. Pair of stereographic scanning electron micro-graphs of surface of developing human enamel. Great depth of focus of this instrument permits visualization of interdigitated nature of this surface. Depressions were occupied by Tomes' processes, which were stripped away with epithelial enamel organ. (Courtesy Dr. A.R. Boyde, London.)

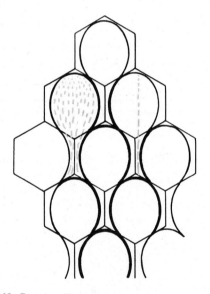

Fig. 3-49. Drawing illustrating one interpretation of rela-tionships between enamel rods and ameloblasts. Cross sections of ameloblasts are indicated by thin lines ar-ranged in regular hexagonal array. Enamel rods are indi-cated by thicker curved black lines, outlining keyhole- or paddle-shaped rods. Gray lines indicate approximate orientation of enamel crystals, which are parallel to long axes of rods in their "bodies" and approach a position perpendicular to long axes in "tails." One can see that each rod is formed by four ameloblasts and that each ameloblast contributes to four different rods. (Modified from Boyde A: In Stack MV and Fearnhead RW, editors: Tooth enamel, Bristol, 1965, John Wright & Sons, Ltd.)

cell proper (Fig. 3-47, *A*). Structurally, they are localized condensations of cytoplasmic substance closely associated with thickened cell membranes. They are observed during the enamel-producing stage of the ameloblasts, but their exact function is not known.

Ameloblasts covering maturing enamel. At the light microscope level one can see that the ameloblasts over maturing enamel are considerably shorter than the ameloblasts over incompletely formed enamel (Fig. 3-50). These short ameloblasts have a villous surface near the enamel, and the ends of the cells are packed with mitochondria (Figs. 3-51 and 3-52). This morphology is

typical of absorptive cells, and it has been demonstrated that ameloblasts are apparently transporting organic components from the matrix. The fact that organic components as well as water are lost in mineralization is a striking difference between enamel and other mineralized tissues. Over 90% of the initially secreted protein is lost during enamel maturation, and that which remains forms envelopes around individual crystals (Fig. 3-10), although there may be a higher content of organic matter in the area of the prism sheath where the abrupt change in crystal orientation occurs. In the electron microscope, several substages can be identified in the transition of amelo-

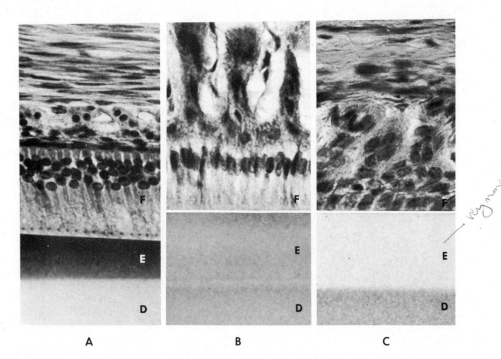

Fig. 3-50. Light micrographs of various stages in life cycle of ameloblasts, *F,* in rat incisor matched with microradiographs of corresponding adjacent enamel, *E,* and dentin, *D.* **A,** Ameloblasts are secreting enamel, which is incompletely formed. Enamel is less radiopaque than dentin, indicating that it is less mineralized. **B,** In area of enamel maturation, ameloblasts are shorter, and enamel matrix is about as heavily mineralized as dentin. **C,** In area in which ameloblasts are in protective stage, enamel is fully mineralized and is much more radiopaque than underlying dentin. (All approximately ×260.)

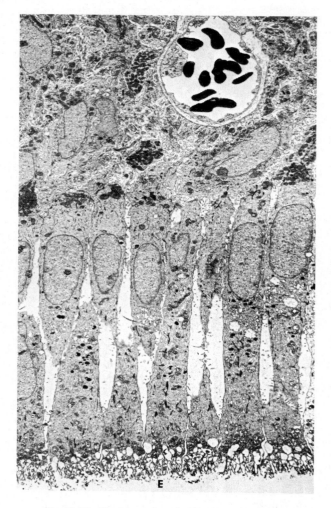

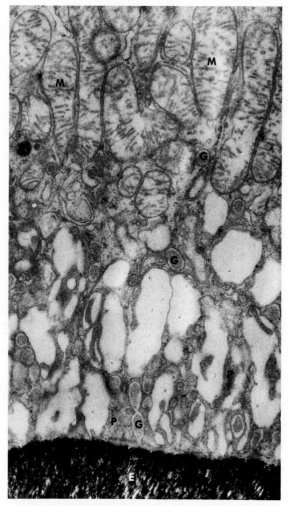

Fig. 3-51. Electron micrograph of ameloblasts during stage of enamel maturation. Enamel has been lost during demineralization. Cells are covered at their surfaces adjoining enamel, *E,* and on their lateral surfaces by numerous microvilli. (Approximately ×3400.) (From Reith EJ: J Biophys Biochem Cytol 9:825, 1961.)

Fig. 3-52. Higher magnification of electron micrograph of ends of ameloblasts during stage of enamel maturation. Adjacent to enamel, *E,* are elaborate cell processes of ameloblasts, *P,* as well as numerous mitochondria within ameloblast cytoplasm, *M.* Granular material, possibly being resorbed, is seen both between cell processes and within ameloblast cytoplasm, *G.* This structure is typical of resorptive cells. (Approximately ×36,000.) (From Reith EJ: J Cell Biol 18:691, 1963.)

blasts from the formative stage through the maturative stage (Fig. 3-53). Shifts are apparent in the cellular organelles from those associated with protein synthesis and secretion to those related to absorption. In addition, a sequence of changes in cell-to-cell contacts and communications between cell layers occurs.

Mineralization and maturation of the enamel matrix

Mineralization of the enamel matrix takes place in two stages, although the time interval between the two appears to be very small. In the first stage an immediate partial mineralization occurs in the matrix segments and the interprismatic substance as they are laid down. Chemical analyses indicate that the initial influx may amount

to 25% to 30% of the eventual total mineral content. It has been shown recently by electron microscopy and diffraction that this first mineral actually is in the form of crystalline apatite (Fig. 3-56, *A*).

The second stage, or *maturation*, is characterized by the gradual completion of mineralization (Fig. 3-50). The process of maturation starts from the height of the crown and progresses cervically (Fig. 3-54). However, at each level, maturation seems to begin at the dentinal end of the rods. Thus there is an integration of two processes: each rod matures from the depth to the surface, and the sequence of maturing rods is from cusps or incisal edge toward the cervical line.

Maturation begins before the matrix has reached its full thickness. Thus it is going

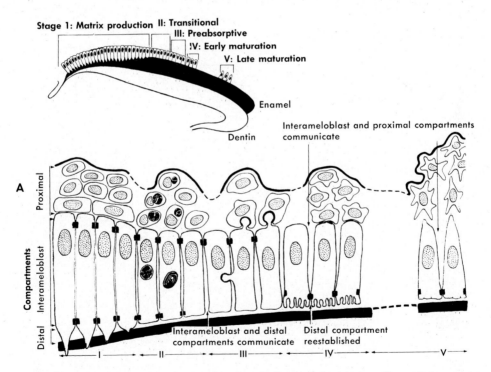

Fig. 3-53. Drawings of electron micrographs of enamel organ of rat incisor. Five substages have been identified from formative to maturative. **A,** Overview of enamel organ.

Continued.

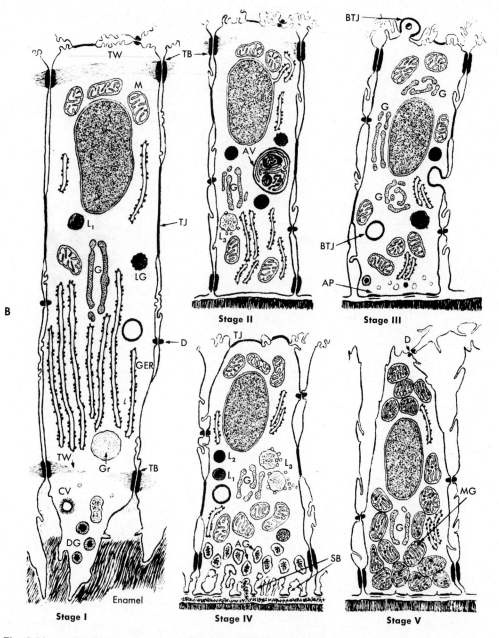

Fig. 3-53, cont'd. B, Individual ameloblasts from five substages. Organelles: *AG,* absorption granules; *AP,* apical contact specialization (hemidesmosomes); *AV,* autophagic vacuoles (lysosomes); *BTJ,* bulb type of contacts; *CV,* coated (absorptive?) vesicles; *D,* desmosomes; *DG,* dense (secretory) granules; *G,* Golgi apparatus; *GER,* granular (rough) endoplasmic reticulum; *Gr,* pale (secretory?) granules; *L₁, L₂, L₃,* lysosomes; *LG,* lipid granules; *M,* mitochondria; *MG,* mitochondrial granules; *SB,* striated border; *TB,* terminal bars; *TJ,* tight junctions; *TW,* terminal web. (From Reith EJ: J Ultrastruct Res 30:111, 1970.)

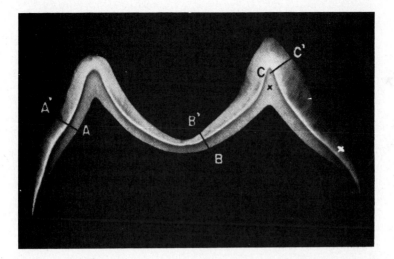

Fig. 3-54. Microradiograph of ground section through developing deciduous molar. From gradation in radiopacity, maturation can be seen to progress from dentinoenamel junction toward enamel surface. Mineralization is more advanced occlusally than in cervical region. Lines *A, B,* and *C* indicate planes in which actual microdensitometric tracings were made. *Black* X, Cusp area. *White* X, Cervical area. (×15.) (From Hammarlund-Essler E: Trans R Schools Dent, Stockholm and Umea 4:15, 1958.)

on in the inner, first-formed matrix at the same time as initial mineralization is taking place in the outer, recently formed matrix. The advancing front is at first parallel to the dentinoenamel junction and later to the outer enamel surface. Following this basic pattern, the incisal and occlusal regions reach maturity ahead of the cervical regions (Fig. 3-55).

At the ultrastructural level, maturation is characterized by growth of the crystals seen in the primary phase (Fig. 3-56, *A*). The original ribbon-shaped crystals increase in thickness more rapidly than in width (Fig. 3-57). Concomitantly the organic matrix gradually becomes thinned and more widely spaced to make room for the growing crystals. Chemical analysis shows that the loss in volume of the organic matrix is caused by withdrawal of a substantial amount of protein as well as water.

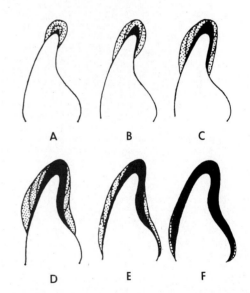

Fig. 3-55. Diagram showing pattern of mineralization of incisor tooth. *Stippled zones,* Consecutive layers of partly mineralized enamel matrix. *Black areas,* Advance of final mineralization during maturation. (From Crabb HSM: Proc R Soc Med 52:118, 1959; and Crabb HSM and Darling AI: Arch Oral Biol 2:308, 1960.)

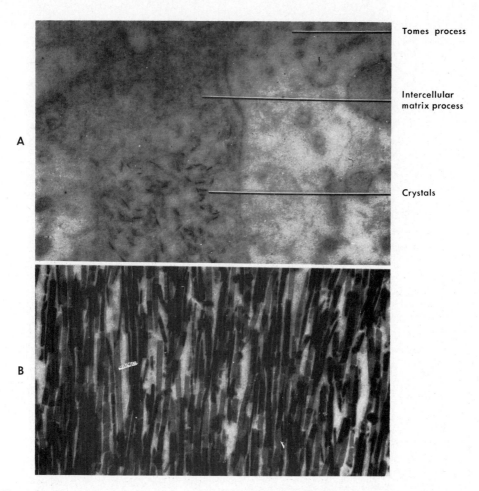

Tomes process

Intercellular
matrix process

Crystals

Fig. 3-56. Electron photomicrographs illustrating difference between short, needlelike crystals laid down in newly deposited enamel matrix **(A)**, and long, ribbonlike crystals seen in mature enamel **(B).** (×70,000.)

Clinical considerations

Clinical interest in amelogenesis is centered primarily on the perfection of enamel formation. Although there is relatively little the dentist can do directly to alter the course of events in amelogenesis, it may be possible to minimize certain factors believed to be associated with the etiology of defective enamel structure. The principal expressions of pathologic amelogenesis are hypoplasia, which is manifested by pitting, furrowing, or even total absence of the enamel, and hypocalcification, in the form of opaque or chalky areas on normally contoured enamel surfaces. The causes of such defective enamel formation can be generally classified as systemic, local, or genetic. The most common systemic influences are nutritional deficiencies, endocrinopathies, febrile diseases, and certain chemical in-

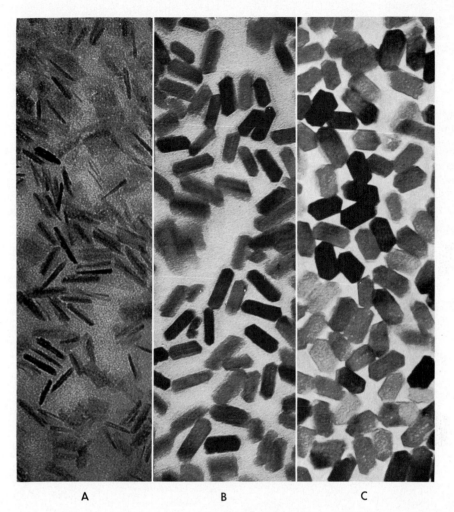

Fig. 3-57. Electron photomicrographs of transverse sections through enamel rods in rat incisor showing three stages in growth of apatite crystals during enamel maturation. From **A** (recently formed enamel) through **C** (more mature enamel) crystals increase in thickness more rapidly than in width. Spaces between crystals will become even smaller as maturation is completed. (×240,000.) (Modified from Nylen MU, Eanes ED, and Omnell K-Å: J Cell Biol 18:109, 1963.)

toxications. It thus stands to reason that the dentist should exert his or her influence to ensure sound nutritional practices and recommended immunization procedures during periods of gestation and postnatal amelogenesis. Chemical intoxication of the ameloblasts is not prevalent and is limited essentially to the ingestion of excessive amounts of water-borne fluoride. Where the drinking water contains fluoride in excess of 1.5 parts per million, chronic endemic fluorosis may occur as a result of continuous use throughout the period of amelogenesis. In such areas it is important to urge substitution of a water with levels of fluoride (about 1 part per million) well below the threshold for fluorosis, yet optimal with regard to protection against dental caries (see discussion of clinical considerations in section on histology).

Since it has been realized that enamel development occurs in two phases, that is, matrix formation and maturation, developmental disturbances of the enamel can be understood more fully. If matrix formation is affected, enamel hypoplasia will ensue. If maturation is lacking or incomplete, hypocalcification of the enamel results. In the case of hypoplasia a defect of the enamel is found. In the case of hypocalcification a deficiency in the mineral content of the enamel is found. In the latter the enamel persists as enamel matrix and is therefore soft and acid insoluble in routine preparation after formalin fixation.

Hypoplasia as well as hypocalcification may be caused by systemic, local, or hereditary factors. Hypoplasia of systemic origin is termed "chronologic hypoplasia" because the lesion is found in the areas of those teeth where the enamel was formed during the systemic (metabolic) disturbance. Since the formation of enamel extends over a longer period and the systemic disturbance is, in most cases, of short duration, the defect is limited to a circumscribed area of the affected teeth. A single narrow zone of hypoplasia (smooth or pitted) may be indicative of a disturbance of enamel formation during a short period in which only those ameloblasts that at that time had just started enamel formation were affected. Multiple hypoplasia develops if enamel formation is interrupted on more than one occasion.

No specific cause of chronologic hypoplasia has been established as yet. Recent investigations have demonstrated that exanthematous diseases are not so fre-

quently a cause of enamel hypoplasia as was heretofore commonly believed. The more frequent causes are said to be rickets and hypoparathyroidism, but hypoplasia cannot be predicted with any reliability even in the most severe forms of those diseases.

The systemic influences causing enamel hypoplasia are, in the majority of cases, active during the first year of life. Therefore the teeth most frequently affected are the incisors, canines, and first molars. The upper lateral incicisor is sometimes found to be unaffected because its development starts later than that of the other teeth mentioned.

Local factors affect single teeth, in most cases only one tooth. If more than one tooth is affected by local hypoplasia, the location of the defects shows no relation to chronology of development. The cause of local hypoplasia may be an infection of the pulp with subsequent infection of the periapical tissues of a deciduous tooth if the irritation occurred during the period of enamel formation of its permanent successor.

The hereditary type of enamel hypoplasia is probably a generalized disturbance of the ameloblasts. Therefore the entire enamel of all the teeth, deciduous as well as permanent, is affected rather than merely a beltlike zone of the enamel of a group of teeth, as in systemic cases. The anomaly is transmitted as a mendelian dominant character. The enamel of such teeth is so thin that is cannot be noticed clinically or in radiographs. The crowns of the teeth of affected family members are yellow-brown, smooth, glossy, and hard, and their shape resembles teeth prepared for jacket crowns.

An example of systemic hypocalcification of the enamel is the so-called mottled enamel. A high fluoride content in the water is the cause of the deficiency in calcification. Fluoride hypocalcification is endemic; that is, it is limited in its distribution to definite areas in which the drinking water contains more than 1 part of fluoride per 1 million parts of water. It has been demonstrated that a small amount of fluoride (about 1 to 1.2 parts per million) reduces susceptibility to dental caries without causing mottling. For this reason many communities are adding small quantities of fluoride to the community water supplies.

The same local causes that might affect the formation of the enamel can disturb maturation. If the injury occurs in the formative stage of enamel development, hypoplasia of the enamel will result. An injury during the maturation stage will cause a deficiency in calcification.

The hereditary type of hypocalcification is characterized by the formation of a normal amount of enamel matrix that, however, does not fully mature. Such teeth, if investigated before or shortly after eruption, show a normal shape. Their surfaces do not have the luster of normal enamel but appear dull. The enamel is opaque. The hypocalcified soft enamel matrix is soon discolored, abraded by mastication, or peeled off in layers. When parts of the soft enamel are lost, the teeth show an irregular, rough surface. When the enamel is altogether lost, the teeth are small and brown, and the exposed dentin is extremely sensitive. In a rare hereditary disturbance of the enamel organ called odontodysplasia, both the apposition and maturation of the enamel are disturbed. Such teeth have irregular, "moth-eaten," poorly calcified enamel.

The discoloration of teeth from administration of tetracyclines during childhood is a very common clinical problem. Whereas usually this discoloration is because of deposition of tetracycline in the dentin, a small amount of the drug may be deposited in the enamel. In mild cases, the use of some of the newly developed surface-binding restorative materials can produce good esthetic results.

REFERENCES
Structure

Arnold FA Jr.: Grand Rapids fluoridation study—results pertaining to the eleventh year of fluoridation, Am J Public Health 47:539, 1957.

Bartelstone HJ, Mandel ID, Oshry E, and Seidlin SM: Use of radioactive iodine as a tracer in the study of the physiology of the teeth, Science 106:132, 1947.

Bergman G, Hammerlund-Essler E, and Lysell L: Studies on mineralized dental tissues. XII. Microradiographic study of caries in deciduous teeth, Acta Odontol Scand 16:113, 1958.

Beust T: Morphology and biology of the enamel tufts with remarks on their relation to caries, J Am Dent Assoc 19:488, 1932.

Bhussry BR and Bibby BG: Surface changes in enamel, J Dent Res 36:409, 1957.

Bibby BG and Van Huysen G: Changes in the enamel surfaces; a possible defense against caries, J Am Dent Assoc 20:828, 1933.

Bodecker CF: Enamel of the teeth decalcified by the celloidin decalcifying method and examined by ultraviolet light, Dent Rev 20:317, 1906.

Bodecker CF: The color of the teeth as an index of their resistance to decay, Int J Orthod 19:386, 1933.

Brabant H and Klees L: Histological contribution to the study of lamellae in human dental enamel, Int Dent J 8:539, 1958.

Brudevold F and Söremark R: Chemistry of the mineral phase of enamel. In Miles AEW, editor: Structural and chemical organization of teeth, vol II, New York, 1967, Academic Press, Inc.

Burgess RC, Nikoforuk G, and Maclaren C: Chromatographic studies of carbohydrate components in enamel, Arch Oral Biol 1:8, 1960.

Chase SW: The number of enamel prisms in human teeth, J Am Dent Assoc 14:1921, 1927.

Crabb HS, and Darling AI: The pattern of progressive mineralization in human dental enamel, Int Ser Monogr Oral Biol 2:1, 1962.

Decker JD: Fixation effects on the fine structure of enamel crystal-matrix relationships, J Ultrastruct Res 44:58, 1973.

Eastoe JE: Organic matrix of tooth enamel, Nature 187:411, 1960.

Eastoe JE: In Stack MV and Fearnhead RW, editors:

Tooth enamel, Bristol, 1965, John Wright & Sons, Ltd.

Eggert FM, Allen GA, and Burgess RC: Amelogenins. Purification and partial characterization of proteins from developing bovine dental enamel, J Biochem 131:471, 1973.

Engel MB: Glycogen and carbohydrate-protein complex in developing teeth of the rat, J Dent Res 27:681, 1948.

Fincham AG, Burkland GA, and Shapiro IM: Lipophilia of enamel matrix. A chemical investigation of the neutral lipids and lipophilic proteins of enamel, Calcif Tissue Res 9:247, 1972.

Frank RM and Brendel A: Ultrastructure of the approximal dental plaque and the underlying normal and carious enamel, Arch Oral Biol 11:883, 1966.

Frank RM, Sognnaes RF, and Kern R: In Sognnaes RF, editor: Calcification in biological systems, Washington, DC, 1960, American Association for the Advancement of Science.

Frazier PD: Adult human enamel: an electron microscopic study of crystallite size and morphology, J Ultrastruct Res 22:1, 1968.

Glas JE and Omnell KA: Studies on the ultrastructure of dental enamel, J Ultrastruct Res 3:334, 1960.

Glimcher MJ, Bonar LC, and Daniel EJ: The molecular structure of the protein matrix of bovine dental enamel, J Mol Biol 3:541, 1961.

Gottlieb B: Dental caries, Philadelphia, 1947, Lea & Febiger.

Gray JA, Schweizer HC, Rosevear FB, and Broge RW: Electron microscopic observations of the differences in the effects of stannous fluoride and sodium fluoride on dental enamel, J Dent Res 37:638, 1958.

Gustafson A-G: A morphologic investigation of certain variations in the structure and mineralization of human dental enamel, Odontal Tidskr 67:361, 1959.

Gustafson G: The structure of human dental enamel, Odontol Tidskr 53(suppl), 1945.

Gustafson G and Gustafson A-G: Human dental enamel in polarized light and contact microradiography, Acta Odontol Scand 19:259, 1961.

Gustafson G and Gustafson A-G: Micro-anatomy and histochemistry of enamel. In Miles AEW, editor: Structural and chemical organization of teeth, vol II, New York, 1967, Academic Press, Inc.

Gwinnett AJ: The ultrastructure of the "prismless" enamel of deciduous teeth, Arch Oral Biol 11:1109, 1966.

Gwinnett AJ: The ultrastructure of the "prismless" enamel of permanent human teeth, Arch Oral Biol 12:381, 1967.

Gwinnett AJ: Human prisimless enamel and its influence on sealant penetration, Arch Oral Biol 18:441, 1973.

Helmcke J-G: Ultrastructure of enamel. In Miles, AEW, editor: Structural and chemical organization of teeth, vol II, New York, 1967, Academic Press, Inc.

Hinrichsen CFL and Engel MB: Fine structure of partially demineralized enamel, Arch Oral Biol 11:65, 1966.

Hodson JJ: An investigation into the microscopic structure of the common forms of enamel lamellae with special reference to their origin and contents, Oral Surg 6:305, 1953.

Houver G and Frank RM: Ultrastructural significance of histochemical reactions on the enamel surface of erupted teeth, Arch Oral Biol 12:1209, 1967.

Leach SA and Saxton CA: An electron microscopic study of the acquired pellicle and plaque formed on the enamel of human incisors, Arch Oral Biol 11:1081, 1966.

Listgarten MA: Phase-contrast and electron microscopic study of the junction between reduced enamel epithelium and enamel in unerupted human teeth, Arch Oral Biol 11:999, 1966.

Listgarten MA: Electron microscopic study of the gingivo-dental junction of man, Am J Anat 119:147, 1966.

Meckel AH: The formation and properties of organic films on teeth, Arch Oral Biol 10:585, 1965.

Meckel AH, Griebstein WJ, and Neal RJ: Structure of mature human dental enamel as observed by electron microscopy, Arch Oral Biol 10:775, 1965.

Muhler JC: Present status of topical fluoride therapy, J Dent Child 26:173, 1959.

Muhler JC and Radike AW: Effect of a dentifrice containing stannous fluoride on adults. II. Results at the end of two years of unsupervised use, J Am Dent Assoc 55:196, 1957.

Nikiforuk G and Sognnaes RF: Dental enamel, Clin Orthop 47:229, 1966.

Orban B: Histology of enamel lamellae and tufts, J Am Dent Assoc 15:305, 1928.

Osborn JW: Three-dimensional reconstructions of enamel prisms, J Dent Res 46:1412,1967.

Osborn JW: Directions and interrelationship of prisms in cuspal and cervical enamel of human teeth, J Dent Res 47:395, 1968.

Osborn JW: A relationship between the striae of Retzius and prism directions in the transverse plane of the human tooth, Arch Oral Biol 16:1061, 1971.

Pautard FGE: An x-ray diffraction pattern from human enamel matrix, Arch Oral Biol 3:217, 1961.

Piez KA: The nature of the protein matrix of human enamel, J Dent Res 39:712, 1960.

Piez KA and Likins RC: The nature of collagen. II. Vertebrate collagens, In Sognnaes RF, editor: Calcification in biological systems, Washington, DC, 1960, American Association for the Advancement of Science.

Ripa LW, Gwinnett AJ, and Buonocore MG: The "prismless" outer layer of deciduous and permanent enamel, Arch Oral Biol 11:41, 1966.

Robinson C, Weatherell JA, and Hallsworth SA: Variation in composition of dental enamel within thin ground tooth sections, Caries Res 5:44, 1971.

Rönnholm E: The amelogenesis of human teeth as revealed by electron microscopy. II. The development of the enamel crystallites, J Ultrastruct Res 6:249, 1962.

Rushton MA: On the fine contour lines of the enamel of milk teeth, Dent Rec 53:170, 1933.

Schmidt WJ and Keil A: Die gesunden und die erkrankten Zahngewebe des Menschen und der Wirbeltiere im Polarisationsmikroskop (Normal and pathological tooth structure of humans and vertebrates in the polarization microscope), Munich, West Germany, 1958, Carl Hanser Verlag.

Schour I: The neonatal line in the enamel and dentin of the human deciduous teeth and first permanent molar, J Am Dent Assoc 23:1946, 1936.

Schour I and Hoffman MM: Studies in tooth development. I. The 16 microns rhythm in the enamel and dentin from fish to man, J Dent Res 18:91, 1939.

Scott DB: The electron microscopy of enamel and dentin. J New York Acad Sci 60:575, 1955.

Scott DB: The crystalline component of dental enamel, Fourth International Conference on Electron Microscopy, Berlin, 1960, Springer Verlag.

Scott DB, Kaplan H, and Wyckoff RWG: Replica studies of changes in tooth surfaces with age, J Dent Res 28:31, 1949.

Scott DB, Ussing MJ, Sognnaes RF, and Wyckoff RWG: Electron microscopy of mature human enamel, J Dent Res 31:74, 1952.

Scott DB and Wyckoff RWG: Typical structures on replicas of apparently intact tooth surfaces, Public Health Rep 61:1397, 1946.

Scott DB and Wyckoff RWG: Studies of tooth surface structure by optical and electron microscopy, J Am Dent Assoc 39:275, 1959.

Selvig KA: The crystal structure of hydroxyapatite in dental enamel as seen with the electron microscope, J Ultrastruct Res 41:369, 1972.

Shaw JH: Fluoridation as a public health measure, Washington, DC, 1954, American Association for the Advancement of Science.

Skillen WC: The permeability of enamel in relation to stain, J Am Dent Assoc 11:402, 1924.

Sognnaes RF: The organic elements of the enamel. III. The pattern of the organic framework in the region of the neonatal and other incremental lines of the enamel, J Dent Res 28:558, 1949.

Sognnaes RF: The organic elements of the enamel. IV. The gross morphology and the histological relationship of the lamellae to the organic framework of the enamel, J Dent Res 29:260, 1950.

Sognnaes RF: Microstructure and histochemical characteristics of the mineralized tisues, J New York Acad Sci 60:545, 1955.

Sognnaes RF, Shaw JH, and Bogoroch R: Radiotracer studies of bone, cementum, dentin and enamel of rhesus monkeys, Am J Physiol 180:408, 1955.

Spiers RL: The nature of surface enamel, Br Dent J 107:209, 1959.

Stack MV: Organic constituents of enamel, J Am Dent Assoc 48:297, 1954.

Stack MV: Chemical organization of the organic matrix of enamel. In Miles AEW, editor: Structural and chemical organization of teeth, vol II, New York, 1967, Academic Press, Inc.

Swancar JR, Scott DB, and Njemirovskij Z: Studies on the structure of human enamel by the replica method, J Dent Res 49:1025, 1970.

Tao L, Pashley DH, and Boyd L: Effect of different types of smear layers on dentin and enamel shear bond strengths, Dent Mat 4:208, 1988.

Wainwright WW and Lemoine FA: Rapid diffuse penetration of intact enamel and dentin by carbon[14]-labeled urea, J Am Dent Assoc 41:135, 1950.

Warshawsky H: A light and electron microscopic study of the nearly mature enamel of rat incisors, Anat Rec 169:559, 1971.

Watson ML: The extracellular nature of enamel in the rat, J Biophys Biochem Cytol 7:489, 1960.

Weber DF and Glick PL: Correlative microscopy of enamel prism orientation. Am J Anat 144:407, 1975.

Yoon SH, Brudwold F, Gardner DE, and Smith FA: Distribution of fluoride in teeth from areas with different levels of fluoride in the water supply, J Dent Res 39:845, 1960.

Development

Allan JH: Investigations into the mineralization pattern of human dental enamel, J Dent Res 38:1096, 1959.

Allan JH: Maturation of enamel. In Miles AEW, editor: Structural and chemical organization of teeth, vol I, New York, 1967, Academic Press, Inc.

Angmar-Måsson B: A quantitative microradiographic study on the organic matrix of developing human enamel in relation to the mineral content, Arch Oral Biol 16:135, 1971.

Bawden JW and Wennberg A: In vitro study of cellular influence on [45]Ca uptake in developing rat enamel, J Dent Res 56:313, 1977.

Boyde A: The structure of developing mamalian dental enamel. In Stack MV and Fearnhead RW, editors: Tooth enamel, Bristol, 1965, John Wright & Sons, Ltd.

Boyde A and Reith EJ: Scanning electron microscopy of the lateral cell surfaces of rat incisor ameloblasts, J Anat 122:603, 1976.

Crabb HSM: The pattern of mineralization of human dental enamel, Proc R Soc Med 52:118, 1959.

Crabb HSM and Darling AI: The gradient of mineralization in developing enamel, Arch Oral Biol 2:308, 1960.

Deakins M: Changes in the ash, water, and organic content of pig enamel during calcification, J Dent Res 21:429, 1942.

Deakins M and Burt RL: The deposition of calcium, phosphorus, and carbon dioxide in calcifying dental enamel, J Biol Chem 156:77, 1944.

Dean HT: Chronic endemic dental fluorosis, JAMA 107:1269, 1936.

Decker JD: The development of a vascular supply to the rat molar enamel organ, Arch Oral Biol 12:453, 1967.

Engel MB: Some changes in the connective tissue ground substance associated with the eruption of the teeth, J Dent Res 30:322, 1951.

Fearnhead RW: Mineralization of rat enamel, Nature 189:509, 1960.

Fosse G: A quantitative analysis of the numerical density and distributional pattern of prisms and ameloblasts in dental enamel and tooth germs. VII. The numbers of cross-sectioned ameloblasts and prisms per unit area in tooth germs, Acta Odontol Scand 26:573, 1968.

Frank RM and Nalbandian J: Ultrastructure of amelogenesis. In Miles AEW, editor: Structural and chemical organization of teeth, vol I, New York, 1967, Academic Press, Inc.

Garant PR and Gillespie R: The presence of fenestrated capillaries in the papillary layer of the enamel organ, Anat Rec 163:71, 1969.

Garant PR and Nalbandian J: The fine structure of the papillary region of the mouse enamel organ, Arch Oral Biol 13:1167, 1968.

Garant PR and Nalbandian J: Observations on the ultrastructure of ameloblasts with special reference to the Golgi complex and related components, J Ultrastruct Res 23:427, 1968.

Glick PL and Eisenmann DR: Electron microscopic and microradiographic investigation of a morphologic basis for the mineralization pattern in rat incisor enamel, Anat Rec 176:289, 1973.

Glimcher MJ, Brickley-Parsons D, and Levine PT: Studies of enamel proteins during maturation, Calcif Tissue Res 24:259, 1977.

Glimcher MJ, Friberg VA, and Levine PT: The isolation and amino acid composition of the enamel proteins of erupted bovine teeth, Biochem J 93:202, 1964.

Gustafson A-G: A morphologic investigation of certain variations in the structure and mineralization of human dental enamel, Odontol Tidskr 67:361, 1959.

Hals E: Fluorescence microscopy of developing and adult teeth, Oslo, 1953, Norwegian Academic Press.

Hammarlund-Essler E: A microradiographic, microphotometric and x-ray diffraction study of human developing enamel, Trans R Schools Dent, Stockholm and Umea 4:15, 1958.

Irving JT: The pattern of sudanophilia in developing rat molar enamel, Arch Oral Biol 18:137, 1973.

Kallenbach E: Fine structure of rat incisor ameloblasts during enamel maturation, J Ultrastruct Res 22:90, 1968.

Kallenbach E: The fine structure of Tomes' process of rat incisor ameloblasts and its relationship to the elaboration of enamel, Tissue Cell 5:501, 1973.

Kallenbach E: Fine structure of rat incisor ameloblasts in transition between enamel secretion and maturation stages, Tissue Cell 6:173, 1974.

Kallenbach E: Fine structure of differentiating ameloblasts in the kitten, Am J Anat 145:283, 1976.

Kallenbach E: Fine structure of ameloblasts in the kitten, Am J Anat 148:479, 1977.

Kreshover SJ and Hancock JA Jr: The pathogenesis of abnormal enamel formation in rabbits inoculated with vaccinia, J Dent Res 35:685, 1936.

Listgarten MA: Phase-contrast and electron microscopic study of the junction between reduced enamel epithelium and enamel in unerupted human teeth, Arch Oral Biol 11:99, 1966.

Matthiessen ME and Møllgard K: Cell junctions of the human enamel organ, Z Zellforsch Mikrosk Anat 146:69, 1973.

Morningstar CH: Effect of infection of the deciduous molar on the permanent tooth germ, J Am Dent Assoc 24:786, 1937.

Nylen MU, Eanes ED, and Omnell K-A: Crystal growth in rat enamel, J Cell Biol 18:109, 1963.

Nylen MU, and Scott DB: An electron microscopic study of the early stages of dentinogenesis, Pub No 613, US Public Health Serivce, Washington, DC, 1958, US Government Printing Office.

Nylen MU and Scott DB: Electron microscopic studies of odontogenesis, J Indiana State Dent Assoc 39:406, 1960.

Orban B, Sicher H, and Weinmann JP: Amelogenesis (a critique and a new concept), J Am Coll Dent 10:13, 1943.

Osborn JW: The mechanism of ameloblast movement: a hypothesis, Calcif Tissue Res 5:344, 1970.

Pannese E: Observations on the ultrastructure of the enamel organ. I. Stellate reticulum and stratum intermedium, J Ultrastruct Res 4:372, 1960.

Pannese E: Observations on the ultrastructure of the enamel organ. II. Involution of the stellate reticulum, J Ultrastruct Res 5:328, 1961.

Pannese E: Observations on the ultrastructure of the enamel organ. III. Internal and external enamel epithelial, J Ultrastruct Res 6:186, 1962.

Reith EJ: The ultrastructure of ameloblasts during matrix formation and the maturation of enamel, J Biophys Biochem Cytol 9:825, 1961.

Reith EJ: The ultrastructure of ameloblasts during early stages of maturation of enamel, J Cell Biol 18:691, 1963.

Reith EJ and Butcher EO: Microanatomy and histochemistry of amelogenesis. In Miles AEW, editor: Structural and chemical organization of teeth, vol I, New York, 1967, Academic Press, Inc.

Reith EJ and Cotty VF: The absorptive activity of ameloblasts during the maturation of enamel, Anat Rec 157:577, 1967.

Reith EJ and Ross MH: Morphological evidence for the presence of contractile elements in secretory ameloblasts of the rat, Arch Oral Biol 18:445, 1973.

Rönnholm E: An electron microscopic study of the amelogenesis in human teeth. I. The fine structure of the ameloblasts, J Ultrastruct Res 6:229, 1962.

Rönnholm E: The amelogenesis of human teeth as revealed by electron microscopy. II. The development of the enamel crystallites, J Ultrastruct Res 6:249, 1962.

Rönnholm E: The amelogenesis of human teeth as revealed by electron microscopy. III. The structure of the organic stroma of human enamel during amelogenesis, J Ultrastruct Res 6:368, 1962.

Sarnat BG and Schour I: Enamel hypoplasia (chronologic enamel aplasia) in relation to systemic disease, J Am Dent Assoc 28:1989, 1941; 29:67, 1942.

Scott DB and Nylen MU: Changing concepts in dental histology, Ann New York Acad Sci 85:133, 1960.

Scott DB and Nylen MU: Organic-incorganic interrelationships in enamel and dentin—a possible key to the mechanism of caries, Int Dent J 12:417, 1962.

Scott DB, Nylen MU, and Takuma S: Electron microscopy of developing and mature calcified tissues, Rev Belg Sci Dent 14:329, 1959.

Slavkin HC, Mino W, and Bringas P Jr: The biosynthesis and secretion of precursor enamel protein by ameloblasts as visualized by autoradiography after tryptophan administration, Anat Rec 185:289, 1976.

Suga S: Amelogenesis—some histological and histochemical observations, Int Dent J 9:394, 1959.

Travis DF and Glimcher MJ: The structure and organization of and the relationship between the organic matrix and the inorganic crystals of embryonic bovine enamel, J Cell Biol 23:447, 1964.

Ussing MJ: The development of the epithelial attachment, Acta Odontol Scand 13:123, 1955; reprinted in J West Soc Periodont 3:71, 1955.

Wasserman F: Analysis of the enamel formation in the continuously growing teeth of normal and vitamin C deficient guinea pigs, J Dent Res 23:463, 1944.

Watson ML: The extracellular nature of enamel in the rat, J Biophys Biochem Cytol 7:489, 1960.

Watson ML and Avery JK: The development of the hamster lower incisor as observed by electron microscopy, Am J Anat 95:109, 1954.

Weber DF and Eisenmann DR: Microscopy of the neonatal line in developing human enamel, Am J Anat 132:375, 1971.

Weinmann JP: Developmental disturbances of the enamel, Bur 43:20, 1943.

Weinmann JP, Svoboda JF, and Woods RW: Hereditary disturbances of enamel formation and calcification, J Am Dent Assoc 32:397, 1945.

Weinmann JP, Wessinger GD, and Reed G: Correlation of chemical and histological investigations on developing enamel, J Dent Res 21:171, 1942.

Weinstock A: Matrix development in mineralizing tissues as shown by radioautography: formation of enamel and dentin. In Slavkin HC and Bavetta LA, editors: Developmental aspects of oral biology, New York, 1972, Academic Press, Inc.

Weinstock A and Leblond CP: Elaboration of the matrix glycoprotein of enamel by the secretory ameloblasts of the rat incisor as revealed by radioautography after galactose-^{3}H injection, J Cell Biol 51:26, 1971.

4
DENTIN

The dentin provides the bulk and general form of the tooth and is characterized as a hard tissue with tubules throughout its thickness. Since it begins to form slightly before the enamel, it determines the shape of the crown, including the cusps and ridges, and the number and size of the roots. As a living tissue it contains within its tubules the processes of the specialized cells, the odontoblasts. Although the cell bodies of the odontoblast are arranged along the pulpal surface of the dentin, the cells are morphologically cells of the dentin, because the odontoblasts produce the dentin as well as the odontoblast processes existing within it. Physically and chemically the dentin closely resembles bone. The main morphologic difference between bone and dentin is that some of the osteoblasts exist on the surface of bone, and when one of these cells becomes enclosed within its matrix, it is called an osteocyte. The odontoblasts' cell bodies remain external to dentin, but their processes exist within tubules in dentin. Both are considered vital tissue because they contain living protoplasm.

PHYSICAL AND CHEMICAL PROPERTIES

In the teeth of young individuals the dentin usually is light yellowish in color, becoming darker with age. Unlike enamel, which is very hard and brittle, dentin is viscoelastic and subject to slight deformation. It is somewhat harder than bone but considerably softer than enamel. Dentin hardness varies slightly between tooth types and between crown and root dentin. Dentin is somewhat harder in its central part than near the pulp or on its periphery. The dentin of primary teeth is slightly less hard than that of permanent teeth. The lower content of mineral salts in dentin renders it more radiolucent than enamel. Dentin consists of 35% organic matter and water and 65% inorganic material. The organic substance consists of collagenous fibrils and a ground substance of mucopolysaccharides (proteoglycans and glycos aminoglycans). The inorganic component has been shown by X-ray diffraction to consist of hydroxyapatite, as in bone, cementum, and enamel. Each hydroxyapatite crystal is composed of several thousand unit cells. The unit cells have a formula of $3Ca_3(PO_4)_2 \cdot Ca(OH)_2$. The crystals are plate shaped and much smaller than the hydroxyapatite crystals in enamel. Dentin also contains small amounts of phosphates, carbonates, and sulfates. Organic and inorganic substances can be separated by either decalcification or incineration. In the process of decalcification the organic constituents can be retained and maintain the shape of the dentin. This is why decalcified teeth and bone can be sectioned and provide clear histologic visualization. The enamel, being over 90% mineral in composition, is lost after decalcification.

STRUCTURE

The dentinal matrix of collagen fibers is arranged in a random network. As dentin calcifies, the hydroxyapatite crystals mask the individual collagen fibers. Collagen fibers are only visible at the electron microscopic level.

The bodies of the odontoblasts are arranged in a layer on the pulpal surface of the dentin, and only their cytoplasmic processes are included in the tubules in the mineralized matrix. Each cell gives rise to one process, which traverses the predentin and calcified dentin within one tubule and terminates in a branching network at the junction with enamel or cementum. Tubules are found throughout normal dentin and are therefore characteristic of it.

Dentinal tubules. The course of the dentinal tubules follows a gentle curve in the crown, less so in the root, where it resembles a gentle S in shape (Fig. 4-1). Starting at right angles from the pulpal surface, the first convexity of this doubly curved course is directed toward the apex of the tooth. These tubules end perpendicular to the dentinoenamel and dentinocementum junctions. Near the root tip and along the in-

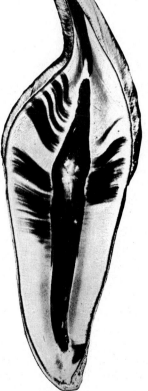

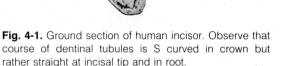

Fig. 4-1. Ground section of human incisor. Observe that course of dentinal tubules is S curved in crown but rather straight at incisal tip and in root.

cisal edges and cusps the tubules are almost straight. Over their entire lengths the tubules exhibit minute, relatively regular secondary curvatures that are sinusoidal in shape. The tubules are longer than the dentin is thick because they curve through dentin. The dentin ranges in thickness from 3 to 10 mm or more.

The ratio between the outer and inner surfaces of dentin is about 5:1. Accordingly, the tubules are farther apart in the peripheral layers and are more closely packed near the pulp (Fig. 4-2). In addition, they are larger in diameter near the pulpal cavity (3 to 4 μm) and smaller at their outer ends (1 μm). The ratio between the numbers of tubules per unit area on the

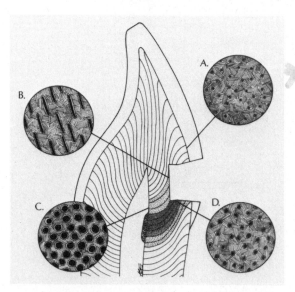

Fig. 4-2. Diagram illustrating the curvature, size, and distance between dentinal tubules in human outer, mid, and inner dentin. The tubules are approximately 1 μm in diameter at the dentinoenamel junction (DEJ), 1.5 to 2 μm midway through dentin, and 1.5 to 3 μm at the pulp. Bacterial penetration (dotted zone) follows line of least resistance to reach the pulp. Note that cut tubules in the floor and walls of a cavity may be different; 1 mm² of cavity exposes 30,000 tubules.

pulpal and outer surfaces of the dentin is about 4:1. Near the pulpal surface of the dentin the number per square millimeter varys between 50,000 and 90,000. There are more tubules per unit area in the crown than in the root. The dentinal tubules have lateral branches throughout dentin, which are termed canaliculi or microtubules. These canaliculi are 1 μm or less in diameter and originate more or less at right angles to the main tubule every 1 to 2 μm along its length (Figs. 4-3, *A* and *B*). Some of them enter adjacent or distant tubules while others end in the intertubular dentin. A few dentinal tubules extend through the dentinoenamel junction into the enamel for several millimeters. These are termed *enamel spindles.*

Peritubular dentin. The dentin that immediately surrounds the dentinal tubules is termed *peritubular dentin.* This dentin forms the walls of the tubules in all but the dentin near the pulp. It is more highly mineralized (about 9%) than intertubular dentin. It is twice as thick in outer dentin (approximately 0.75 μm) than in inner dentin (0.4 μm). By its growth, it constricts the dentinal tubules to a diameter of 1 μm near the dentinoenamel junction. Studies with soft roentgen rays and with electron microscopy show the increased mineral density in the peritubular dentin (Fig. 4-4). A very delicate organic matrix has been demonstrated in this dentin that along with the mineral is lost after decalcification (Fig. 4-4, *B*). After decalcification the odontoblast process appears to be surrounded by an empty space. In demineralized dentin visualized with a light microscope the tubule diameter will therefore appear similar in inner and outer dentin because of the loss of the peritubular dentin. This is important clinically, as etching of a cavity floor will open up the tubules. When peritubular dentin is visualized ultrastructurally in a

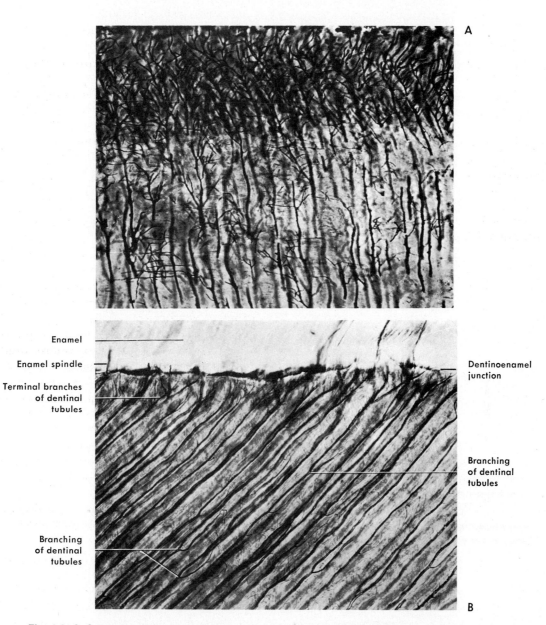

Enamel

Enamel spindle

Terminal branches
of dentinal
tubules

Dentinoenamel
junction

Branching
of dentinal
tubules

Branching
of dentinal
tubules

Fig. 4-3. A, Secondary branching of human dentinal tubules in mid dentin. Note that branches join neighboring as well as distant tubules. **B,** Secondary branches of human dentinal tubules in outer dentin. Note relationships of these tubules to adjacent tubules and their occasional anastomoses. (Courtesy Dr. Gerrit Bevelander, Houston.)

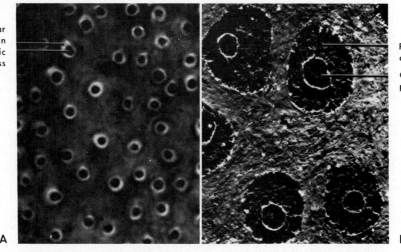

Peritubular
dentin
Odontoblastic
process

Peritubular
dentin

Odontoblastic
process

A

B

Fig. 4-4. Microscopic appearance of peritubular dentin. **A,** Undermineralized ground section of soft roentgen ray showing increased mineral density in peritubular zone. (×1000.) **B,** Electron micrograph of demineralized section of dentin showing loss of mineral in peritubular zone. Organic matrix in peritubular zone is sparse. (Approximately ×4000.)

calcified section of a tooth, the densely mineralized peritubular dentin appears structurally different than the intertubular dentin. The collagen fibers in the tubule wall are masked in peripheral dentin (Fig. 4-5, *A*). A comparison of the tubule wall in inner and outer dentin is shown in Figs. 4-5 and 4-6. Several investigators believe the calcified tubule wall has an inner organic lining termed the *lamina limitans*. This is described as a thin organic membrane, high in glycosaminoglycan (GAG) and similar to the lining of lacunae in cartilage and bone. Other investigators believe this lining in the tubules is absent or limited and that instead only the plasma membrane of the odontoblast is present there.

Intertubular dentin. The main body of dentin is composed of intertubular dentin. It is located between the dental tubules or, more specifically, between the zones of peritubular dentin. Although it is highly mineralized, this matrix, like bone and ce-

mentum, is retained after decalcification, whereas peritubular dentin is not. About one half of its volume is organic matrix, specifically collagen fibers, which are randomly oriented around the dentinal tubules (Figs. 4-5 and 4-6). The fibrils range from 0.5 to 0.2 μm in diameter and exhibit crossbanding at 64 μm (640 Å) intervals, which is typical for collagen (Fig. 4-6, *A*). Hydroxyapatite crystals, which average 0.1 μm in length, are formed along the fibers with their long axes oriented parallel to the collagen fibers.

Predentin. The predentin is located adjacent to the pulp tissue and is 2 to 6 μm wide, depending on the extent of activity of the odontoblast. It is the first-formed dentin and is not mineralized (Figs. 4-7 and 4-2). As the collagen fibers undergo mineralization at the predentin-dentin junction, the predentin becomes dentin and a new layer of predentin forms circumpulpally.

Odontoblast process. The odontoblast pro-

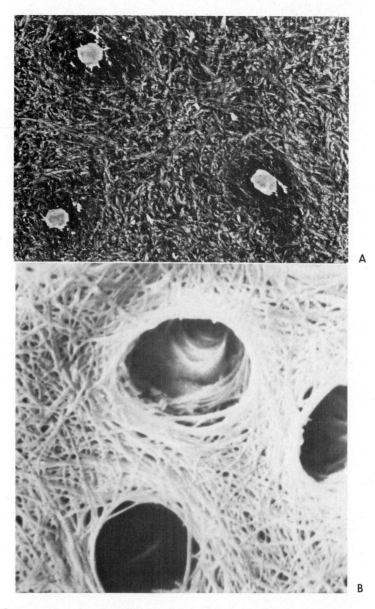

A

B

Fig. 4-5. A, Cross section of undecalcified peripheral human dentin, showing crisscross arrangement of collagen matrix fibers. Observe the more densely calcified peritubular dentin. **B,** Scanning electron microscope picture of pulpal surface of dentin illustrating random arrangement of calcifying collagen fibers of matrix surrounding the dentinal tubules. ($\times$15,000.) (Courtesy A. Boyde, London.)

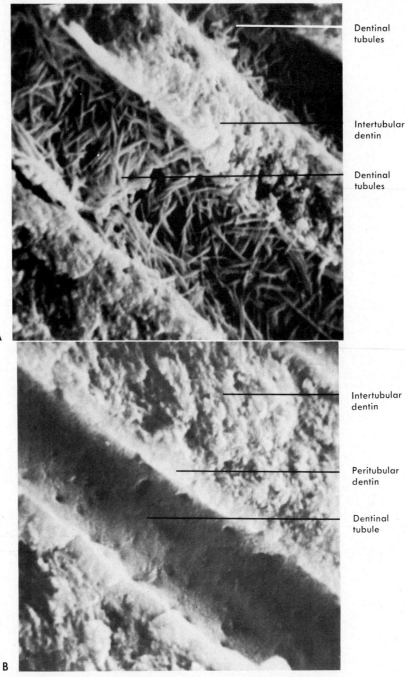

Dentinal
tubules

Intertubular
dentin

Dentinal
tubules

Intertubular
dentin

Peritubular
dentin

Dentinal
tubule

A

B

Fig. 4-6. A, Dentinal tubule representative of inner dentin near formative front as seen by scanning electron microscopy. Collagen fibers are evident, composing the walls of the dentinal tubules. (×18,000.) **B,** Same dentinal tubule as in **A,** further peripheral in calcified dentin viewed by scanning electron microscopy. Peritubular dentin masks collagen fibers in the tubule wall. Observe numerous side branches (canaliculi) of dentinal tubule. (×15,000.) (From Boyde A: Beitr Electronmikroskop Direktabb Oberfl 1[S]:213, 1968.)

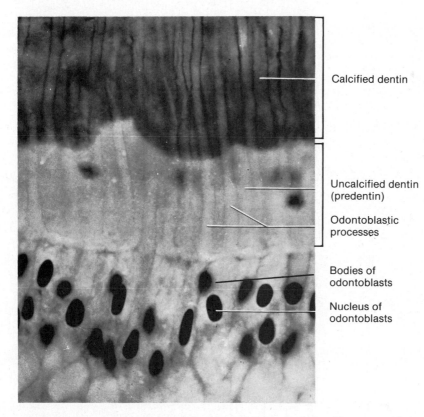

Calcified dentin

Uncalcified dentin
(predentin)

Odontoblastic
processes

Bodies of
odontoblasts

Nucleus of
odontoblasts

Fig. 4-7. Odontoblast processes (Tomes' fibers) within dentinal tubules. They extend from the cell body below at the pulp-predentin junction into the dentin above.

cesses are the cytoplasmic extensions of the odontoblasts. The odontoblast cells reside in the peripheral pulp at the pulp-predentin border and their processes extend into the dentinal tubules (Fig. 4-7). The processes are largest in diameter near the pulp (3 to 4 μm) and taper to approximately 1 μm further into the dentin. The odontoblast cell bodies are approximately 7 μm in diameter and 40 μm in length. Consequently the processes narrow to about half the size of the cell as they enter the tubules (Fig. 4-7). There is disagreement among investigators whether the odontoblast processes extend through the thickness of mature human dentin. Good evidence is shown by transmission electron microscopy that dentinal tubules 200 to 300 μm from the pulp contain processes (Fig. 4-8, *A*). Other investigators, using scanning electron microscopy, have shown what appear to be processes at the dentinoenamel junctions (Fig. 4-8, *B*). Recently cryofractured human teeth revealed the odontoblast process to extend to the dentinoenamel junction (Fig. 4-9). The initial group of investigators believe the findings in Fig. 4-8 and 4-9 represent the organic lining membrane of the tubule (lamina limitans) and not the living process of the odontoblast. Further investigations using immunofluorescent techniques revealed tubulin

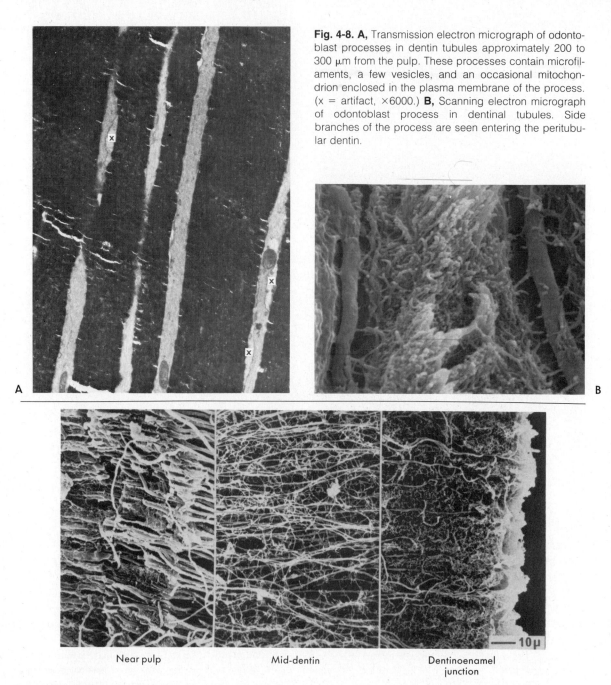

Fig. 4-8. A, Transmission electron micrograph of odontoblast processes in dentin tubules approximately 200 to 300 μm from the pulp. These processes contain microfilaments, a few vesicles, and an occasional mitochondrion enclosed in the plasma membrane of the process. (x = artifact, ×6000.) **B,** Scanning electron micrograph of odontoblast process in dentinal tubules. Side branches of the process are seen entering the peritubular dentin.

Near pulp   Mid-dentin   Dentinoenamel junction

Fig. 4-9. Low magnification scanning electron micrograph of the human odontoblast processes in intact crown dentin. The odontoblasts and their processes are seen in the pulp predentin *(left)* extending through mid-dentin *(center),* and reaching the dentinoenamel junction *(right).* (×1000.) (Courtesy Dr. Toshimoto Yamada.)

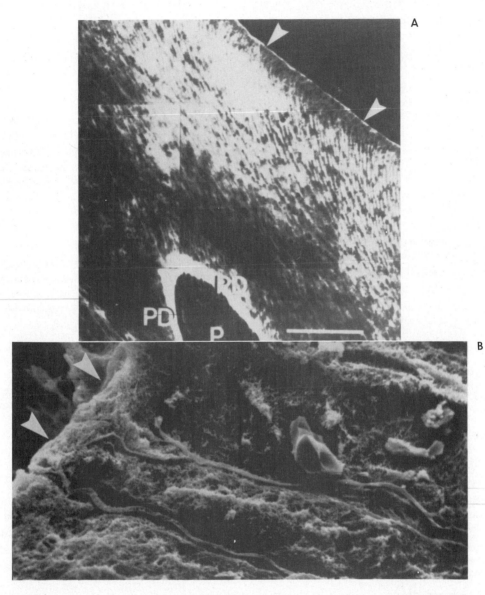

Fig. 4-10. A, Photomicrograph of immunofluorescence labeling of tubulin. This is a subunit protein of the microtubules present in the odontoblast process. *P,* pulp, *Pd,* predentin, *arrows,* dentinoenamel junction (DEJ). **B,** Scanning EM picture of odontoblast processes at DEJ *(arrowheads).* One of the processes displays terminal branching near the DEJ. (Courtesy Drs. J.E. Aubin, A.R. Ten Cate, and S. Pitaru, Medical Research Council Group in Periodontal Physiology and Faculty of Dentistry.)

(an intracellular protein of microtubules) throughout the thickness of dentin (Fig. 4-10, A). It is appropriate to consider that some odontoblast processes traverse the thickness of dentin. In other areas a shortened process may be characteristic in tubules that are narrow or obliterated by mineral deposit.

The odontoblast process is composed of microtubules of 20 μm (200 to 250 Å) in diameter and small filaments 5 to 7.5 μm (50 to 75 Å) in diameter. Occasionally mitochondria, dense bodies resembling lysosomes, microvesicles, and coated vesicles that may open to the extracellular space are also seen (Fig. 4-8, A). The odontoblast processes divide near the dentinoenamel junction and may indeed extend into enamel in the *enamel spindles*. Periodically along the course of the processes side branches appear that extend laterally into adjacent tubules (Fig. 4-9).

PRIMARY DENTIN

Mantle dentin is the name of the first-formed dentin in the crown underlying the dentinoenamel junction. It has also been described in the root underlying the granular layer. It is thus the outer or most peripheral part of the primary dentin and is about 20 μm thick. It is bounded by the dentinoenamel junction and the zone of interglobular dentin. The fibrils formed in this zone are perpendicular to the dentinoenamel junction, and the organic matrix is composed of larger collagen fibrils than are present in the rest of the primary dentin (circumpulpal dentin). Mantle dentin also has fewer defects than circumpulpal dentin.

Circumpulpal dentin forms the remaining primary dentin or bulk of the tooth. It is the circumpulpal dentin that represents all of the dentin formed before root completion. The collagen fibrils in circumpul-

pal dentin are much smaller in diameter (0.05 μm) and are more closely packed together compared to the mantle. The circumpulpal dentin may contain slightly more mineral than mantle dentin.

SECONDARY DENTIN

Secondary dentin is a narrow band of dentin bordering the pulp and representing that dentin formed after root completion. This dentin contains fewer tubules than primary dentin. There is usually a bend in the tubules where primary and secondary dentin interface (Fig. 4-11). Many believe that secondary dentin is formed more slowly than primary dentin and that it looks similar to primary dentin but contains fewer tubules. Secondary dentin is not formed uniformly and appears in greater amounts on the roof and floor of the coronal pulp chamber, where it protects the pulp from exposure in older teeth.

TERTIARY DENTIN

Tertiary dentin is reparative, response, or reactive dentin. This is localized formation of dentin on the pulp-dentin border, formed in reaction to trauma such as caries or restorative procedures. This type of dentin is described in greater detail under reparative dentin, page 124.

INCREMENTAL LINES

The incremental lines (von Ebner), or imbrication lines, appear as fine lines or striations in dentin. They run at right angles to the dentinal tubules and correspond to the incremental lines in enamel or bone (Fig. 4-12). These lines reflect the daily rhythmic, recurrent deposition of dentin matrix as well as a hesitation in the daily formative process. The distance between lines varies from 4 to 8 μm in the crown to much less in the root. The daily increment decreases after a tooth reaches functional

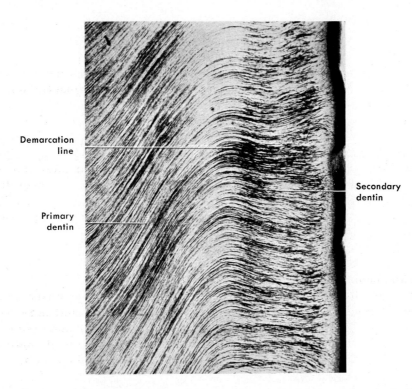

Demarcation line

Primary dentin

Secondary dentin

Fig. 4-11. Dentinal tubules bend sharply as they pass from primary into secondary dentin. The dentinal tubules are somewhat irregular in secondary dentin. Pulpal surface on the right. Ground section human dentin. (Courtesy Dr. Gerrit Bevelander, Houston.)

occlusion. The course of the lines indicates the growth pattern of the dentin.

Occasionally some of the incremental lines are accentuated because of disturbances in the matrix and mineralization process. Such lines are readily demonstrated in ground sections and are known as *contour lines* (Owen), (Fig. 4-13). Analysis with soft x-ray has shown these lines to represent hypocalcified bands.

In the deciduous teeth and in the first permanent molars, where dentin is formed partly before and partly after birth, the prenatal and postnatal dentin are separated by an accentuated contour line. This is termed the *neonatal line* and is seen in enamel as

well as dentin (Fig. 4-14). This line reflects the abrupt change in environment that occurs at birth. The dentin matrix formed prior to birth is usually of better quality than that formed after birth, and the neonatal line may be a zone of hypocalcification.

INTERGLOBULAR DENTIN

Sometimes mineralization of dentin begins in small globular areas that fail to coalesce into a homogenous mass. This results in zones of hypomineralization between the globules. These zones are known as *globular dentin* or *interglobular spaces*. This dentin forms in the crowns of teeth in the circumpulpal dentin just below the

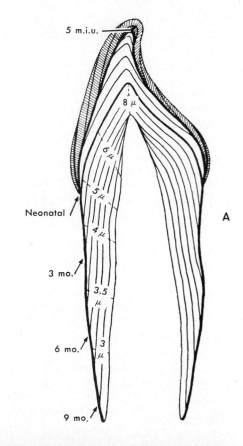

Fig. 4-12. **A,** Diagram of incremental appositional pattern in dentin in a human deciduous central incisor in a 5-month fetus. In the crown as much as 8 μm/day was deposited and in the root 3 to 4 μm. **B,** Incremental lines in dentin. Also known as imbrication lines or incremental lines of von Ebner. Ground section human tooth. (**A** from Schour I and Massler M: J Am Dent Assoc 23:1946, 1936.)

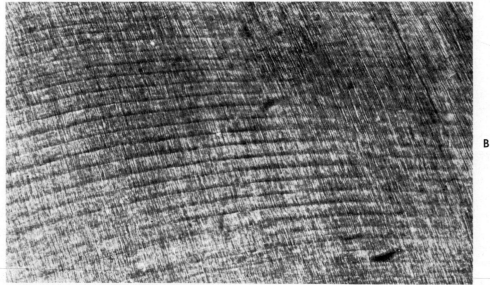

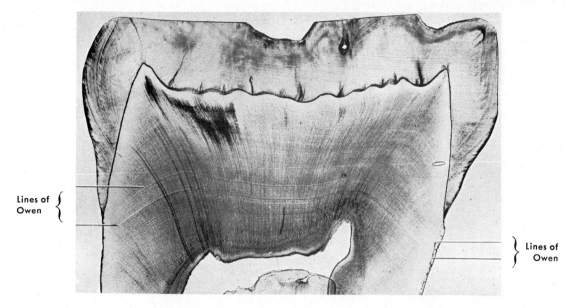

Lines of
Owen

Lines of
Owen

Fig. 4-13. Accentuated incremental lines are termed contour lines (of Owen). Ground section human tooth.

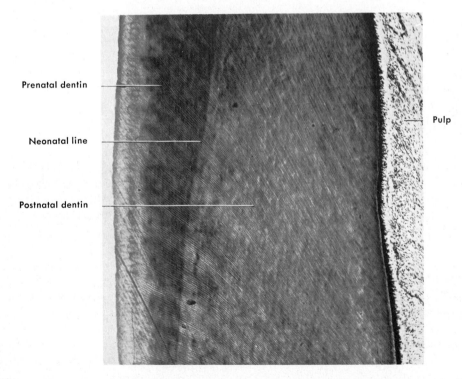

Prenatal dentin

Neonatal line

Postnatal dentin

Pulp

Fig. 4-14. Postnatal formed dentin is separated from prenatal formed dentin by an accentuated incremental line termed the neonatal line. (From Schour I and Poncher HG: Am J Dis Child 54:757, 1937.)

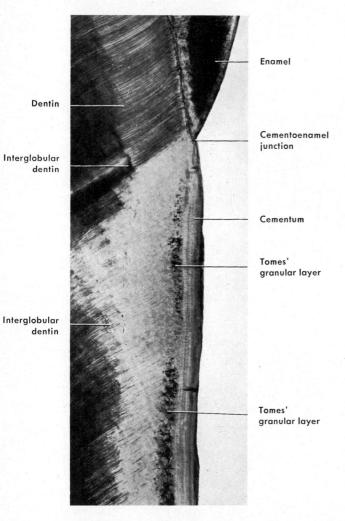

Dentin

Interglobular dentin

Interglobular dentin

Enamel

Cementoenamel junction

Cementum

Tomes' granular layer

Tomes' granular layer

Fig. 4-15. Granular layer (Tomes') appears in root dentin a short distance from the cementodentinal junction. The spaces are air filled and appear black in transmitted light in a ground section.

mantle dentin, and it follows the incremental pattern (Fig. 4-15). The dentinal tubules pass uninterruptedly through interglobular dentin, thus demonstrating more defect of mineralization and not of matrix formation (Fig. 4-16). In dry ground sections some of the globular dentin may be lost, and a space results that appears black in transmit-

ted light (Fig. 4-17). However, spaces in interglobular dentin are not believed to be present, only hypominalized areas.

GRANULAR LAYER

When dry ground sections of the root dentin are visualized in transmitted light, a zone adjacent to the cementum appears granular (Fig. 4-15). This is known as (Tomes') granular layer. This zone increases slightly in amount from the cementoenamel junction to the root apex and is believed to be caused by a coalescing and looping of the terminal portions of the dentinal tubules. Such a process is considered possible as a result of the odontoblasts turning on themselves during early dentin formation. The cause of development of this zone is probably similar to the branching and beveling of the tubules at the dentinoenamel junction. In any case the differentiating odontoblast initially interacts with ameloblasts or the root sheath cells through the basal lamina. In the crown extensive branching of the odontoblast process occurs, and in the root there is branching and coalescing of adjacent processes.

INNERVATION OF DENTIN

Intratubular nerves. Dentinal tubules contain numerous nerve endings in the predentin and inner dentin no farther than 100 to 150 μm from the pulp. Most of these small vesiculated endings are located in tubules in the coronal zone, specifically in the pulp horns. The nerves and their terminals are found in close association with the odontoblast process within the tubule. There may be single terminals (Fig. 4-18) or several dilated and constricted portions (Fig. 4-19). In either case, the nerve endings are packed with small vesicles, either electron dense or lucent, which probably depends on whether there has been dis-

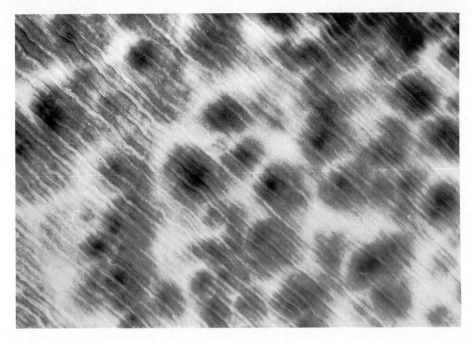

Fig. 4-16. Globular dentin with interglobular spaces as seen in decalcified section of dentin. Dentin tubules pass uninterrupted through uncalcified and hypocalcified areas.

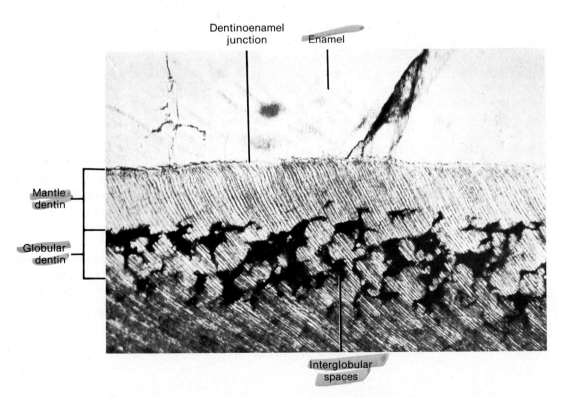

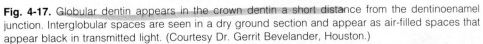

Fig. 4-17. Globular dentin appears in the crown dentin a short distance from the dentinoenamel junction. Interglobular spaces are seen in a dry ground section and appear as air-filled spaces that appear black in transmitted light. (Courtesy Dr. Gerrit Bevelander, Houston.)

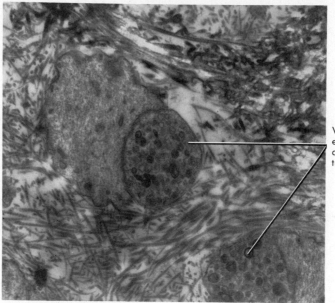

Vesiculated nerve
endings in
adjacent
tubules

Fig. 4-18. Nerve endings in dentinal tubules in region of predentin. The vesiculated endings are
seen in adjacent tubules lying in contact with the odontoblast processes.

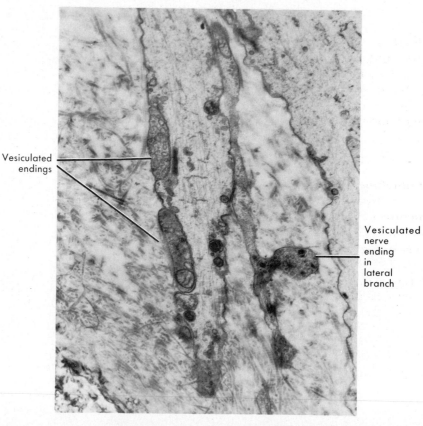

Vesiculated
endings

Vesiculated
nerve
ending
in
lateral
branch

Fig. 4-19. On the left two nerve endings in a dentinal tubule along with an odontoblast process. On
the right a nerve ending extends into the side branch of a dentinal tubule in region of predentin.
(Transmission electron micrograph.)

charge of their neurotransmitter substance. In any case, they interdigitate with the odontoblast process, indicating an intimate relationship to this cell. It is believed that most of these are terminal processes of the myelinated nerve fibers of the dental pulp. The primary afferent somatosensory nerves of the dentin and pulp project to the descending trigeminal nuclear complex (subnucleus caudalis).

Theories of pain transmission through dentin. There are three basic theories of pain conduction through dentin. The first is that of *direct neural stimulation,* meaning that stimuli, in some manner as yet unknown, reach the nerve endings in the inner dentin. There is little scientific support of this theory. The second and most popular theory is the fluid or *hydrodynamic theory.* Various stimuli such as heat, cold, air blast desiccation, or mechanical or osmotic pressure affect fluid movement in the dentinal tubules. This fluid movement, either inward or outward, stimulates the pain mechanism in the tubules by mechanical disturbance of the nerves closely associated with the odontoblast and its process. Thus these endings may act as mechanoreceptors as they are affected by mechanical displacement of the tubular fluid. The third theory is the *transduction theory,* which presumes that the odontoblast process is the primary structure excited by the stimulus and that the impulse is transmitted to the nerve endings in the inner dentin. This is not a popular theory since there are no neurotransmitter vesicles in the odontoblast process to facilitate the synapse or synaptic specialization. The three theories are further explained in Fig. 4-20.

AGE AND FUNCTIONAL CHANGES

Vitality of dentin. Since the odontoblast and its process are an integral part of the dentin, there is no doubt that dentin is a vital tissue. Again, if vitality is understood to be the capacity of the tissue to react to physiologic and pathologic stimuli, dentin must be considered a vital tissue. Dentin is laid down throughout life, although after the teeth have erupted and have been functioning for a short time, dentinogenesis slows, and further dentin formation is at a much slower rate. This is the secondary dentin described earlier in this chapter.

Pathologic effects of dental caries, abra-

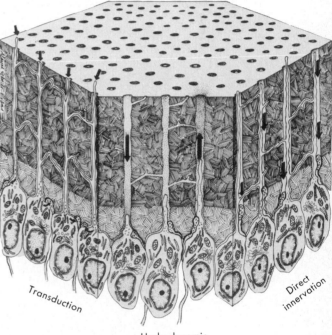

Fig. 4-20. A diagram of the three main explanations of pain transmission through dentin. On the left is shown the *transduction* theory in which the membrane of the odontoblast process conducts an impulse to the nerve endings in the predentin, odontoblast zone, and pulp. In the center is the *hydrodynamic* theory. Stimuli cause an inward or outward movement of fluid in the tubule, which in turn produces movement of the odontoblast and its process. This in turn stimulates the nerve endings. On the right is the *direct conduction* theory in which stimuli directly affect the nerve endings in the tubules.

sion, attrition, or the cutting of dentin of operative procedures cause changes in dentin. These are described as the development of *dead tracts, sclerosis,* and the addition of *reparative dentin.* The formation of reparative dentin pulpally underlying an area of injured odontoblast processes can be explained on the basis of increased dentinogenic activity of the odontoblasts. The mechanisms underlying the series of events that occur in the development of reparative dentin, dead tracts, and sclerosis are not yet fully understood although the histology has been clearly described.

Reparative dentin. If by extensive abrasion, erosion, caries, or operative procedures the odontoblast processes are exposed or cut, the odontoblasts die or, if they live, deposit reparative dentin. The majority of odontoblasts in this situation degenerate, but a few may continue to form dentin. Those odontoblasts that are killed

are replaced by the migration of undifferentiated cells arising in deeper regions of the pulp to the dentin interface. It is believed that the origin of the new odontoblast is from cells in the cell-rich zone or from undifferentiated perivascular cells deeper in the pulp. Both the remaining and the newly differentiated odontoblasts then begin deposition of reparative dentin. This action to seal off the zone of injury occurs as a healing process initiated by the pulp, resulting in resolution of the inflammatory process and removal of dead cells. The hard tissue thus formed is best termed reparative dentin although the terms tertiary dentin, response, or reactive dentin are also used. Reparative dentin is characterized as having fewer and more twisted tubules than normal dentin (Fig. 4-21). Dentin-forming cells are often included in the rapidly produced intercellular substance. In other instances a combination of osteodentin and tubular dentin are seen (Fig. 4-

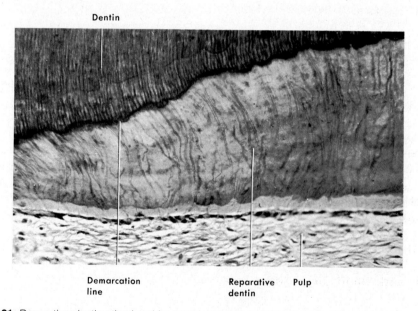

Dentin

Demarcation line   Reparative dentin   Pulp

Fig. 4-21. Reparative dentin stimulated by penetration of caries into dentin. Dentinal tubules are irregular and less numerous than in regular dentin. Decalcified section.

REPARATIVE DENTIN

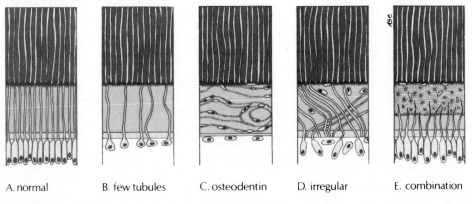

A. normal   B. few tubules   C. osteodentin   D. irregular   E. combination

Fig. 4-22. Diagrammatic illustration of normal *(A)* and other types of reparative dentin *(B to E)*. Reparative dentin contains fewer than normal tubules *(B)*, or it includes cells within its matrix *(C)*, shows irregularly arranged tubules *(D)*, or is a combination of different types *(E)*.

22). It is believed that bacteria, living or dead, or their toxic products, as well as chemical substances from restorative materials, migrate down the tubules to the pulp and stimulate pulpal response, leading to reparative dentin formation. All of the events in this process are not yet known.

Dead tracts. In dried ground sections of normal dentin the odontoblast processes disintegrate, and the empty tubules are filled with air. They appear black in transmitted and white in reflected light (Fig. 4-23). Loss of odontoblast processes may also occur in teeth containing vital pulp as a result of caries, attrition, abrasion, cavity preparation, or erosion (Figs. 4-23 and 4-24). Their degeneration is often observed in the area of narrow pulpal horns (Fig. 4-24) because of crowding of odontoblasts. Again, where reparative dentin seals dentinal tubules at their pulpal ends, dentinal tubules fill with fluid or gaseous substances. In ground sections such groups of tubules may entrap air and appear black in transmitted and white in reflected light.

Dentin areas characterized by degenerated odontoblast processes give rise to dead tracts. These areas demonstrate decreased sensitivity and appear to a greater extent in older teeth. Dead tracts are probably the initial step in the formation of sclerotic dentin.

Sclerotic or transparent dentin. Stimuli may not only induce additional formation of reparative dentin but also lead to protective changes in the existing dentin. In cases of caries, attrition, abrasion, erosion, or cavity preparation, sufficient stimuli are generated to cause collagen fibers and apatite crystals to begin appearing in the dentinal tubules. This condition is prevalent in older individuals. In such cases blocking of the tubules may be considered a defensive reaction of the dentin. Apatite crystals are initially only sporadic in a dentinal tubule but gradually the tubule becomes filled with a fine meshwork of crystals (Fig. 4-25). Gradually, the tubule lumen is obliterated with mineral, which appears very much like the peritubular dentin (Fig. 4-26). The

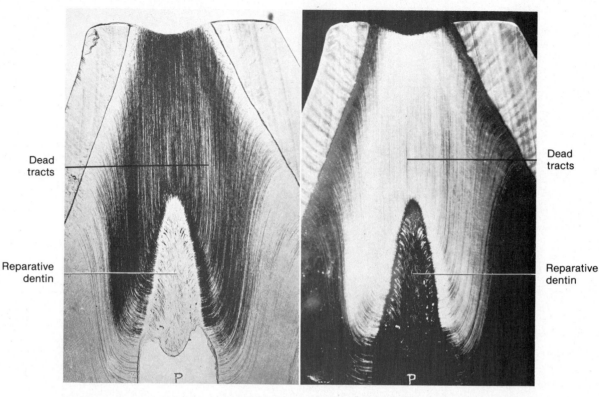

Dead tracts

Reparative dentin

Dead tracts

Reparative dentin

Fig. 4-23. Dead tracts in vital tooth caused by attrition and exposure of dentin. **A,** They appear black in transmitted light and, **B,** white in reflected light. Reparative dentin underlies exposed dentinal tubules and, because of the absence of tubules, appears light in transmitted and dark in reflected light. *P,* pulp. (Courtesy Dr. Gerrit Bevelander, Houston.)

refractive indices of dentin in which the tubules are occluded are equalized, and such areas become *transparent*. Transparent or sclerotic dentin can be observed in the teeth of elderly people, especially in the roots (Fig. 4-27). Sclerotic dentin may also be found under slowly progressing caries (Fig. 4-28). Sclerosis reduces the permeability of the dentin and may help prolong pulp vitality. Mineral density is greater in this area of dentin, as shown both by radiography and permeability studies. It ap-

pears transparent or light in transmitted light and dark in reflected light (Fig. 4-28).

DEVELOPMENT

Dentinogenesis. Dentinogenesis begins at the cusp tips after the odontoblasts have differentiated and begin collagen production. As the odontoblasts differentiate they change from an ovoid to a columnar shape, and their nuclei become basally oriented at this early stage of development (Fig. 4-29). One or several processes arise from the api-

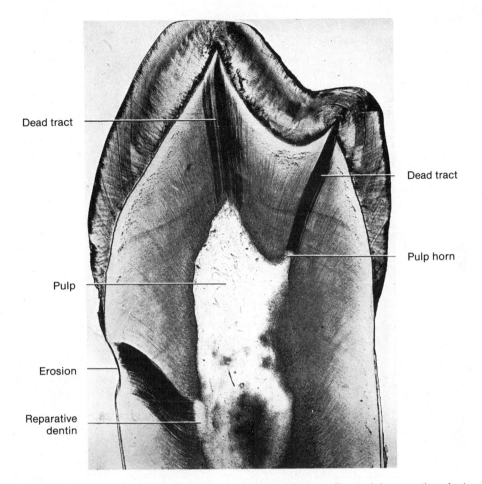

Dead tract

Dead tract

Pulp horn

Pulp

Erosion

Reparative
dentin

Fig. 4-24. Dead tracts in dentin of vital human tooth caused by crowding and degeneration of odontoblasts in narrow pulpal horns and by exposure of tubules to erosion.

cal end of the cell in contact with the basal lamina. The length of the odontoblast then increases to approximately 40 μm, although its width remains constant (7 μm). Proline appears in the rough surface endoplasmic reticulum and Golgi apparatus. The proline then migrates into the cell process in dense granules and is emptied into the extracellular collagenous matrix of the predentin. As the cell recedes it leaves behind a single extension, and the several initial processes join into one, which becomes enclosed in a tubule. As the matrix formation continues, the odontoblast process lengthens, as does the dentinal tubule. Initially daily increments of approximately 4 μm of dentin are formed. This continues until the crown is formed and the teeth erupt and move into occlusion. After this time dentin production slows to about 1 μm/day. After root development is complete, dentin formation may decrease further, although reparative

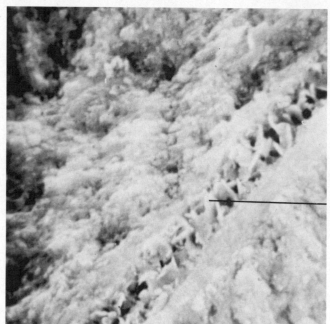

Fig. 4-25. Scanning electron micrograph of partially sclerosed longitudinal sectioned dentin tubules. Platelike crystals form a meshwork occluding tubule lumen. (×9700). (From Lester KS and Boyde A: Virchows Arch [Zell-pathol] 344:196, 1968.)

Tubule

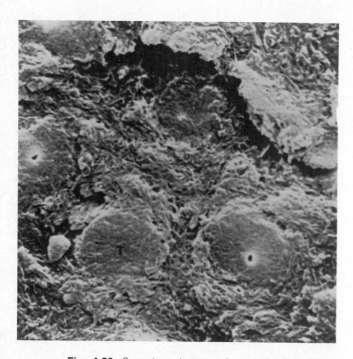

Fig. 4-26. Scanning electron micrograph of fractured cross section of dentin located between attrited surface and the pulp. Various degrees of closure of the tubule lumen are seen. Complete obliteration *(T)* is seen as well as a minute lumen in other tubules. (×5800). (From Brannstrom M: Dentin and pulp in restorative dentistry, London, 1982, Wolfe Medical Publications, Ltd.)

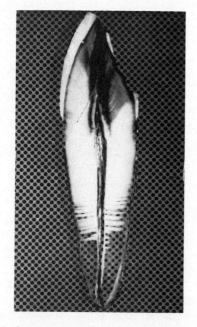

Fig. 4-27. Sclerotic dentin in apical area of root dentin from a section of tooth. Absence of the tubules causes transparent appearance of the dentin. (Courtesy Dr. A.E.W. Miles.)

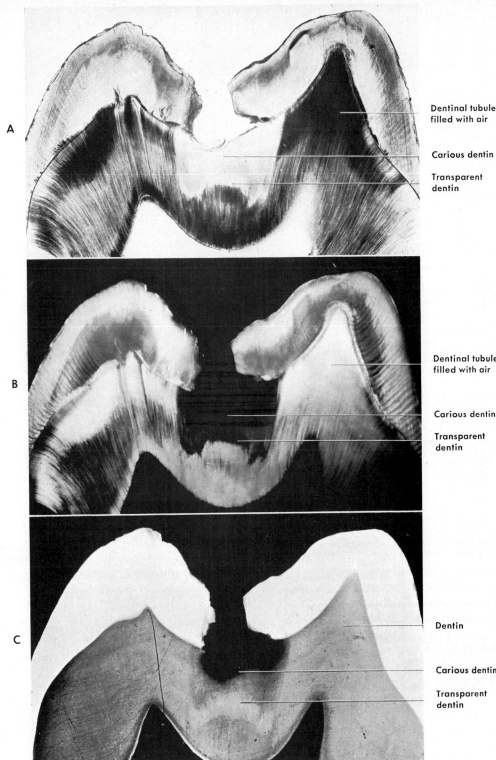

Labels in figure:
A
Dentinal tubules filled with air
Carious dentin
Transparent dentin

B
Dentinal tubules filled with air
Carious dentin
Transparent dentin

C
Dentin
Carious dentin
Transparent dentin

Fig. 4-28. Sclerotic dentin under carious area viewed by, **A,** transmitted light, **B,** reflected light and, **C,** radiograph (grenz ray). Dentinal tubules in dried ground section may be filled with air and appear black in transmitted light **(A),** and white in reflected light, **(B).** Sclerotic dentin with mineral-filled tubules will appear transparent in transmitted light, dark in reflected light, and white in radiographs. (Courtesy Dr. E. Applebaum, New York.)

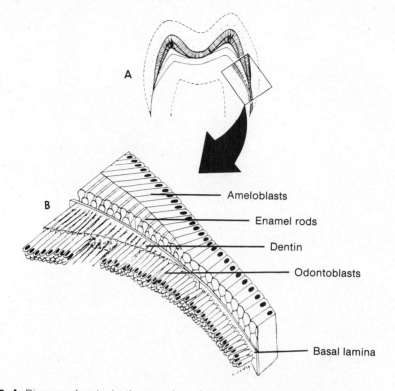

Ameloblasts

Enamel rods

Dentin

Odontoblasts

Basal lamina

Fig. 4-29. A, Diagram of early dentinogenesis and amelogenisis. Lower right, on **B,** is site of differentiation of odontoblasts and ameloblasts. As the odontoblasts move away from the dentinoenamel junction, increments of dentin are formed.

dentin may form at a rate of 4 μm/day for several months after a tooth is restored. Dentinogenesis is a two-phase sequence in that collagen matrix is first formed and then calcified. As each increment of predentin is formed along the pulp border, it remains a day before it is calcified and the next increment of predentin forms (Fig. 4-30). *Korff's fibers* have been described as the initial dentin deposition along the cusp tips. Because of the argyrophilic reaction (stain black with silver) it was long believed that bundles of collagen formed among the odontoblasts (Fig. 4-31). Recently, ultrastructural studies revealed that the staining is of the ground substance among the cells and not collagen. Consequently, all predentin is formed in the apical end of the cell and along the forming tubule wall (Fig. 4-30). The finding of formation of collagen fibers in the immediate vicinity of the apical ends of the cells is in agreement with the general concept of collagen synthesis in connective tissue and bone. The odontoblasts secrete both collagen and other components of the extracellular matrix.

Mineralization. The mineralization sequence in dentin appears to be as follows. The earliest crystal deposition is in the form of very fine plates of hydroxyapatite

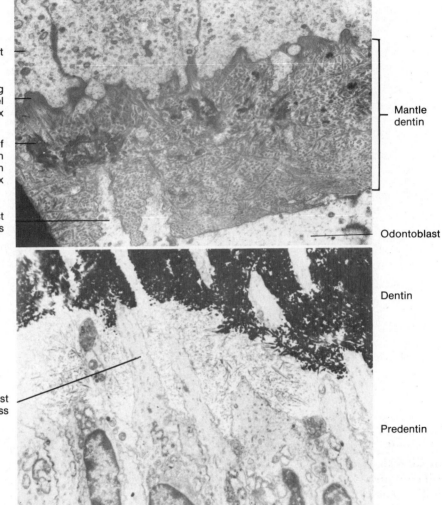

Ameloblast

Forming
enamel
matrix

First sites of
calcification
of dentin
matrix

Odontoblast
process

Mantle
dentin

Odontoblast

Dentin

Odontoblast
process

Predentin

Fig. 4-30. A, First-formed dentin, showing cytoplasm of apical zone of ameloblast, above, and first-formed enamel matrix at the dentinoenamel junction. Below the junction collagen fibers of dentin matrix are seen with calcification sites appearing near the first-formed enamel. Predentin zone is seen below these sites with the odontoblast process extending from the odontoblasts at bottom of field. **B,** Predentin and dentin as visualized in a later developing tooth. Observe calcified (black) dentin above, predentin composed of collagen fibers below, odontoblast processes, and the cell body. (Transmission electron micrographs.)

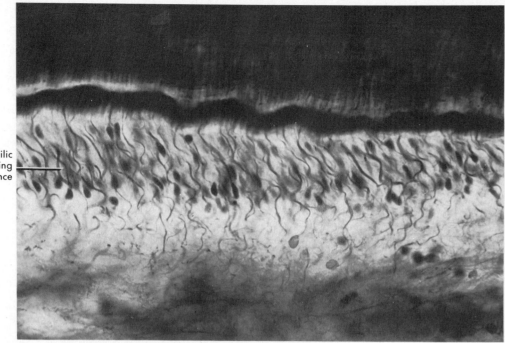

Argyrophilic
staining
substance

Fig. 4-31. Light micrograph of a silver-stained section of early forming dentin. The argyrophilic nature of the ground substances among the odontoblasts appears like bundles of collagen fibers. Fig. 4-30, *B*, illustrates that the collagen formed by the odontoblast is apical to the cell body in the area of the forming predentin.

on the surfaces of the collagen fibrils and in the ground substance (Fig. 4-30, *A*). Subsequently, crystals are laid down within the fibrils themselves. The crystals associated with the collagen fibrils are arranged in an orderly fashion, with their long axes paralleling the fibril long axes, and in rows conforming to the 64 nm (640 Å) striation pattern. Within the globular islands of mineralization, crystal deposition appears to take place radially from common centers, in a so-called spherulite form. These are seen as the first sites of calcification of dentin (Fig. 4-30, *A*).

The general calcification process is gradual, but the peritubular region becomes highly mineralized at a very early stage. Although there is obviously some crystal growth as dentin matures, the ultimate crystal size remains very small, about 3 nm (30 Å) in thickness and 100 nm (1000 Å) in length. The apatite crystals of dentin resemble those found in bone and cementum. They are 300 times smaller than those formed in enamel (Fig. 4-32). It is interesting that two cells so closely allied at the dentinoenamel junction produce crystals of such a size difference but at the same time produce chemically the same hydroxyapatite crystals. Calcospherite mineralization is seen occasionally along the pulp-predentin-forming front (Fig. 4-33).

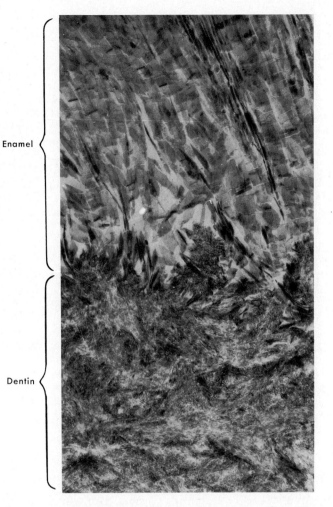

Fig. 4-32. Dentinoenamel junction. Enamel is above and dentin below. Note difference in size and orientation between crystallites of enamel and dentin. Whereas crystals of human enamel may be 90 nm (900 Å) in width and 0.5 to 1 μm in length, those of dentin are only 3nm (30 Å) in width and 100 nm (1000 Å) in length. Crystals of dentin are similar in size to bone. (Electron microphotograph; ×35,000.)

CLINICAL CONSIDERATIONS

The cells of the exposed dentin should not be insulted by bacterial toxins, strong drugs, undue operative trauma, unnecessary thermal changes, or irritating restorative materials. One should bear in mind that when 1 mm^2 of dentin is exposed, about 30,000 living cells are damaged. It is advisable to seal the exposed dentin surface with a nonirritating, insulating substance.

The rapid penetration and spread of car-

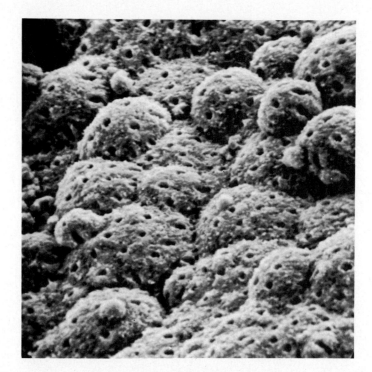

Fig. 4-33. Scanning electron micrograph of globular dentin (calcospherite mineralization) formation at predentin-forming front. Later-forming dentin may be linear, causing interglobular spaces to appear among earlier-formed globular dentin. Treated with ethylene diamine to remove organic material. (Courtesy A. Boyde, London.)

ies in the dentin is the result of the tubule system in the dentin (Fig. 4-2). The enamel may be undermined at the dentinoenamel junction, even when caries in the enamel is confined to a small surface area. This is due in part to the spaces created at the dentinoenamel junction by enamel tufts, spindles, and open and branched dentinal tubules. The dentinal tubules provide a passage for invading bacteria and their products through either a thin or thick dentinal layer.

Electron micrographs of carious dentin show regions of massive bacterial invasion of dentinal tubules (Fig. 4-34). The tubules are enlarged by the destructive action of the microorganisms. Dentin sensitivity of pain, unfortunately, may not be a symptom of caries until the pulp is infected and responds by the process of inflammation, leading to toothache. Thus patients are surprised at the extent of damage to their teeth with little or no warning from pain. Undue trauma from operative instruments also may damage the pulp. Air-driven cutting instruments cause dislodgement of the odontoblasts from the periphery of the pulp and their "aspiration" within the dentinal tubule. This could be an important factor in survival of the pulp if the pulp is already inflamed. Repair requires the mobilization of the macrophage system as healing takes

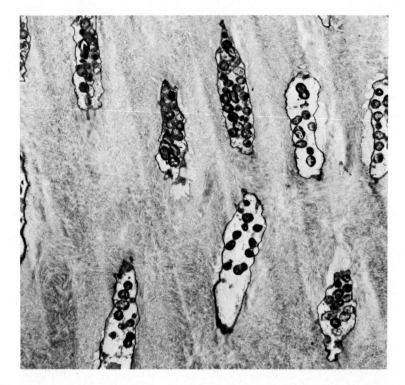

Fig. 4-34. Electron micrograph of dentin underlying carious lesion. Coccoid bacteria are present in the tubules. The peritubular dentin has been destroyed causing the enlargement of the tubules. (×10,000).

place; as this progresses there is the contribution of deeper pulpal cells, through cytodifferentiation into odontoblasts, which will be active in formation of reparative dentin.

The sensitivity of the dentin has been explained by the hydrodynamic theory, that alteration of the fluid and cellular contents of the dentinal tubules causes stimulation of the nerve endings in contact with these cells (Fig. 4-20). This theory explains pain throughout dentin since fluid movement will occur at the dentinoenamel junction as well as near the pulp.

Because we know that reparative dentin is stimulated by cavity lining materials and that dentin forms throughout the life of a tooth, it is now possible to save teeth that previously were lost by extraction or treated by endodontic therapy. Again, teeth with deep, penetrating, carious lesions can be treated by only partial removal of carious dentin and insertion of a "dressing" containing calcium hydroxide for a period of a few weeks or months. During this period the odontoblasts form new dentin along the pulpal surface underlying the carious lesion, and the dentist can then re-open the cavity and remove the remaining bacteria-laden decay without endangering the pulp. This treatment is termed indirect pulp capping. Today there is considerable research on the permeability of dentin. Fluid flow caused by hydrostatic pressure is directly proportional to the number of tubules and radii of tubules per unit surface area of the dentin. Thus coronal dentin is most permeable over the pulp horns. The permeability of radicular dentin near the pulp is only about 20% that of coronal dentin, and the permeability of outer radicular dentin is about 2% of coronal dentin. This suggests that the outer dentin of the root acts as a barrier to fluid movement across dentin in normal circumstances and recalls the correlation between root planing and hypersensitivity. A number of factors have been noted to interfere with fluid flow in

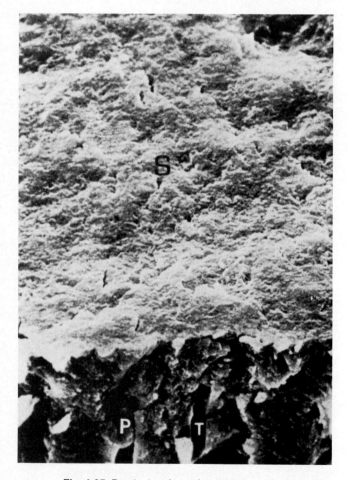

Fig. 4-35. Dentinal surface of prepared cavity with smear layer *(S)* covering ends of tubules. Below surface are dentinal tubules *(T)* and in one tubule a debris plug *(P)*. (Courtesy of Dr. Martin Brännström, Karolinskā Institute, Stockholm.)

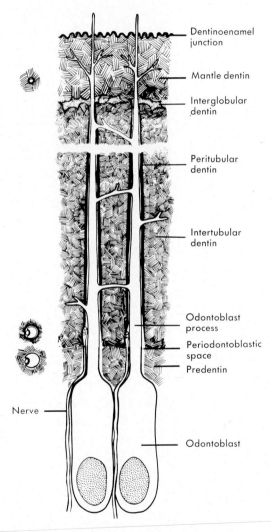

Fig. 4-36. Diagram of the odontoblast and its process in the dental tubule. Note the relationship of the process to the periodontoblastic space and the pertitubular dentin.

the tubules, such as when protein and apatite crystals are present in the tubules. Perhaps the most surprising is the effect of the smear layer on the cavity floor created during cavity preparation (Fig. 4-35). Although it reduces permeability temporarily, it is a bacteria-laden mass and it is important to remove it because toxic products will migrate to the pulp. A cavity liner is then recommended to line the cavity.

A summary diagram illustrating the relationship of the odontoblast and its process to the dentin matrix is shown in Fig. 4-36.

REFERENCES

Anderson DJ and Ronning GA: Osmotic excitants of pain in human dentine, Arch Oral Biol 7:513, 1962.

Applebaum E, Hollander F, and Bodecker CF: Normal and pathological variations in calcification of teeth as shown by the use of soft x-rays, Dent Cosmos 75:1097, 1933.

Arwill T: Innervation of the teeth, Stockholm, 1958, Ivar Haeggströms Boktryckeri AB.

Bergman G and Engfeldt B: Studies on mineralized dental tissues. II. Microradiography as a method for studying dental tissue and its application to the study of caries, Acta Odontol Scand 12:99, 1954.

Bernick S: Innervation of the human tooth, Anat Rec 101:81, 1948.

Bevelander G: The development and structure of the fiber system of dentin, Anat Rec 81:79, 1941.

Bhaskar SN and Lilly GE: Intrapulpal temperature during cavity preparation, J Dent Res 44:644, 1965.

Boyde A: Scanning electron microscopy of collagen-free calcified connective tissues. Beitr elektronenikroskop, direktabb. Oberfl. 1[s]:213-222, Munster, 1968.

Boyde A and Lester KS: An electron microscope study of fractured dentinal surfaces, Calcif Tissue Res 1:122, 1967.

Bradford EW: The maturation of the dentine, Br Dent J 105:212, 1958.

Brannstrom M: Dentin and pulp in restorative dentistry, London, 1982, Wolfe Medical Publications, Ltd.

Brannstrom M and Garberoglio R: Occlusion of dentinal tubules under superficial attrited dentine, Swed Dent J 4:87, 1980.

Ebner V von: Ueber die Entwicklung der leimgebenden Fibrillen im Zahnbein (Development of collagenous fibrils in the dentin), Sitzungsber Akad Wissensch Vienna 115:281, 1906; Anat Anz 29:137, 1906.

Fearnhead RW: Histological evidence for the innervation of human dentine, J Anat 91:267, 1957.

Fogel M, Marshall FJ, and Pashley DH: Effects of distance from the pulp and thickness on the hydraulic conductance of human radicular dentin, J Dent Res 67, 11:1381, 1988.

Frank RM: Electron microscopy of undecalcified sections of human adult dentine, Arch Oral Biol 1:29, 1959.

Harcourt JK: Further observations on the peritubular translucent zone in human dentine, Aust Dent J 9:387, 1964.

Hess WC, Leo DY, and Peckham SC: The lipid content of enamel and dentin, J Dent Res 35:273, 1956.

Holland GR: The dentinal tubule and odontoblast process in the cat, J Anat 12:1169, 1975.

von Korff K: Die Entwicklung der Zahnbein Grundsubstanz der Säugetiere (The development of the dentin matrix in mammals), Arch Mikrosk Anat 67:1, 1905.

von Korff K: Wachstum der Dentingrundsubstanz verschiedener Wirbeltiere (Growth of the dentin matrix of different vertebrates), Z Mikrosk Anat Forsch 22:445, 1930.

Kramer IRH: The distribution of collagen fibrils in the dentine matrix, Br Dent J 91:1, 1951.

Jessen H: The ultrastructure of odontoblasts in perfusion fixed, demineralized incisors of adult rats, Acta Odontol Scand 25:491, 1967.

Lester KS and Boyde A: Electron microscopy of predentinal surfaces, Calcif Tissue Res 1:44, 1967.

Lester KS and Boyde A: Some preliminary observations on caries ("remineralization") crystals in enamel and dentine by surface electron microscopy, Virchows Arch [Pathol Anat] 344:196-212, 1968.

Martens PJ, Bradford EW, and Frank RM: Tissue changes in dentine, Int Dent J 9:330, 1959.

Nalbandian J, Gonzales F, and Sognnaes RF: Sclerotic age changes in root dentin of human teeth as observed by optical, electron, and x-ray microscopy, J Dent Res 39:598, 1960.

Nylen MU and Scott DB: An electron microscopic study of the early stages of dentinogenesis, Pub No 613, US Public Health Service, Washington, DC, 1958, US Government Printing Office.

Nylen MU and Scott DB: Basic studies in calcification, J Dent Med 15:80, 1960.

Orban B: The development of the dentin, J Am Dent Assoc 16:1547, 1929.

Pashley DH: Consideration of dentin permeability in cytotoxicity testing, Int Endo J 21:143, 1988.

Pashley DH, Kepler EE, Williams EC, and O'Meara

JA: The effect on dentine permeability of time following cavity preparation in dogs, Arch Oral Biol 29:1, 65, 1984.

Schour I and Massler M: The neonatal line in enamel and dentin of the human deciduous teeth and first permanent molar, J Am Dent Assoc 23:1946, 1936.

Schour I and Massler M: Studies in tooth development: the growth pattern of the human teeth, J Am Dent Assoc 27:1778, 1940.

Schour I and Poncher HG: The rate of apposition of human enamel and dentin as measured by the effects of acute fluorosis, Am J Dis Child 54:757, 1937.

Scott DB and Nylen MU: Changing concepts in dental histology, Ann New York Acad Sci 85:133, 1960.

Selvig KA: Ultrastructural changes in human dentine exposed to a weak acid, Arch Oral Biol 13:719, 1968.

Shroff FR: Further electron microscope studies on dentin: the nature of the odontoblast process, Oral Surg 9:432, 1956.

Shroff FR, Williamson KI, and Bertaud WS: Electron microscope studies of dentin, Oral Surg 7:662, 1954.

Sicher II: The biology of dentin, Bur 46:121, 1946.

Sognnaes RF: Microstructure and histochemical characteristics of the mineralized tissues, J New York Acad Sci 60:545, 1955.

Takuma S: Electron microscopy of the structure around the dentinal tubule, J Dent Res 39:973, 1960.

Takuma S and Kurahashi Y: Electron microscopy of various zones in the carious lesion in human dentine, Arch Oral Biol 7:439, 1962.

Ten Cate AR: An analysis of Tomes' granular layer, Anat Rec 172(2):137, 1972.

Ten Cate AR, Melcher AH, Pudy G, and Wagner D: The non-fibrous nature of the von Korff fibers in developing dentine. A light and electron microscope study, Anat Rec 168(4):491, 1970.

Watson ML and Avery JK: The development of the hamster lower incisor as observed by electron microscopy, Am J Anat 95:109, 1954.

Yamada T, Nakamura K, Iwaku M, and Fusayama T: The extent of the odontoblast process in normal and carious human dentin, J Dent Res 62(7):798, 1983.

5
PULP

ANATOMY

General features. The dental pulp occupies the center of each tooth and consists of soft connective tissue. Every person normally has a total of 52 pulp organs, 32 in the permanent and 20 in the primary teeth. Each of these organs has a shape that conforms to that of the respective tooth. They have a number of morphologic characteristics that are similar. Each pulp organ resides in a pulp chamber surrounded by dentin containing the peripheral extensions of the cells that formed it. The total volumes of all the permanent teeth pulp organs is 0.38 cc, and the mean volume of a single adult human pulp is 0.02 cc. Molar pulps are three to four times larger than incisor pulps (Fig. 5-1). Table 2 gives the variation in the size of pulp organs in different permanent teeth.

The gross description of the pulps of the maxillary and the mandibular teeth is as follows.

PULPS OF MAXILLARY TEETH

Central incisor: It is somewhat shovel shaped coronally with three short horns on the coronal roof, tapering down to a triangle root in cross section, with the point of the triangle pointing lingually.

Lateral incisor: It is a small and spoon shaped coronally changing to a round evenly tapering root to the apex.

Cuspid: It is the longest pulp with an elliptical cross section buccolingually and a distally inclined apex.

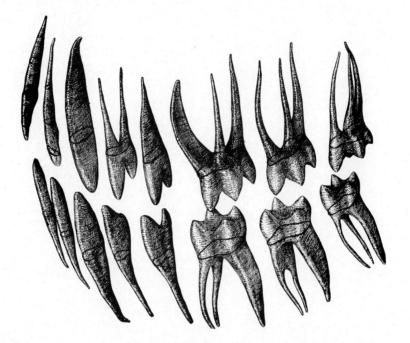

Fig. 5-1. Pulp organs of permanent human teeth. *Upper row,* Maxillary arch; left central incisor through third molar. *Lower row,* Mandibular arch; left central incisor through third molar.

First premolar: It has a large occlusocervical pulp chamber with a mesial concavity extending from the root surface onto the cervical third of the pulp chamber. The coronal chamber divides into two smooth funnel-shaped roots.

Second premolar: It is similar coronally to the first premolar, except it has only one root, which begins to taper at about its midpoint.

Molars: The molars are generally all similar, having a roughly rectangular cervical cross section with the greatest dimension buccolingually and demonstrating a mesiobuccal prominence. There are three roots; the lingual is longest, the distobuccal is shortest and straight, and the mesiobuccal is curved and flattened buccolingually with its mesial surface convex. From the first to third molars the coronal pulp chambers get smaller and the roots get closer together.

PULPS OF MANDIBULAR TEETH

Central incisor: It is one of the smallest pulps in the dentition and is long and narrow with a flattened elliptical shape in cross section buccolingually.

Lateral incisor: It is the same as the central incisor, only smaller in all dimensions.

Cuspid: It is similar to, but shorter than, the maxillary canine, and its root begins tapering at about its midpoint, ending in a distally inclined apex.

First premolar: It looks like a small mandibular canine with an insignificant or missing lingual pulp horn.

Second premolar: The lingual horn is much smaller than the buccal horn and is about the dimension of the mandibular canine. In cross section it is often roundly triangular or sometimes rectangular.

Molars: The mandibular molars are all similar. The coronal cross section is usually rectangular with the mesiodistal dimension greatest, and it also displays a mesiobuccal prominence. The horn heights from highest to lowest are mesiobuccal, mesiolingual, distobuccal, distolingual. There are two roots, the distal being shorter and straighter and singular

Table 2. Pulp volumes for the permanent human teeth from a preliminary investigation of 160 teeth*

	Maxillary (cubic centimeters)	Mandibular (cubic centimeters)
Central incisor	0.012	0.006
Lateral incisor	0.011	0.007
Canine	0.015	0.014
First premolar	0.018	0.015
Second premolar	0.017	0.015
First molar	0.068	0.053
Second molar	0.044	0.032
Third molar	0.023	0.031

*Figures for volumes from Fanibunda KB: Personal communication, University of Newcastle upon Tyne, Department of Oral Surgery, Newcastle upon Tyne, England.

whereas the mesial is longer, curved, and often double. From first to third, the roots get smaller and closer together.

Coronal pulp. Each pulp organ is composed of a coronal pulp located centrally in the crowns of teeth and a root or radicular pulp. The coronal pulp in young individuals resembles the shape of the outer surface of the crown dentin. The coronal pulp has six surfaces: the roof or occlusal, the mesial, the distal, the buccal, the lingual, and the floor. It has pulp horns, which are protrusions that extend into the cusps of each crown. The number of these horns thus depends on the cuspal number. The cervical region of the pulp organs constricts as does the contour of the crown, and at this zone the coronal pulp joins the radicular pulp (Fig. 5-1). Because of continuous deposition of dentin, the pulp becomes smaller with age. This is not uniform through the coronal pulp but progresses faster on the floor than on the roof or side walls.

Radicular pulp. The radicular or root pulp is that pulp extending from the cervical region of the crown to the root apex. In the anterior teeth the radicular pulps are single and in posterior ones multiple. They are not always straight and vary in size, shape, and number. The radicular portions of the pulp organs are continuous with the periapical connective tissues through the apical foramen or foramina. The dentinal walls taper, and the shape of the radicular pulp is tubular. During root formation the apical root end is a wide opening limited by an epithelial diaphragm (Fig. 5-2, A). As growth proceeds, more dentin is formed, so that when the root of the tooth has matured the radicular pulp is narrower. The apical pulp canal becomes smaller also because of apical cementum deposition (Fig. 5-2, B).

Apical foramen. The average size of the apical foramen of the maxillary teeth in the adult is 0.4 mm. In the mandibular teeth it is slightly smaller, being 0.3 mm in diameter.

The location and shape of the apical foramen may undergo changes as a result of functional influences on the teeth. A tooth may be tipped from horizontal pressure, or it may migrate mesially, causing the apex to tilt in the opposite direction. Under these conditions the tissues entering the pulp through the apical foramen may exert pressure on one wall of the foramen, causing resorption. At the same time, cementum is laid down on the opposite side of the apical root canal, resulting in a relocation of the original foramen (Fig. 5-3, A).

Sometimes the apical opening is found on the lateral side of the apex (Fig. 5-3, B), although the root itself is not curved. Frequently, there are two or more foramina separated by a portion of dentin and cementum or by cementum only.

Accessory canals. Accessory canals leading from the radicular pulp laterally through the root dentin to the periodontal tissue may be seen anywhere along the root but are most numerous in the apical third of the root (Fig. 5-4, A). They are clinically significant in spread of infection, either from the pulp to the periodontal ligament or vice versa. The mechanism by

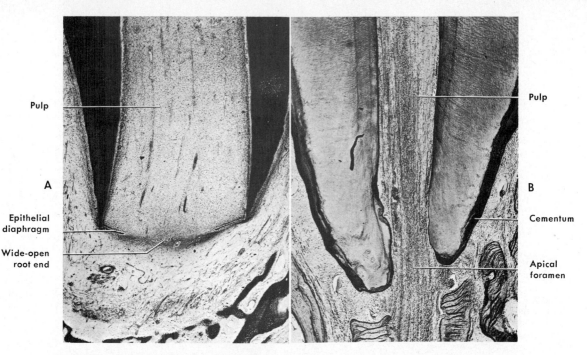

Pulp

A

Epithelial
diaphragm

Wide-open
root end

Pulp

B

Cementum

Apical
foramen

Fig. 5-2. Development of apical foramen. **A,** Undeveloped root end. Wide opening at end of root, partly limited by epithelial diaphragm. **B,** Apical foramen fully formed. Root canal straight. Apical foramen surrounded by cementum. (From Coolidge ED: J Am Dent Assoc 16:1456, 1929.)

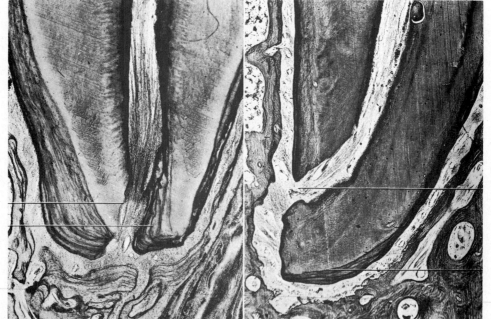

Resorption
of dentin

Apposition
of ce-
mentum

Apical
foramen

Apex

A

B

Fig. 5-3. Variations of apical foramen. **A,** Shift of apical foramen by resorption of dentin and cementum on one surface and apposition of cementum on the other. **B,** Apical foramen on side of apex. (From Coolidge ED: J Am Dent Assoc 16:1456, 1929.)

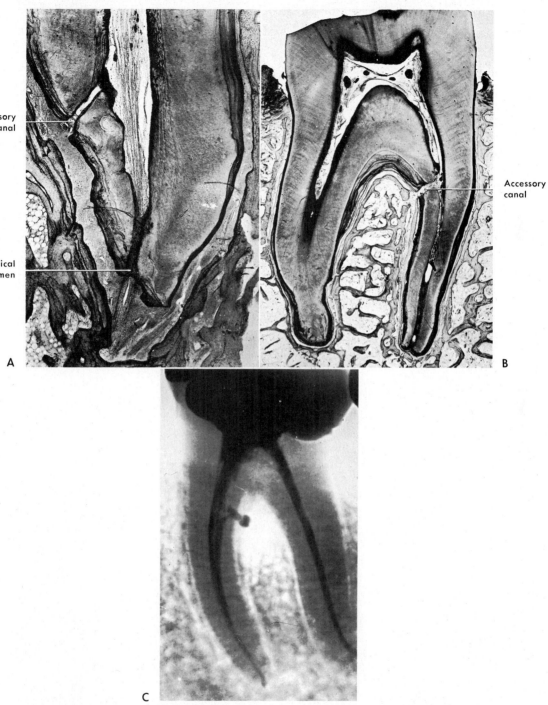

Accessory
canal

Apical
foramen

Accessory
canal

A

B

C

Fig. 5-4. A *and* **B,** Sections through teeth with accessory canals. **A,** Close to apex. **B,** Close to bifurcation. **C,** Roentgenogram of lower molar with accessory canal filled. (**C** from Johnston HB and
Orban B: J Endodont 3:21, 1948.)

which they are formed is not known, but it is likely that they occur in areas where there is premature loss of root sheath cells because these cells induce the formation of the odontoblasts which form the dentin. Accessory canals may also occur where the developing root encounters a blood vessel. If the vessel is located in the area where the dentin is forming, the hard tissue may develop around it, making a lateral canal from the radicular pulp.

STRUCTURAL FEATURES

The central region of both the coronal and the radicular pulp contains large nerve trunks and blood vessels. Peripherally, the pulp is circumscribed by the specialized *odontogenic* region composed of (1) the od-

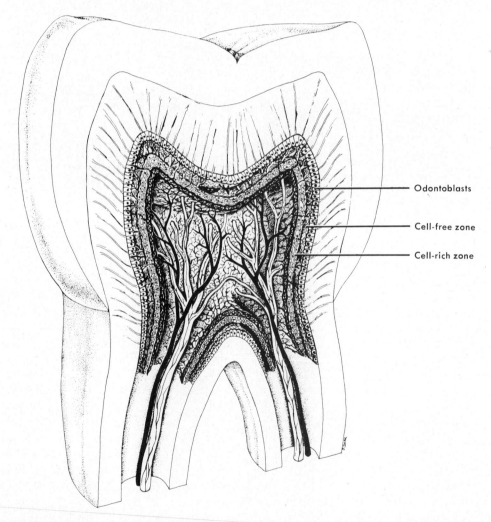

Odontoblasts

Cell-free zone

Cell-rich zone

Fig. 5-5. Diagram of pulp organ, illustrating architecture of large central nerve trunks *(dark)* and vessels *(light)* and peripheral cell-rich, cell-free, and odontoblast rows. Observe small nerves on blood vessels.

ontoblasts (the dentin-forming cells), (2) the cell-free zone (Weil's zone), and (3) the cell-rich zone (Fig. 5-5). The cell-free zone is a space in which the odontoblast may move pulpward during tooth development and later to a limited extent in functioning teeth. This may be why the zone is inconspicuous during early stages of rapid dentinogenesis since odontoblast migration would be greatest at that time. The cell-rich layer is composed principally of fibroblasts and undifferentiated mesenchymal cells. The latter are distinctive because they lack a ribosome-studded endoplasmic reticulum and have mitochrondria with readily discernible cristernae. During early dentinogenesis there are also many young collagen fibers in this zone.

Intercellular substance. The intercellular substance is dense and gellike in nature, varies in appearance from finely granular to fibrillar, and appears more dense in some areas, with clear spaces left between various aggregates. It is composed of both acid mucopolysaccharides and protein polysaccharide compounds (glycosaminoglycans and proteoglycans). During early development, the presence of chondroitin A, chondroitin B, and hyaluronic acid has been demonstrated in abundance. Glycoproteins are also present in the ground substance. The aging pulp contains less of all of these substances. The ground substance lends support to the cells of the pulp while it also serves as a means for transport of nutrients from the blood vessels to the cells, as well as for transport of metabolites from cells to blood vessels.

Fibroblasts. The pulp organ is said to consist of specialized connective tissue because it lacks elastic fibers. Fibroblasts are the most numerous cell type in the pulp. As their name implies, they function in collagen fiber formation throughout the pulp during the life of the tooth. They have the typical stellate shape and extensive processes that contact and are joined by intercellular junctions to the processes of other fibroblasts (Fig. 5-6, *A*). Under the light microscope the fibroblast nuclei stain deeply with basic dyes, and their cytoplasm is lighter stained and appears homogeneous. Electron micrographs reveal abundant rough-surfaced endoplasmic reticulum, mitochondria, and other organelles in the fibroblast cytoplasm (Fig. 5-6, *B*). This indicates these cells are active in pulpal collagen production. There is some difference in appearance of these cells depending on the age of the pulp organ. In the young pulp the cells divide and are active in protein synthesis, but in the older pulp they appear rounded or spindle shaped with short processes and exhibit fewer intracellular organelles. They are then termed *fibrocytes*. In the course of development the relative number of cellular elements in the dental pulp decreases, whereas the fiber population increases (Fig. 5-7). In the embryonic and immature pulp the cellular elements predominate, while in the mature pulp the fibrous components predominate. The fibroblasts of the pulp, in addition to forming the pulp matrix, also have the capability of ingesting and degrading this same matrix. These cells thus have a dual function with pathways for both synthesis and degradation in the same cell.

Fibers. The collagen fibers in the pulp exhibit typical cross striations at 64 nm (640Å) and range in length from 10 to 100 nm or more (Fig. 5-8). Bundles of these fibers appear throughout the pulp. In very young pulp fine fibers ranging in diameter from 10 to 12 nm (100 to 120 Å) have been observed. Their significance is unknown. Pulp collagen fibers do not contribute to dentin matrix production, which is the function of the odontoblast. After root completion the pulp matures and bundles

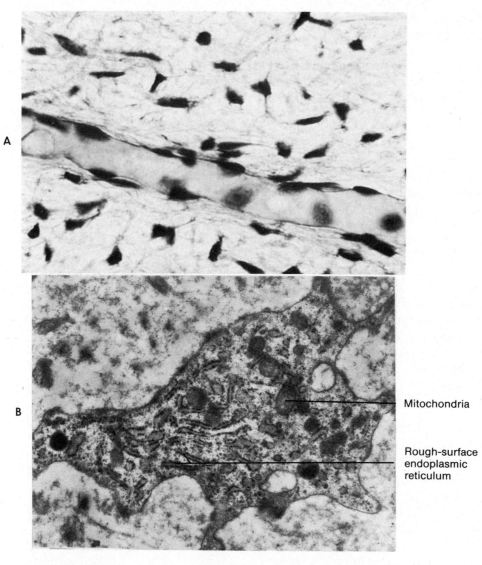

Fig. 5-6. A, Typical fibroblasts of pulp are stellate in shape with long processes. **B,** Electron micrograph of pulp fibroblast.

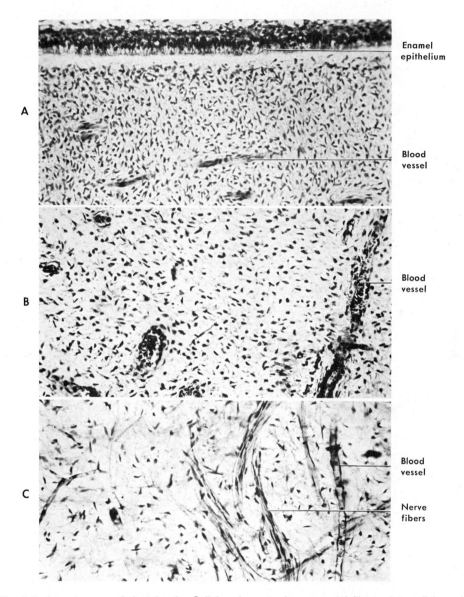

Fig. 5-7. Age changes of dental pulp. Cellular elements decrease and fibrous intercellular substance increases with advancing age. **A,** Newborn infant, **B,** Infant 9 months of age. **C,** Adult.

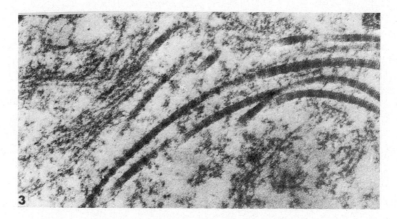

Fig. 5-8. Typical collagen fibers of the pulp with 640 Å banding.

of collagen fibers increase in number. They may appear scattered throughout the coronal or radicular pulp, or they may appear in bundles. These are termed *diffuse* or *bundle collagen* depending on their appearance, and their presence may relate to environmental trauma. Fiber bundles are most prevalent in the root canals, especially near the apical region.

Undifferentiated mesenchymal cells. Undifferentiated mesenchymal cells are the primary cells in the very young pulp, but a few are seen in the pulps after root completion. They appear larger than fibroblasts and are polyhedral in shape with peripheral processes and large oval staining nuclei. They are found along pulp vessels, in the cell-rich zone and scattered throughout the central pulp. Viewed from the side, they appear spindle shaped (Fig. 5-9). They are believed to be a totipotent cell and when need arises they may become odontoblasts, fibroblasts, or macrophages. They decrease in number in old age.

Odontoblasts. Odontoblasts, the second most prominent cell in the pulp, reside adjacent to the predentin with cell bodies in the pulp and cell processes in the dentinal tubules. They are approximately 5 to 7 μm

in diameter and 25 to 40 μm in length. They have a constant location adjacent to the predentin, in what is termed the "odontogenic zone of the pulp" (Fig. 5-10). The cell bodies of the odontoblasts are columnar in appearance with large oval nuclei, which fill the basal part of the cell (Fig. 5-10). Immediately adjacent to the nucleus basally is rough-surfaced endoplasmic reticulum and the Golgi apparatus. The cells in the odontoblastic row lie very close to each other, and the plasma membranes of adjacent cells exhibit junctional complexes, (Fig. 5-11). Further toward the apex of the cell appears an abundance of rough-surfaced endoplasmic reticulum. Near the pupal-predentin junction the cell cytoplasm is devoid of organelles. The clear terminal part of the cell body and the adjacent intercellular junction is described by some as the terminal bar apparatus of the odontoblast. At this zone the cell constricts to a diameter of 3 to 4 μm, where the cell process enters the predentinal tubule (Fig. 5-10). The process of the cell contains no endoplasmic reticulum, but during the early period of active dentinogenesis it does contain occasional mitochondria and vesicles. During the later stages of dentinogenesis

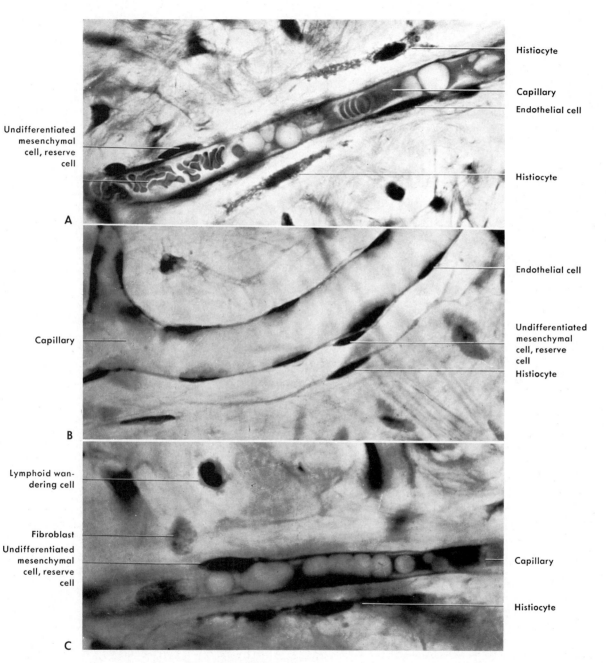

Histiocyte

Capillary

Endothelial cell

Undifferentiated
mesenchymal
cell, reserve
cell

Histiocyte

A

Endothelial cell

Undifferentiated
mesenchymal
cell, reserve
cell

Capillary

Histiocyte

B

Lymphoid wan-
dering cell

Fibroblast

Undifferentiated
mesenchymal
cell, reserve
cell

Capillary

Histiocyte

C

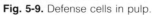

Fig. 5-9. Defense cells in pulp.

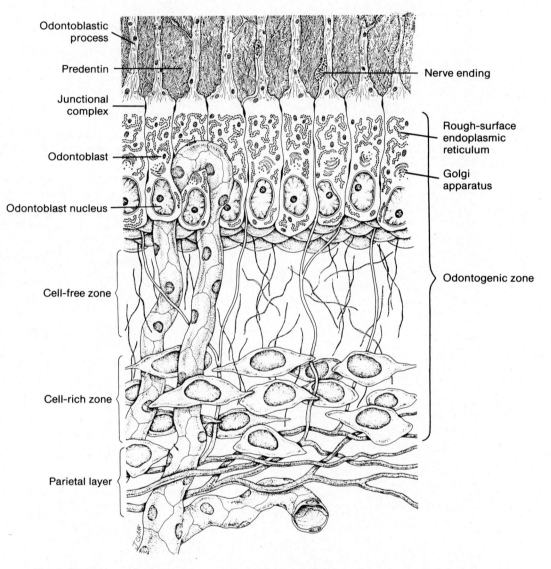

Odontoblastic process

Predentin

Junctional complex

Odontoblast

Odontoblast nucleus

Cell-free zone

Cell-rich zone

Parietal layer

Nerve ending

Rough-surface endoplasmic reticulum

Golgi apparatus

Odontogenic zone

Fig. 5-10. Diagram of odontogenic zone illustrating odontoblast, cell-free, and cell-rich zones, with blood vessels and nonmyelinated nerves among odontoblasts.

these are less frequently seen. There is also a striking difference in the cytoplasm of the young cell body, active in dentino-genesis, and the older cell. During this early active phase the Golgi apparatus is more prominent, the rough-surfaced endo-plasmic reticulum is more abundant, and numerous mitochondria appear throughout the odontoblast. A great number of vesicles are seen along the periphery of the process where there is evidence of protein synthe-sis along the tubule wall. The cell actually increases in size as its process lengthens during dentin formation. When the cell process becomes 2 mm long, it is then many times greater in volume than the cell body. The form and arrangement of the bodies of the odontoblasts are not uniform throughout the pulp. They are more cylin-drical and longer (tall columnar) in the crown (Fig. 5-12, *A*) and more cuboid in the middle of the root (Fig. 5-12, *B*). Close to the apex of an adult tooth the odonto-blasts are ovoid and spindle shaped, ap-pearing more like osteoblasts than odonto-blasts, but they are recognized by their pro-cesses extending into the dentin. In areas close to the apical foramen the dentin is ir-regular in appearance (Fig. 5-12, *C*).

Defense cells. In addition to fibroblasts, odontoblasts, and the cells that are a part of the neural and vascular systems of the pulp, there are cells important to the de-fense of the pulp. These are histiocytes, or macrophages, mast cells, and plasma cells. In addition, there are the blood vascular el-ements such as the neutrophils (PMNs), eo-sinophils, basophils, lymphocytes, and monocytes. These latter cells emigrate from the pulpal blood vessels and develop characteristics in response to inflammation.

The histiocyte, or macrophage, is an ir-regularly shaped cell with short blunt pro-cesses (Figs. 5-9 and 5-13). In the light mi-croscope the nucleus is somewhat smaller,

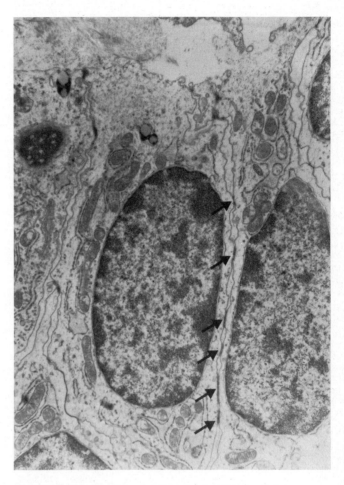

Fig. 5-11. Close relation of adjacent odontoblasts. Note junctional complexes between cells *(arrows)*.

more rounded, and darker staining than that of fibroblasts, and it exhibits granular cytoplasm. When the macrophages are in-active and not in the process of ingesting foreign materials, one has difficulty distin-guishing them from fibroblasts. In the case of a pulpal inflammation these cells exhibit granules and vacuoles in their cytoplasm, and their nuclei increase in size and ex-hibit a prominent nucleolus. Their pres-ence is disclosed by intravital dyes such as

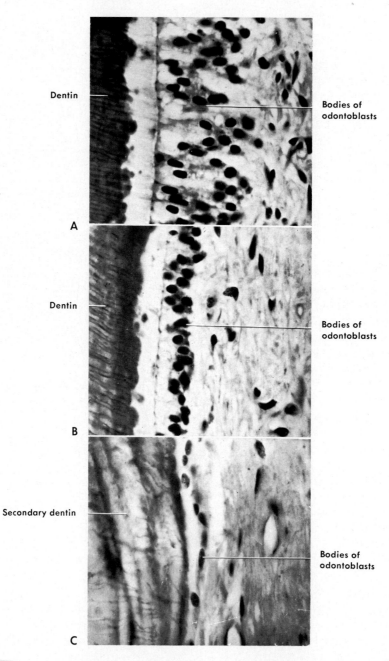

Dentin

Bodies of
odontoblasts

A

Dentin

Bodies of
odontoblasts

B

Secondary dentin

Bodies of
odontoblasts

C

Fig. 5-12. Variation of odontoblasts in different regions of one tooth. **A,** High columnar odontoblasts in pulp chamber. **B,** Low columnar odontoblasts in root canal. **C,** Flat odontoblasts in apical region.

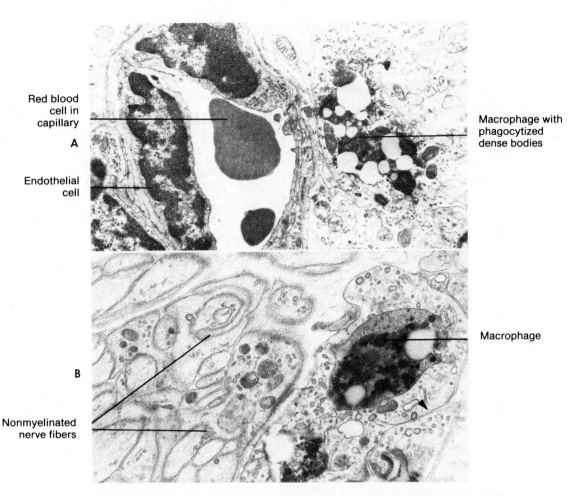

Red blood
cell in
capillary

A

Endothelial
cell

Macrophage with
phagocytized
dense bodies

B

Nonmyelinated
nerve fibers

Macrophage

Fig. 5-13. A, This histiocyte or macrophage is located adjacent to capillary in peripheral pulp. Characteristic aggregation of vesicles, vacuoles, and phagocytized dense bodies is seen to right of capillary wall. **B,** Multivesiculated body characteristic of macrophage. Note typical invagination of cell plasma membrane *(arrow).* This cell is located adjacent to group of nonmyelinated nerve fibers seen on left.

toluidin blue. These cells are usually associated with small blood vessels and capillaries. Ultrastructurally the macrophage exhibits a rounded outline with short, blunt processes (Fig. 5-13). Invaginations of the plasma membrane are noted, as are mitochondria, rough-surfaced endoplasmic reticulum, free ribosomes, and also a moder-ately dense nucleus. The distinguishing feature of macrophages is aggregates of vesicles, or phagosomes, which contain phagocytized dense irregular bodies (Fig. 5-13).

Both lymphocytes and eosinophils are found extravascularly in the normal pulp (Fig. 5-14), but during inflammation they

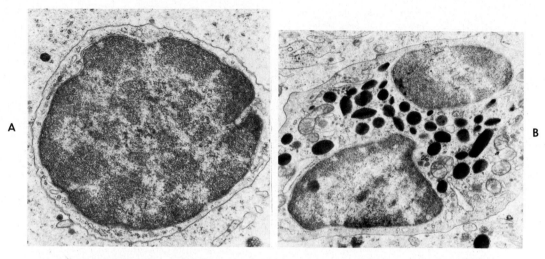

A

B

Fig. 5-14. A, Small lymphocyte located in pulp. Cytoplasm forms narrow rim around large oval-to-round nucleus. **B,** Eosinophil in extravascular location in pulp organ. Nucleus is polymorphic, and granules in cytoplasm are characteristically banded.

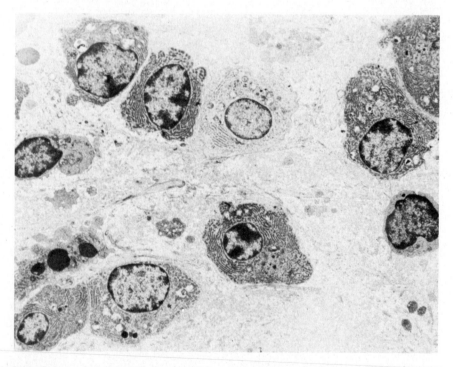

Fig. 5-15. Cluster of plasma cells in pulp with early caries pulpitis. Observe dense peripheral nuclear chromatin and cytoplasm with cisternae of rough endoplasmic reticulum. (Courtesy C. Torneck, University of Toronto Dental School.)

increase noticeably in number. Mast cells are also seen along vessels in the inflamed pulp. They have a round nucleus and contain many dark-staining granules in the cytoplasm, and their number increases during inflammation.

The plasma cells are seen during inflammation of the pulp (Fig. 5-15). With the light microscope the plasma cell nucleus appears small and concentric in the cytoplasm. The chromatin of the nucleus is adherent to the nuclear membrane and gives the cell a cartwheel appearance. The cytoplasm of this cell is basophilic with a light-stained Golgi zone adjacent to the nucleus.

Under the electron microscope these cells have a densely packed, roughsurfaced endoplasmic reticulum. Both immature and mature cells may be found. The mature type exhibits a typical small eccentric nucleus and more abundant cytoplasm (Fig. 5-15). The plasma cells function in the production of antibodies.

Blood vessels. The pulp organ is extensively vascularized. It is known that the blood vessels of both the pulp and the periodontium arise from the inferior or superior alveolar artery and also drain by the same veins in both the mandibular and maxillary regions. The communication of the vessels

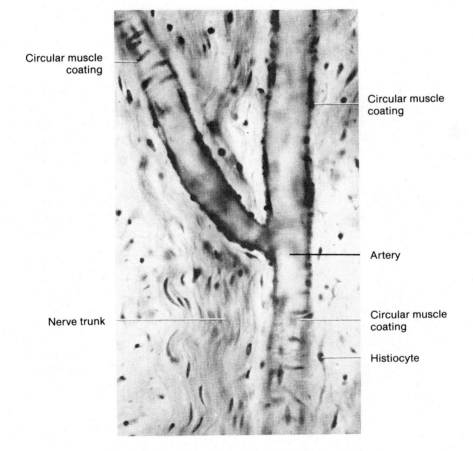

Fig. 5-16. Branching artery and nerve trunk in the pulp.

of the pulp with the periodontium, in addition to the apical connections, is further enhanced by connections through the accessory canals. These relationships are of considerable clinical significance in the event of a potential pathologic condition in either the periodontium or the pulp, because the infection has a potential to spread through the accessory and apical canals. Although branches of the alveolar arteries supply both the tooth and its supporting tissues, those periodontal vessels entering the pulp change their structure from the branches to the periodontium and become considerably thinner walled than those surrounding the tooth.

Small arteries and arterioles enter the apical canal and pursue a direct route to the coronal pulp (Fig. 5-16). Along their course they give off numerous branches in the radicular pulp that pass peripherally to form a plexus in the odontogenic region (Fig. 5-17). Pulpal blood flow is more rapid than in most areas of the body. This is perhaps attributable to the fact that the pulpal pressure is among the highest of body tissues. The flow of blood in arterioles is 0.3 to 1 mm per second, in venules approximately 0.15 mm per second, and in capillaries about 0.08 mm per second. The largest arteries in the human pulp are 50 to 100 μm in diameter, thus equaling in size arterioles found in most areas of the body. These vessels possess three layers. The first, the tunica intima, consists of squamous or cuboid endothelial cells surrounded by a closely associated basal lamina. Where the endothelial cells contact,

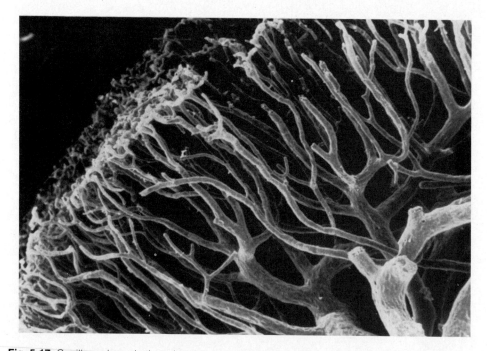

Fig. 5-17. Capillary plexus in the odontogenic region. These casts of vessels illustrate how they penetrate the odontoblastic cell row and loop back to join venules of central pulp. (The odontoblasts are lost in the preparation of the capillary loops.) (Courtesy K. Takahashi, Kanagawa Dental College, Kanagawa, Japan.)

they appear overlapped to varying degrees. The second layer, the tunica media, is approximately 5 μm thick and consists of one to three layers of smooth muscle cells (Figs. 5-18 and 5-19). A basal lamina surrounds and passes between these muscle cells and separates the muscle cell layer from the intima. Occcasionally the endothelial cell wall is in contact with the muscle cells. This is termed a myoendothelial junction. The third and outer layer, the tunica adventitia, is made up of a few collagen fibers forming a loose network around the larger arteries. This layer becomes more conspicuous in vessels in older pulps. Arterioles with diameters of 20 to 30 μm with one or occasionally two layers of smooth muscle cells are common throughout the coronal pulp (Fig. 5-18). The tunica adventita blends with the fibers of the surrounding intercellular tissue. Terminal arterioles with diameters of 10 to 15 μm appear peripherally in the pulp. The endothelial cells of these vessels contain numerous micropinocytotic vesicles, which function in transendothelial fluid movement. A single layer of smooth muscle cells surrounds these small vessels. Occasionally a fibroblast or pericyte lies on the surface of these vessels. Pericytes are capillary-associated fibroblasts, and their nuclei can be distiguished as round or slightly oval bodies closely associated with the outer surface of the terminal arterioles or precapil-

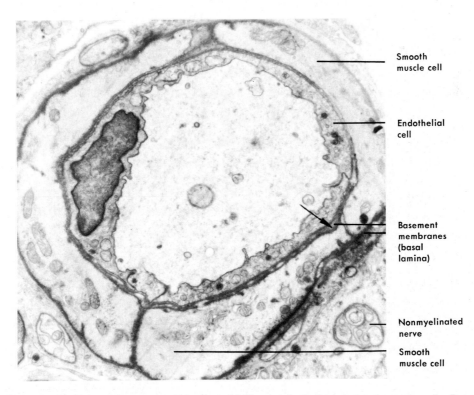

Smooth muscle cell

Endothelial cell

Basement membranes (basal lamina)

Nonmyelinated nerve

Smooth muscle cell

Fig. 5-18. Small arteriole near central pulp exhibiting relatively thick layer of muscle cells. Dense basement membrane interspersed between endothelial and muscle cells *(arrow).*

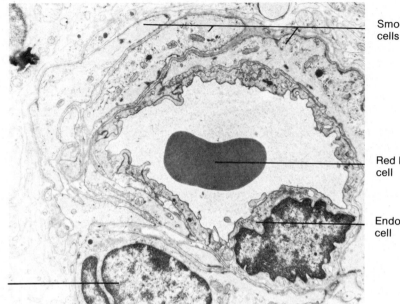

Smooth muscle cells

Red blood cell

Endothelial cell

Pericyte

Fig. 5-19. Peripheral pulp and small arteriole or precapillary exhibiting two thin layers of smooth muscle cells surrounding the endothelial cell lining of vessel. Nucleus at bottom left of figure belongs to a pericyte.

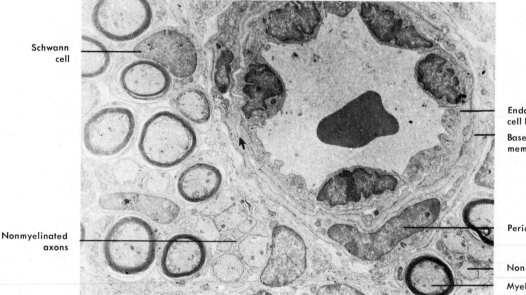

Schwann cell

Nonmyelinated axons

Endothelial cell lining

Basement membrane

Pericyte

Nonmyelinated axon

Myelinated axon

Fig. 5-20. Area near subodontoblastic plexus showing both myelinated and nonmyelinated axons adjacent to large capillary or precapillary. Endothelial cell lining is surrounded by basement membrane *(arrow)* and pericytes.

laries (Figs. 5-19 and 5-20). Some authors call the smaller diameter arterioles "precapillaries." They are slightly larger than the terminal capillaries and exhibit a complete or incomplete single layer of muscle cells surrounding the endothelial lining. These range in size from 8 to 12 μm.

Veins and venules that are larger than the arteries also appear in the central region of the root pulp. They measure 100 to 150 μm in diameter, and their walls appear less regular than those of the arteries because of bends and irregularities along their course. The microscopic appearance of the veins is similar to that of the arteries except that they exhibit much thinner walls in relation to the size of the lumen. The endothelial cells appear more flattened, and

their cytoplasm does not project into the lumen. Fewer intracytoplasmic filaments appear in these cells than in the arterioles. The tunica media consists of a single layer or two of thin smooth muscle cells that wrap around the endothelial cells and appear discontinuous or absent in the smaller venules. The basement membranes of these vessels are thin and less distinct than those of arterioles. The adventitia is lacking or appears as fibroblasts and fibers continuous with the surrounding pulp tissue. Occasionally two venous loops will be seen connected by an anastomosing branch (Fig. 5-21). Both venous-venous anastomosis and arteriole-venous anastomosis occur in the pulp. The arteriole-venous shunts may have an important role in regulation of pul-

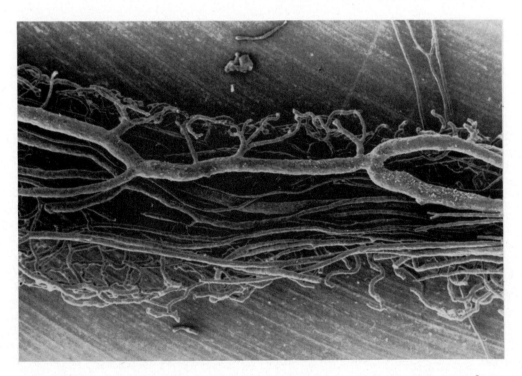

Fig. 5-21. Venous loops seen at the left and right of the field with connecting branch in center. Scanning electron micrograph. (Courtesy K. Takahashi, Kanagawa Dental College, Kanagawa, Japan.)

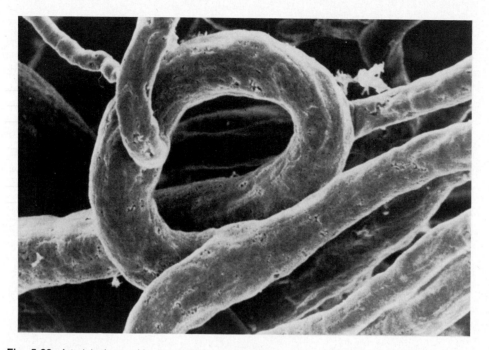

Fig. 5-22. Arteriole loop with associated capillaries located in subodontoblastic zone. Scanning electron micrograph. (Courtesy K. Takahashi, Kanagawa Dental College, Kanagawa, Japan.)

pal blood flow. Frequently arteriole or pre-capillary loops with capillaries are found underlying the odontogenic zone in the coronal pulp (Fig. 5-22).

Blood capillaries, which appear as endothelium-lined tubes, are 8 to 10 μm in diameter. The nuclei of these cells may be lobulated and have cytoplasmic projections into the luminal surface. The terminal network of capillaries in the coronal pulp appears nearly perpendicular to the main trunks. The vascular network passes among the odontoblasts and underlies them as well (Fig. 5-17). A few peripheral capillaries found among the odontoblasts have fenestrations in the endothelial cells. These pores are located in the thin part of the capillary wall and are spanned only by the thin diaphragm of contacting inner and

outer plasma membranes of endothelial cells, (Fig. 5-23). These fenestrated capillaries are assumed to be involved in rapid transport of metabolites at a time when the odontoblasts are active in the process of dentinal matrix formation and its subsequent calcification. Both fenestrated and continuous terminal capillaries are found in the odontogenic region. During active dentinogenesis capillaries appear among the odontoblasts adjacent to the predentin (Fig. 5-17). Later, after the teeth have reached occlusion and dentinogenesis slows down, these vessels usually retreat to a subodontoblastic position.

Lymph vessels. The presence of lymph vessels in the dental pulp is questioned by some and agreed upon by other investigators. Support for this system stems from in-

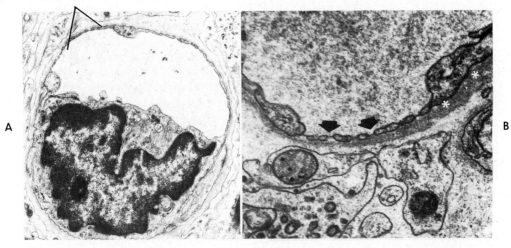

Fig. 5-23. A, Terminal capillary loops located among odontoblasts may be fenestrated. These capillaries have both thick and thin segments in their walls. **B,** Endothelial cell wall bridges pores *(arrows)* and is supported only by basement membrane (**).

vestigators who use injection of fine particulate substances into the dentin or peripheral pulp, which are subsequently reported present in some of the thin-walled vessels that exit through the apical foramen. Lymph capillaries are described as endothelium-lined tubes that join thin-walled lymph venules or veins in the central pulp. The larger vessels have an irregular-shaped lumen composed of endothelial cells surrounded by an incomplete layer of pericytes or smooth muscle cells or both. They are further characterized by absence of red blood cells and presence of lymphocytes. Absence of basal lamina adjacent to the endothelium has also been reported (Fig. 5-30). Lymph vessels draining the pulp and periodontal ligament have a common outlet. Those draining the anterior teeth pass to the submental lymph nodes; those of the posterior teeth pass to the submandibular and deep cervical lymph nodes.

Nerves. The abundant nerve supply in the pulp follows the distribution of the blood vessels. The majority of the nerves that enter the pulp are nonmyelinated. Many of these gain a myelin sheath later in life. The nonmyelinated nerves are found in close association with the blood vessels of the pulp and many are sympathetic in nature. They have terminals on the muscle cells of the larger vessels and function in vasoconstriction (Fig. 5-18). Thick nerve bundles enter the apical foramen and pass along the radicular pulp to the coronal pulp where their fibers separate and radiate peripherally to the parietal layer of nerves (Fig. 5-24). The number of fibers in these bundles varies greatly, from as few as 150 to more than 1200. The larger fibers range between 5 and 13 μm, although the majority are smaller than 4 μm. The large myelinated fibers mediate the sensation of pain that may be caused by external stimuli. The peripheral axons form a network of nerves located adjacent to the cell-rich

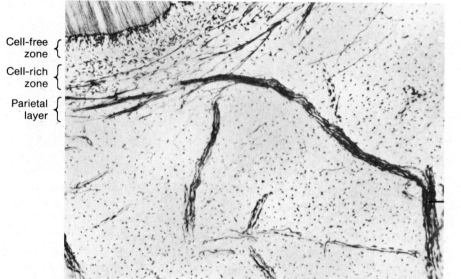

Cell-free zone {

Cell-rich zone {

Parietal layer {

Central trunk

Fig. 5-24. Major nerve trunks branch in pulp and pass to parietal layer, which lies adjacent to cell-rich zone. Cell-rich zone curves upward to right.

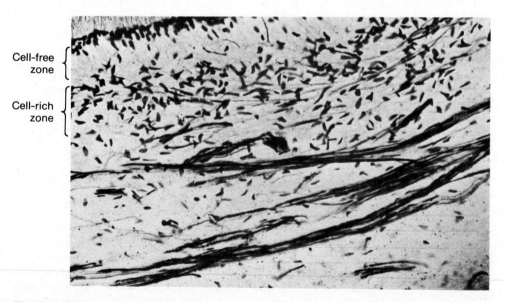

Cell-free zone {

Cell-rich zone {

Fig. 5-25. Parietal layer of nerves is composed of myelinated nerve fibers. Cell-rich zone curves upward to right.

zone. This is termed the *parietal layer of nerves,* also known as the plexus of Rashkow (Figs. 5-24 and 5-25). Both myelinated axons, ranging from 2 to 5 μm in diameter, and minute nonmyelinated fibers of approximately 200 to 1600 μm (2000 to 16,000 Å) in size make up this layer of nerves. The parietal layer develops gradually, becoming prominent when root formation is complete.

Nerve endings. Nerve axons from the parietal zone pass through the cell-rich and cell-free zones and either terminate among or pass between the odontoblasts to terminate adjacent to the odontoblast processes at the pulp-predentin border or in the dentinal tubules (Fig. 5-26). Nerve terminals consisting of round or oval enlargements of the terminal filaments contain microvesicles, small, dark, granular bodies, and mitochondria (Fig. 5-27). These terminals are very close to the odontoblast plasma membrane, separated only by a 20 μm (200 Å) cleft (Fig. 5-28). Many of these indent the odontoblast surface and exhibit a special

relationship to these cells. Most of the nerve endings located among the odontoblasts are believed to be sensory receptors. Some sympathetic endings are found in this location as well. Whether they have some function relative to the capillaries or the odontoblast in dentinogenesis is not known. The nerve axons found among the odontoblasts and in the cell-free and cell-rich zones are nonmyelinated but are enclosed in a Schwann cell covering. It is presumed that these fibers lost their myelin sheath as they passed peripherally from the parietal zone. More nerve fibers and endings are found in the pulp horns than in other peripheral areas of the coronal pulp (Fig. 5-5).

Recently a great deal of information has been reported regarding the types of potential neurotransmitters that are present in the nerves of the dental pulp. Substances such as substance P, 5-hydroxytryptamine, vasoactive intestinal peptide, somatostatin, and prostaglandins, as well as acetylcholine and norepinephrine have been found

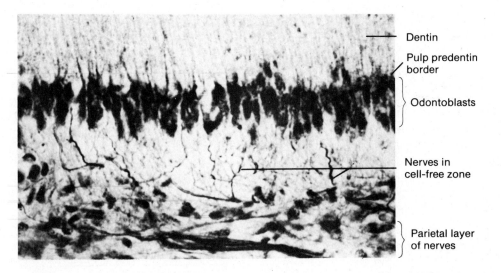

Dentin

Pulp predentin border

Odontoblasts

Nerves in cell-free zone

Parietal layer of nerves

Fig. 5-26. Terminal nerve endings located among odontoblasts. These arise from subjacent parietal layer.

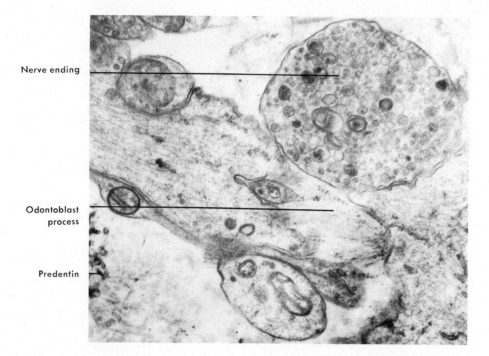

Nerve ending

Odontoblast process

Predentin

Fig. 5-27. Vesiculated nerve endings in predentin in zone adjacent to odontoblast process.

throughout the pulp. The majority of these putative transmitters have been shown to affect vascular tone and subsequently modify the excitability of the nerve endings. Further, it has been suggested that these changes in vascular tone can also affect the incremental growth of dentin.

It is a feature unique to dentin receptors that environmental stimuli always elicit pain as a response. Sensory response in the pulp cannot differentiate between heat, touch, pressure, or chemicals. This is because the pulp organs lack those types of receptors that specifically distinguish these other stimuli.

FUNCTIONS

Inductive. The primary role of the pulp anlage is to interact with the oral epithelial cells, which leads to differentiation of the dental lamina and enamel organ formation. The pulp anlage also interacts with the developing enamel organ as it determines a particular type of tooth.

Formative. The pulp organ cells produce the dentin that surrounds and protects the pulp. The pulpal odontoblasts develop the organic matrix and function in its calcification. Through the development of the odontoblast processes, dentin is formed along the tubule wall as well as at the pulp-predentin front.

Nutritive. The pulp nourishes the dentin through the odontoblasts and their processes and by means of the blood vascular system of the pulp.

Protective. The sensory nerves in the tooth respond with pain to all stimuli such as heat, cold, pressure, operative cutting procedures, and chemical agents. The

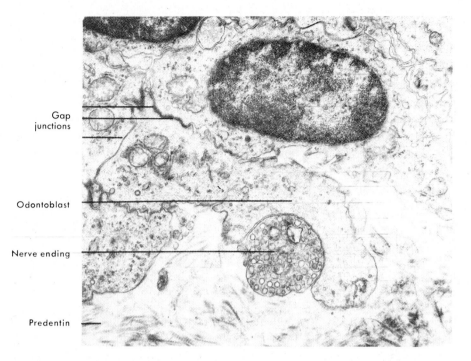

Gap
junctions

Odontoblast

Nerve ending

Predentin

Fig. 5-28. Vesiculated nerve ending partially surrounded by an odontoblast process located adjacent to predentin. Note the uniform cleftlike space between the nerve ending and the odontoblast process. Gap junction appears between odontoblasts.

nerves also initiate reflexes that control circulation in the pulp. This sympathetic function is a reflex, providing stimulation to visceral motor fibers terminating on the muscles of the blood vessels.

Defensive or reparative. The pulp is an organ with remarkable reparative abilities. It responds to irritation, whether mechanical, thermal, chemical, or bacterial, by producing reparative dentin and mineralizing any affected dentinal tubules. Both the reparative dentin created in the pulp and the calcification of the tubules (sclerosis) are attempts to wall off the pulp from the source of irritation. Also, the pulp may become inflamed due to bacterial infection or by cutting action and placement of an irritating restorative material. The pulp has macrophages, lymphocytes, neutrophils, monocytes, and plasma and mast cells, all of which aid in the process of repair of the pulp. Although the rigid dentinal wall has to be considered as a protection of the pulp, it also endangers its existence under certain conditions. During inflammation of the pulp, hyperemia and edema may lead to the accumulation of excess fluid outside the capillaries. An imbalance of this type, limited by the unyielding enclosure, can lead to pressure on apical vessels and ischemia, resulting in necrosis of the pulp. In most cases, if the inflammation is not too severe, however, the pulp will heal since it has excellent regenerative properties.

PRIMARY AND PERMANENT PULP ORGANS

Primary pulp organs. The primary pulp organs function for a shorter period of time than do the permanent pulps. The average length of time a primary pulp functions in the oral cavity is only about 8.3 years. This amount of time may be divided into three time periods—that of *pulp organ growth,* which takes place during the time the crown and roots are developing; that period of time after the root is completed until root resorption begins, which is termed the time of *pulp maturation;* and finally the period of *pulp regression,* which is the time from beginning root resorption until the time of exfoliation. Let us consider the average time of pulp life based on figures for the entire primary dentition. These three periods (growth, maturation, and regression) are not of equal lengths. Tooth eruption to root completion is about 1 year (11.85 months), and the time of root completion to beginning root loss (based on completion of the permanent crown) is 45.3 months, or 3 years, 9 months. Finally, the time of pulp regression based on the beginning of root resorption to exfoliation is 3 years, 6 months. The amount of time the primary pulp is undergoing changes relative to growth based on both the *prenatal* crown formation and the postnatal root completion is about 4 years, 2 months, 11 months of which are involved in crown completion from the time of beginning of crown calcification to its completion. The period of time the primary radicular pulp is regressing is based on the time from when the permanent crown is completed till the time of permanent tooth eruption. In some cases, root loss commences before the root is entirely complete. The maximum life of the primary pulp including both prenatal and postnatal times of development and the period of regression is approximately 9.6 years.

Permanent pulp organs. During crown formation the pulps of primary and permanent teeth are morphologically nearly identical. In the permanent teeth this is a process requiring about 5 years. During this time the organs are highly cellular, exhibiting a high mitotic rate especially in the cervical region. The young differentiating odontoblasts exhibit few organelles until dentin formation begins; then they rapidly change into protein-synthesizing cells. Both the primary and the permanent pulps are highly vascularized; however, the primary teeth never attain the extent of neural development that occurs in the permanent teeth. This is caused in part by the loss of neural elements during the root-resorption period. The greater the extent of root resorption, the greater the degenerative changes seen in the primary pulps. The architecture of the primary and permanent pulps is similar in appearance to the cell-free and cell-rich zones, parietal layer, and the large nerve trunks and vessels in the central pulp.

The periods of development for the pulps of the permanent teeth are, as might be expected, longer than those required for completion of the same processes in the primary teeth. As mentioned above, crown completion, based on the time during which the crown is completing formation and calcification, averages 5 years, 5 months. From the time of crown completion to eruption the time in both arches averages 3 years, 6 months. The time from eruption to root completion is 3 years, 11 months. Thus the pulp of the permanent teeth undergoes development for about 12 years, 4 months (based on the time from beginning prenatal crown calcification to root completion). This is in contrast to the 4 years, 2 months it takes in the primary teeth. Furthermore, the permanent roots take over twice as long to reach completion

(7 years, 5 months) as do those of the primary pulps (average 3 years, 3 months).

The period of pulp aging is much accelerated in the primary teeth and occupies the time from root completion to exfoliation, or about 7 years, 5 months. Aging of the pulp in the permanent teeth, on the other hand, requires much of the adult life span.

Finally, one should note in passing that for both the primary and permanent teeth the maxillary arches require slightly longer to complete each process of development than do the mandibular arches.

REGRESSIVE CHANGES (AGING)

Cell changes. In addition to the appearance of fewer cells in the aging pulp, the cells are characterized by a decrease in size and number of cytoplasmic organelles. The typical active pulpal fibrocyte or fibroblast has abundant rough-surfaced endoplasmic reticulum, notable Golgi complex, and numerous mitochondria with well-developed

cristae. The fibroblasts in the aging pulp exhibit less perinuclear cytoplasm and possess long, thin cytoplasmic processes. The intracellular organelles are reduced in number and size; the mitochondria and endoplasmic reticulum are good examples of this.

Fibrosis. In the aging pulp accumulations of both diffuse fibrillar components as well as bundles of collagen fibers usually appear. Fiber bundles may appear arranged longitudinally in bundles in the radicular pulp, and in a random more diffuse arrangement in the coronal area. This condition is variable, with some older pulps showing surprisingly small amounts of collagen accumulation, whereas others display considerable amounts (Fig. 5-29). The increase in fibers in the pulp organ is gradual and is generalized throughout the organ. Any external trauma such as dental caries or deep restorations usually causes a localized fibrosis or scarring effect. Collagen increase is noted in the medial and adventi-

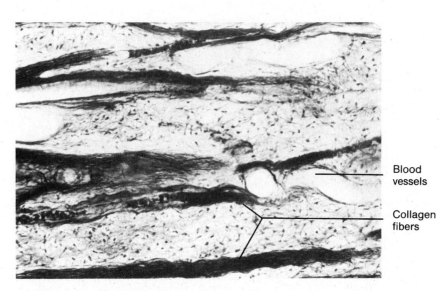

Blood vessels

Collagen fibers

Fig. 5-29. Bundles of collagen fibers around and among blood vessels of pulp.

tial layers of blood vessels as well. The increase in collagen fibers may be more apparent than actual, being attributable to the decrease in the size of the pulp, which makes the fibers present occupy less space, and hence they become more concentrated without increasing in total volume.

Vascular changes occur in the aging pulp organ as they do in any organ. Atherosclerotic plaques may appear in pulpal vessels. In other cases the outer diameter of vessel walls becomes greater as collagen fibers increase in the medial and adventitial layers. Also calcifications are found that surround vessels (Fig. 5-30). Calcification in the walls of blood vessels is found most often in the region near the apical foramen.

Pulp stones (denticles). Pulp stones, or denticles, are nodular, calcified masses appearing in either or both the coronal and root portions of the pulp organ. They often develop in teeth that appear to be quite normal in other respects. They usually are asymptomatic unless they impinge on nerves or blood vessels. They have been seen in functional as well as embedded unerupted teeth.

Pulp stones are classified, according to their structure as **true denticles** or **false denticles.** True denticles are similar in

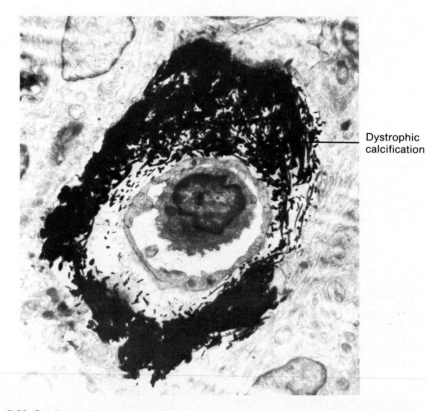

Dystrophic calcification

Fig. 5-30. Small vessel containing lymphocyte. Its wall exhibits no basement membrane around endothelial cells. It is probably a lymphatic capillary. Calcification appears around periphery of vessel.

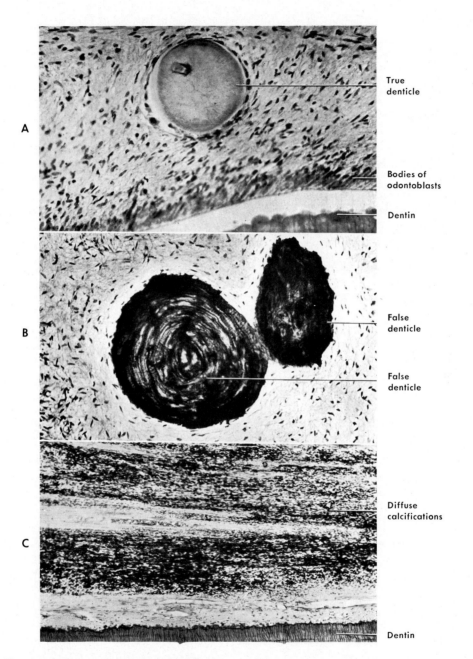

Fig. 5-31. Calcifications in the pulp. **A,** True denticle. **B,** False denticle. **C,** Diffuse calcifications.

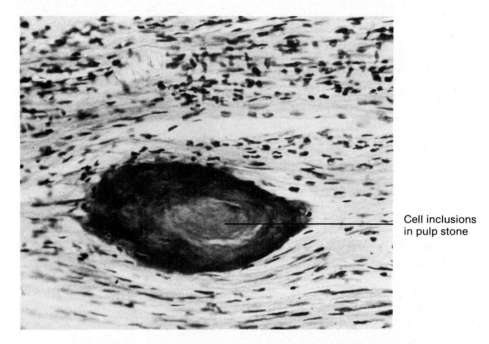

Cell inclusions
in pulp stone

Fig. 5-32. Free, false pulp stone within collagen bundle of coronal pulp.

structure to dentin in that they have dental tubules and contain the processes of the odontoblasts that formed them and that exist on their surface (Fig. 5-31, *A*). True denticles are comparatively rare and are usually located close to the apical foramen. A theory has been advanced that the development of the true denticle is caused by the inclusion of remnants of the epithelial root sheath within the pulp. These epithelial remnants induce the cells of the pulp to differentiate into odontoblasts, which then form the dentin masses called true pulp stones.

False denticles do not exhibit dentinal tubules but appear instead as concentric layers of calcified tissue (Fig. 5-31, *B*). In some cases these calcification sites appear within a bundle of collagen fibers (Fig. 5-32). Other times they appear in a location in the pulp free of collagen accumulations

(Fig. 5-31, *B*). Some false pulp stones undoubtedly arise around vessels as seen in Fig. 5-30. In the center of these concentric layers of calcified tissue there may be remnants of necrotic and calcified cells (Fig. 5-32). Calcification of thrombi in blood vessels, called phleboliths, may also serve as nidi for false denticles. All denticles begin as small nodules but increase in size by incremental growth on their surface. The surrounding pulp tissue may appear quite normal. Pulp stones may eventually fill substantial parts of the pulp chamber. Pulp stones may be classified as free, attached, or embedded, depending on their relation to the dentin of the tooth (Fig. 5-33). The free denticles are entirely surrounded by pulp tissue, attached denticles are partly fused with the dentin, and embedded denticles are entirely surrounded by dentin. All are believed to be formed free in the

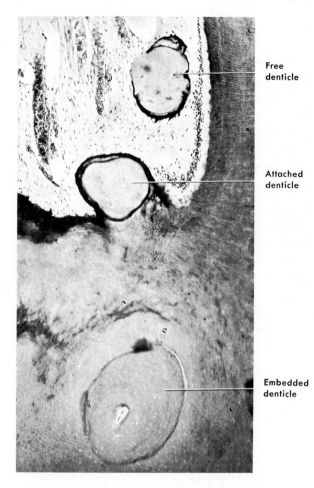

Free
denticle

Attached
denticle

Embedded
denticle

Fig. 5-33. Examples of the typical appearance of pulp stones as free, attached, and embedded.

pulp and later to become attached or embedded as dentin formation progresses. Pulp stones may appear close to blood vessels and nerve trunks (Fig. 5-34). This is believed to be because they are large and grow so that they impinge on whatever structures are in their paths. The occurrence of pulp stones appears more prevalent through histologic study of human teeth than found by radiographic study. It is believed that only a relatively small number of them are sufficiently large

enough to be detected in roentgenograms. The incidence as well as the size of pulp stones increases with age. According to one estimate, 66% of teeth in persons 10 to 30 years of age, 80% in those between 30 and 50 years, and 90% in those over 50 years of age contain calcifications of some type.

Diffuse calcifications. Diffuse calcifications appear as irregular calcific deposits in the pulp tissue, usually following collagenous fiber bundles or blood vessels (Fig. 5-31, C). Sometimes they develop into larger

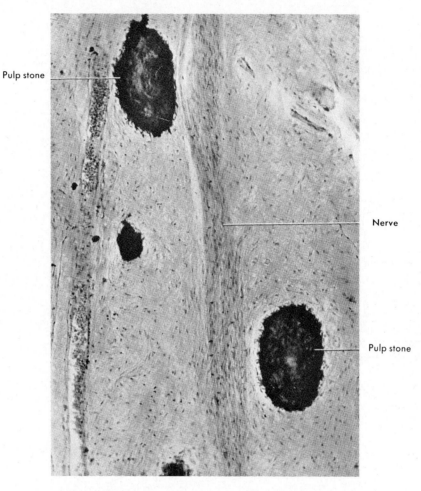

Pulp stone

Nerve

Pulp stone

Fig. 5-34. Pulp stones in proximity to nerve.

masses but usually persist as fine calcified spicules. The pulp organ may appear quite normal in its coronal portion without signs of inflammation or other pathologic changes but may exhibit these calcifications in the roots. Diffuse calcifications are usually found in the root canal and less often in the coronal area, whereas denticles are seen more frequently in the coronal pulp. Diffuse calcification surrounds blood vessels, as in Fig. 5-30. These calcifications may be classified as dystrophic calcification.

DEVELOPMENT

The tooth pulp is initially called the dental papilla. This tissue is designated as "pulp" only after dentin forms around it. The dental papilla controls early tooth formation. In the earliest stages of tooth development it is the area of the proliferating future papilla that causes the oral epithelium to invaginate and form the enamel organs. The enamel organs then enlarge to enclose the dental papillae in their central portions (Fig. 5-35, *A*). The dental papilla may play a role whether the forming enamel organ is to be an incisor or a molar. Recent information indicates that the epithelium may have that information. At the location of the future incisor the development of the dental pulp begins at about the eighth week of embryonic life in the human. Soon thereafter the more posterior tooth organs begin differentiating. The cell density of the dental papilla is great because of proliferation of the cells within it (Fig. 5-35, *A*). The young dental papilla is highly vascularized, and a well-organized network of vessels appears by the time dentin formation begins (Fig. 5-35, *B*). Capillaries crowd among the odontoblasts during this period of active dentinogenesis. The cells of the dental papilla appear as undifferentiated mesenchymal cells. Gradually these cells differentiate into stellate-shaped fibroblasts. After the inner and enamel organ cells differentiate into ameloblasts, the odontoblasts then differentiate from the peripheral cells of the dental papilla and dentin production begins. As this occurs, the tissue is no longer called dental papilla but is now designated the pulp organ. Few large myelinated nerves are found in the pulp until the dentin of the crown is well advanced. At that time nerves reach the odontogenic zone in the pulp horns. The sympathetic nerves, however, follow the blood vessels into the dental papilla as the pulp begins to organize.

CLINICAL CONSIDERATIONS

For all operative procedures the shape of the pulp chamber and its extensions into the cusps, the pulpal horns, is important to remember. The wide pulp chamber in the tooth of a young person will make a deep

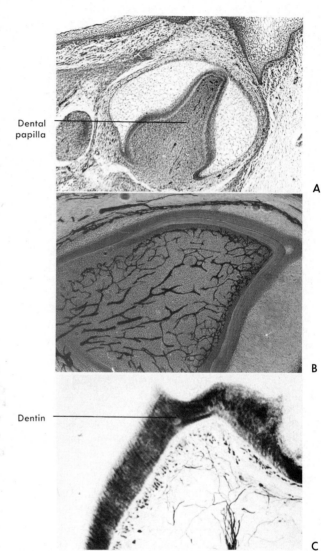

Dental
papilla

A

B

Dentin

C

Fig. 5-35. A, Young tooth bud exhibiting highly cellular dental papilla. Compare dense cell population to that of adjacent connective tissue. **B,** Young tooth with blood vessels injected with india ink to demonstrate extent of vascularity of pulp. Large vessels located centrally and smaller ones peripherally among odontoblasts. Pulp surrounded by dentin and enamel. **C,** Young tooth stained with silver to demonstrate neural elements. Myelinated nerves appear in pulp horn only after considerable amount of dentin has been laid down.

Fig. 5-36. These four diagrams depict pulp organ throughout life. Observe first the decrease in size of pulp organ. **A** to **D,** Dentin is formed circumpulpally but especially in bifurcation zone. Note decrease in cells and increase in fibrous tissue. Blood vessels *(white)* organize early into odontoblastic plexus and later are more prominent in subodontoblastic zone, indicating decrease in active dentinogenesis. Observe sparse number of nerves in young pulp, organization of pariental layer of nerves. They are less prominent in aging pulp. Reparative dentin and pulp stones are apparent in oldest pulp, at lower right, **D.**

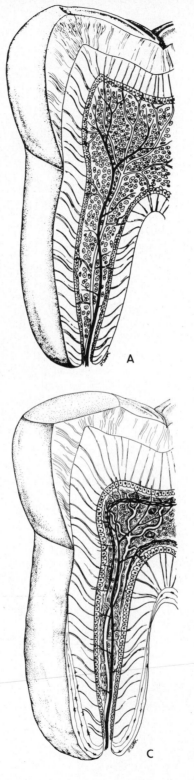

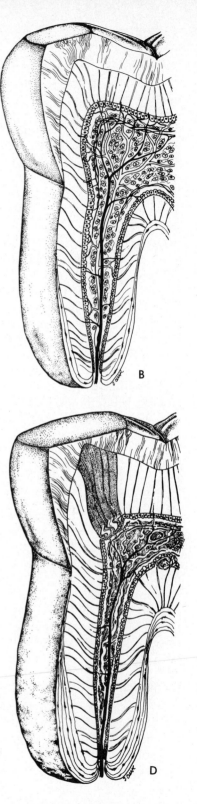

cavity preparation hazardous, and it should be avoided, if possible. In some instances of developmental disturbances the pulpal horns project high into the cusps, and the exposure of a pulp can occur when it is least anticipated. Sometimes a roentgenogram will help to determine the size of a pulp chamber and the extent of the pulpal horns.

If opening a pulp chamber for treatment becomes necessary, its size and variation in shape must be taken into consideration. With advancing age, the pulp chamber becomes smaller (Fig. 5-36), and because of excessive dentin formation at the roof and floor of the chamber, it is sometimes difficult to locate the root canals. In such cases it is advisable when one opens the pulp chamber to advance toward the distal root in the lower molar and toward the lingual root in the upper molar. In this region one is most likely to find the opening of the pulp canal without risk of perforating the floor of the pulp chamber. In the anterior teeth the coronal part of the pulp chamber may be filled with secondary dentin; thus locating the root canal is made difficult. Pulp stones lying at the opening of the root canal may cause considerable difficulty when an attempt is made to locate the canals.

The shape of the apical foramen and its location may play an important part in the treatment of root canals. When the apical foramen is narrowed by cementum, it is more readily located because further progress of the broach will be stopped at the foramen. If the apical opening is at the side of the apex, as shown in Fig. 5-3, *B*, not even roentgenograms will reveal the true length of the root canal, and this may lead to misjudgment of the length of the canal and the root canal filling.

Since accessory canals are rarely seen in roentgenograms, they are not treated in root canal therapy. In any event it would be mechanically difficult or impossible to reach them. Fortunately, however, the majority of them do not affect the success of endodontic therapy.

When accessory canals are located near the coronal part of the root or in the bifurcation area (Fig. 5-4, *B*), a deep periodontal pocket may cause inflammation of the dental pulp. Thus periodontal disease can have a profound influence on pulp integrity. Conversely, a necrotic pulp can cause spread of disease to the periodontium through an accessory canal. It is recognized that pulpal and periodontal disease may spread by their common blood supply.

Until recently, some clinicians believed that an exposed pulp meant a lost pulp. This is no longer necessarily so. The fact that defense cells have been recognized in the pulp and that new odontoblasts can differentiate and form reparative dentin has changed this concept. Extensive experimental work has shown that exposed pulps can be preserved if proper pulp capping procedures are applied. This is especially true in noninfected or minimally infected, accidentally exposed pulps in individuals of any age. In these instances dentin is formed at the site of the exposure; thus a dentin barrier or bridge is developed and the pulp retains vitality. Pulp capping of primary teeth has been shown to be remarkably successful.

All operative procedures cause an initial response in the pulp, which is dependent on the severity of the insult. The pulp is highly responsive to stimuli. Even a slight stimulus will cause inflammatory cell infiltration (Fig. 5-37). A severe reaction is characterized by increased inflammatory cell infiltration adjacent to the cavity site, hyperemia, or localized abscesses. Hemorrhage may be present, and the odontoblast layer is either destroyed or greatly dis-

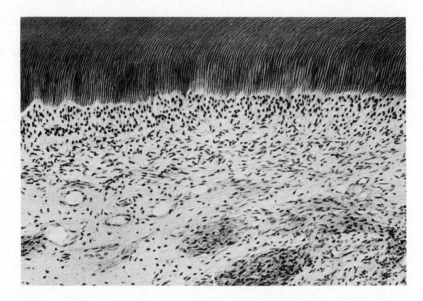

Fig. 5-37. Mild pulp response with loss of odontoblast identity and inflammatory cells obliterating cell-free zone.

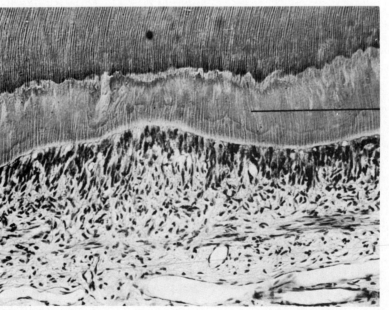

Reparative
dentin

Fig. 5-38. Moderate cell response with formation of reparative dentin underlying cavity. Note viable odontoblasts have deposited tubular, reparative dentin.

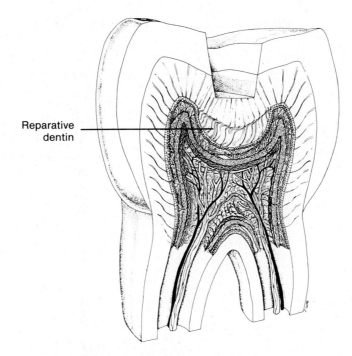

Reparative
dentin

Fig. 5-39. Diagram of reparative function of pulp organ to cavity preparation and subsequent restoration. Reparative dentin is limited to zone of stimulation.

rupted. It is of interest that most compounds containing calcium hydroxide readily induce reparative dentin underlying a cavity (Fig. 5-38). Most restorative materials also induce reparative dentin formations (Fig. 5-39). Usually the closer a restoration is to the pulp organ the greater will be the pulp response.

Since dehydration causes pulpal damage, operative procedures producing this condition should be avoided. When filling materials contain harmful chemicals (e.g., acid in silicate cements and monomer in the composites), an appropriate cavity liner should be used prior to the insertion of restorations. Most important is the effect of bacteria and bacterial toxins on the health of the pulp.

A vital pulp is essential to good dentition. Although modern endodontic procedures can prolong the usefulness of a tooth, a nonvital tooth becomes brittle and is subject to fractures. Therefore, every precaution should be taken to preserve the vitality of a pulp.

In clinical practice, instruments called vitalometers, which test the reaction of the pulp to electrical stimuli, or thermal stimuli (heat and cold) are often used to test the "vitality" of the pulp. These methods provide information about the status of the nerves supplying the pulpal tissue and therefore check the "sensitivity" of the pulp and not its "vitality." The vitality of the pulp depends on its blood supply, and one can have teeth with damaged nerve but normal blood supply (as in cases of traumatized teeth). Such pulps do not respond to electrical or thermal stimuli but are completely viable in every respect.

The preservation of a healthy pulp during operative procedures and successful management in cases of disease are two of the most important challenges to the clinical dentist.

REFERENCES

Avery JK: Structural elements of the young normal human pulp. In Siskin M, editor: The biology of the human dental pulp, St Louis, 1973, The CV Mosby Co. (Available only through American Association of Endodontists, Atlanta, Ga.)

Avery JK and Han SS: The formation of collagen fibrils in dental pulp, J Dent Res 40(6):1248, 1961.

Beveridge EE and Brown AC: The measurement of human dental intrapulpal pressure and its response to clinical variables, Oral Surg 19(5):655, 1965.

Bhussry BR: Modification of the dental pulp organ during development and aging. In Finn SB, editor: Biology of the dental pulp organ: a symposium, University of Alabama, 1968, University of Alabama Press.

Corpron RE and Avery JK: The ultrastructure of intradental nerves in developing mouse molars, Anat Rec 175(3):585, 1973.

Corpron RE, Avery JK, and Lee SD: Ultrastructure of terminal pulpal blood vessels in mouse molars, Anat Rec 179(4):527, 1974.

Dahl E and Mjör IA: The fine structure of the vessels in the human dental pulp, Acta Odontol Scand 31(4):223, 1973.

Fanibunda KB: Volume of the dental pulp cavity-method of measurement. British IADR Abstr No 150, J Dent Res 52(suppl.):971, 1973.

Fanibunda KB: A preliminary study of the volume of the pulp in the permanent human teeth. Unpublished personal communication, 1975.

Fearnhead RW: The histological demonstration of nerve fibers in human dentin. In Anderson DJ, editor: Sensory mechanisms in dentin, Oxford, England, 1963, Pergamon Press.

Finn SB: Biology of the dental pulp organ: a symposium, University of Alabama, 1968, University of Alabama Press.

Green DA: Stereoscopic study of the root apices of 400 maxillary and mandibular anterior teeth, Oral Surg 9:1224, 1956.

Griffin CJ and Harris R: The ultrastructure of the blood vessels of the human dental pulp following injury, Aust Dent J 17:303, 1972.

Griffin CJ and Harris R: The ultrastructure of the blood vessels of the human dental pulp following injury, Aust Dent J 18:88, 1973.

Han SS and Avery JK: The ultrastructure of capillaries and arterioles of the hamster dental pulp, Anat Rec 145(4):549, 1963.

Han SS and Avery JK: The fine structure of intercellular substances and rounded cells in the incisor pulp of the guinea pig, Anat Rec 151(1):41, 1965.

Han SS, Avery JK, and Hale LE: The fine structure of differentiating fibroblasts in the incisor pulp of the guinea pig, Anat Rec 153(2):187, 1965.

Harrop TJ and MacKay B: Electron microscopic observations of healing in dental pulp in the rat, Arch Oral Biol 13(43):365, 1968.

Kim S: Regulation of blood flow of the dental pulp of dogs: macrocirculation and microcirculation studies, Thesis, 1981, Columbia University, New York.

Kollar EJ and Baird GR: The influence of the dental papilla on the development of tooth shape in embryonic mouse tooth germs, J Embryol Exp Morphol 21:131, 1969.

Kollar EJ and Baird GR: Tissue interactions in embryonic mouse tooth germs. II. The indicative role of the dental papilla, J Embryol Exp Morphol 24:173, 1970.

Kollar EJ and Baird GR: Tissue interactions in embryonic mouse tooth germs. I. Reorganization of the dental epithelium during tooth-germ reconstruction, J Embryol Exp Morphol 24:159, 1970.

Kovacs I: A systematic description of dental roots. In Dahlberg AA, editor: Dental morphology and evaluation, Chicago, 1971, University of Chicago Press.

Mjör IA and Pindborg JJ: Histology of the human tooth, Copenhagen, 1973, Munksgaard, International Booksellers & Publishers, Ltd.

Nishijima S, Imanishi I, and Aka M: An experimental study on the lymph circulation in dental pulp, J Osaka Dent School 5:45, 1965.

Nygaard-Ostby B and Hjortdal O: Tissue formation in the root canal following pulp removal, Scand J Dent Res 79:333, 1971.

Ogilvie AL and Ingle JE: An atlas of pulpal and periapical biology, Philadelphia, 1965, Lea & Febiger.

Orban BJ: Contribution to the histology of the dental pulp and periodontal membrane, with special reference to the cells of "defense" of these tissues, J Am Dent Assoc 16(6):965, 1929.

Rapp R, Avery JK, and Rector RA: A study of the distribution of nerves in human teeth, J Can Dent Assoc 23:447, 1957.

Rapp R, Avery JK, and Strachan DS: The distribution of nerves in human primary teeth, Anat Rec 159(1):89, 1967.

Saunders RL de CH and Röckert HÖE: Vascular supply of dental tissues, including lymphatics. In Miles AEW, editor: Structural and chemical organization of teeth, vol 1, New York, 1967, Academic Press, Inc.

Schroff FR: Physiologic path of changes in the dental pulp, Oral Surg 6:1455, 1953.

Stanley HR and Rainey RR: Age changes in the human dental pulp, Oral Surg 15:1396, 1962.

Takahashi K, Yoshiaki K, and Kim S.: A scanning electron microscope study of the blood vessels of dog pulp using corrosion resin casts, J Endod 8(3):131, 1982.

Ten Cate AR: Oral histology: development, structure, and function, ed 2, St Louis, 1985, The CV Mosby Co.

Torneck CD: Changes in the fine structure of the dental pulp in human caries pulpitis. I. Nerves and blood vessels, J Oral Pathol 3:71, 1974.

Torneck CD: Changes in the fine structure of the dental pulp in human caries pulpitis. II. Inflammatory infiltration, J Oral Pathol 3:83, 1974.

Weinstock M and Leblond CP: Formation of collagen, Fed Proc 33(5):1205, 1974.

Weinstock M and Leblond CP: Synthesis migration and release of precursor collagen by odontoblasts as visualized by radioautography after [3H] proline administration, J Cell Biol 60:92, 1974.

Zachrisson BV: Mast cells in human dental pulp, Arch Oral Biol 16:555, 1971.

Zerlotti E: Histochemical study of the connective tissue of the dental pulp, Arch Oral Biol 9:149, 1964.

6

CEMENTUM

Cementum is the mineralized dental tissue covering the anatomic roots of human teeth. It was first demonstrated microscopically in 1835 by two pupils of Purkinje. It begins at the cervical portion of the tooth at the cementoenamel junction and continues to the apex. Cementum furnishes a medium for the attachment of collagen fibers that bind the tooth to surrounding structures. It is a specialized connective tissue that shares some physical, chemical, and structural characteristics with compact bone. Unlike bone, however, human cementum is avascular.

PHYSICAL CHARACTERISTICS

The hardness of fully mineralized cementum is less than that of dentin. Cementum is light yellow in color and can be distinguished from enamel by its lack of luster and its darker hue. Cementum is somewhat lighter in color than dentin. The difference in color, however, is slight, and under clinical conditions it is not possible to distinguish cementum from dentin based on color alone. Under some experimental conditions cementum has been shown to be permeable to a variety of materials.

CHEMICAL COMPOSITION

On a dry weight basis, cementum from fully formed permanent teeth contains about 45% to 50% inorganic substances and 50% to 55% organic material and water. The inorganic portion consists mainly of calcium and phosphate in the form of hydroxyapatite. Numerous trace elements are found in cementum in varying amounts. It is of interest that cementum has the highest fluoride content of all the mineralized tissues.

The organic portion of cementum consists primarily of type I collagen and protein polysaccharides (proteoglycans). Amino acid analyses of collagen obtained from the cementum of human teeth indicate close similarities to the collagens of dentin and alveolar bone. The chemical nature of the protein polysaccharides or ground substance of cementum is virtually unknown.

CEMENTOGENESIS

Cementum formation in the developing tooth is preceded by the deposition of dentin along the inner aspect of Hertwig's epithelial root sheath. Once dentin formation is under way, breaks occur in the epithelial root sheath allowing the newly formed dentin to come in direct contact with connective tissue of the dental follicle (Fig. 6-1). Cells derived from this connective tissue are responsible for cementum formation.

At the ultrastructural level, breakdown of Hertwig's epithelial root sheath involves degeneration or loss of its basal lamina on the cemental side. Loss of continuity of the basal lamina is soon followed by the appearance of collagen fibrils and cementoblasts between epithelial cells of the root sheath. Some sheath cells migrate away from the dentin toward the dental sac,

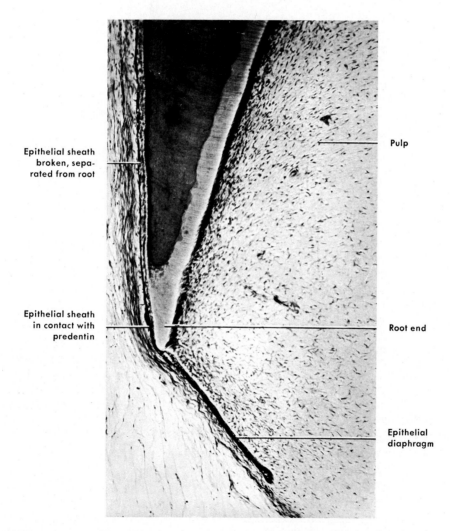

Epithelial sheath broken, separated from root

Epithelial sheath in contact with predentin

Pulp

Root end

Epithelial diaphragm

Fig. 6-1. Hertwig's epithelial root sheath at end of forming root. At side of root, sheath is broken up, and cementum formation begins. (From Gottlieb B: J Periodontol 13:13, 1942.)

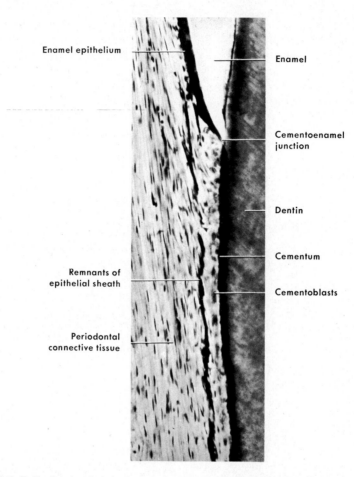

Enamel epithelium

Enamel

Cementoenamel junction

Dentin

Cementum

Cementoblasts

Remnants of epithelial sheath

Periodontal connective tissue

Fig. 6-2. Epithelial sheath is broken and separated from root surface by connective tissue.

whereas others remain near the developing tooth and ultimately are incorporated into the cementum. Sheath cells that migrate toward the dental sac become the epithelial rests of Malassez found in the periodontal ligament of fully developed teeth.

Cementoblasts. Soon after Hertwig's sheath breaks up, undifferentiated mesenchymal cells from adjacent connective tissue differentiate into cementoblasts (Fig. 6-2). Cementoblasts synthesize collagen and protein polysaccharides, which make up the organic matrix of cementum. These

cells have numerous mitochondria, a well-formed Golgi apparatus, and large amounts of granular endoplasmic reticulum (Fig. 6-3). These ultrastructural features are not unique to cementoblasts and can be observed in other cells actively producing proteins and polysaccharides.

After some cementum matrix has been laid down, its mineralization begins. The uncalcified matrix is called cementoid. Calcium and phosphate ions present in tissue fluids are deposited into the matrix and are arranged as unit cells of hydroxyapatite.

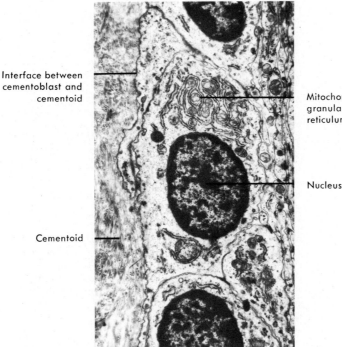

Interface between
cementoblast and
cementoid

Mitochondria and
granular endoplasmic
reticulum

Nucleus

Cementoid

Fig. 6-3. Cementoblasts on surface of cementoid. Mitochondria and granular endoplasmic reticulum are visible. (Electron micrograph; ×8000.) (Courtesy S.D. Lee, Ann Arbor, Mich.)

Mineralization of cementoid is a highly ordered event and not the random precipitation of ions into an organic matrix.

Cementoid tissue. Under normal conditions growth of cementum is a rhythmic process, and as a new layer of cementoid is formed, the old one calcifies. A thin layer of cementoid can usually be observed on the cemental surface (Fig. 6-4). This cementoid tissue is lined by cementoblasts. Connective tissue fibers from the periodontal ligament pass between the cementoblasts into the cementum. These fibers are embedded in the cementum and serve to attach the tooth to surrounding bone. Their embedded portions are known as Sharpey's fibers (Fig. 6-5). Each Sharpey's fiber is composed of numerous collagen fibrils that pass well into the cementum (Fig. 6-6).

STRUCTURE

With the light microscope two kinds of cementum can be differentiated: acellular and cellular. The term "acellular cementum" is unfortunate. As a living tissue, cells are an integral part of cementum at all times. However, some layers of cementum do not *incorporate* cells, the spiderlike cementocytes, whereas other layers do contain such cells in their lacunae. It is probably best to view cementum as a unit consisting of cementoblasts, cementoid, and fully mineralized tissue.

Acellular cementum may cover the root

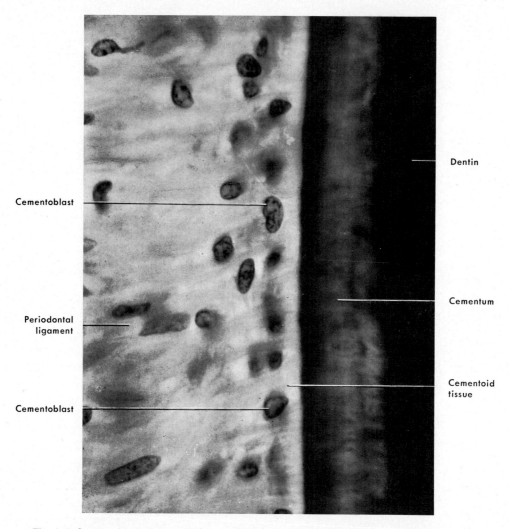

Dentin

Cementoblast

Cementum

Periodontal
ligament

Cementoid
tissue

Cementoblast

Fig. 6-4. Cementoid tissue on surface of calcified cementum. Cementoblasts between fibers.

dentin from the cementoenamel junction to the apex but is often missing on the apical third of the root. Here the cementum may be entirely of the cellular type. Cementum is thinnest at the cementoenamel junction (20 to 50 μm) and thickest toward the apex (150 to 200 μm). The apical foramen is surrounded by cementum. Sometimes cementum extends to the inner wall of the dentin

for a short distance, and so a lining of the root canal is formed.

In decalcified specimens of cementum, collagen fibrils make up the bulk of the organic portion of the tissue. Interspersed between some collagen fibrils are electron-dense reticular areas, which probably represent protein polysaccharide materials of the ground substance (Fig. 6-7). Collagen

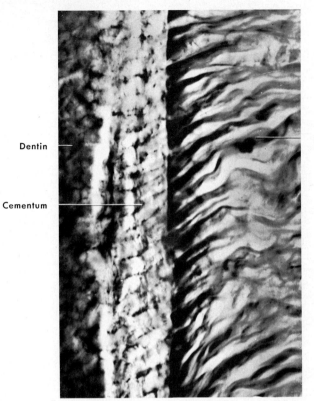

Dentin

Cementum

Fibers of
periodontal
ligament

Fig. 6-5. Fibers of periodontal ligament continue into surface layer of cementum as Sharpey's fibers.

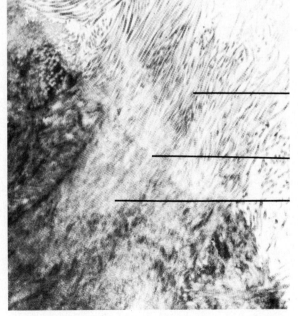

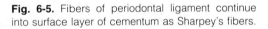

Collagen fibrils
of periodontal
ligament

Surface of
cementum

Collagen fibrils
embedded in
cementum

Fig. 6-6. Collagen fibrils from periodontal ligament continue into cementum. Numerous collagen fibrils embedded in cementum are collectively referred to as Sharpey's fibers. (Decalcified human molar; electron micrograph; ×17,000.)

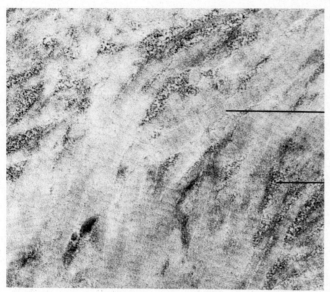

Collagen
fibrils

Ground
substance

Fig. 6-7. Electron micrograph of human cementum showing ground substance interspersed between collagen fibrils. (Decalcified specimen; ×42,000.)

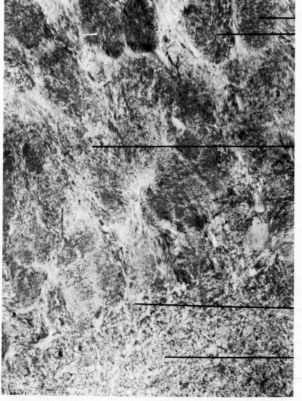

Sharpey's
fibers

Cementum

Cementodentinal
junction

Dentin

Fig. 6-8. Ultrastructural view of cementodentinal junction of human incisor. In this tangential section, Sharpey's fibers are visible as discrete bundles of collagen fibrils. (Decalcified specimen; electron micrograph; ×5000.)

fibrils of both acellular and cellular cementum are arranged in a very complex fashion with little discernible pattern. In some areas, however, relatively discrete bundles of collagen fibrils can be seen, particularly in tangential sections (Fig. 6-8). These bundles are Sharpey's fibers, which make up a substantial portion of the cementum.

In mineralized specimens it has been observed that cemental collagen is not totally mineralized. This is particularly true in a zone 10 to 50 μm wide near the cementodentinal junction where unmineralized areas about 1 to 5 μm in diameter are seen. These areas probably represent poorly mineralized cores of Sharpey's fibers.

The cells incorporated into cellular cementum, cementocytes, are similar to osteocytes. They lie in spaces designated as lacunae. A typical cementocyte has numerous cell processes, or canaliculi, radiating from its cell body. These processes may branch, and they frequently anastomose with those of a neighboring cell. Most of the processes are directed toward the periodontal surface of the cementum. The full extent of these processes does not show up in routinely prepared histologic sections. They are best viewed in mineralized ground sections (Fig. 6-9). The cytoplasm of cementocytes in deeper layers of cementum contains few organelles, the endoplasmic reticulum appears dilated, and mitochondria are sparse. These characteristics indicate that cementocytes are either degenerating or are marginally active cells. At a depth of 60 μm or more cementocytes show definite signs of degeneration such as cytoplasmic clumping and vesiculation. At the light microscopic level, lacunae in the deeper layers of cementum appear to be empty, suggesting complete degeneration of cementocytes located in these areas (Fig. 6-10).

Both acellular and cellular cementum are

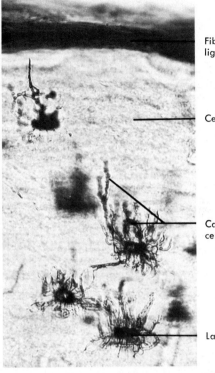

Fibers of periodontal ligament

Cellular cementum

Canaliculi of cementocyte

Lacuna of cementocyte

Fig. 6-9. Cellular cementum from human premolar. Note lacunae of spiderlike cementocytes with numerous canaliculi or cell processes. (Ground section; ×480.)

separated by incremental lines into layers, which indicate periodic formation (Figs. 6-10 and 6-11). Incremental lines can be seen best in decalcified specimens prepared for lightmicroscopic observation. They are difficult to identify at the ultrastructural level. Histochemical studies indicate that incremental lines are highly mineralized areas with less collagen and more ground substance than other portions of the cementum.

When cementum remains relatively thin, Sharpey's fibers cross the entire thickness of the cementum. With further apposition of cementum, a larger part of the fibers is incorporated in the cementum. The attach-

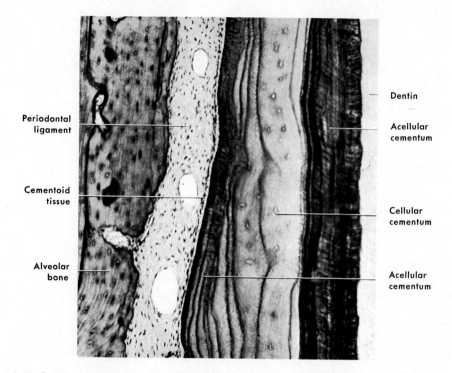

Periodontal ligament

Cementoid tissue

Alveolar bone

Dentin

Acellular cementum

Cellular cementum

Acellular cementum

Fig. 6-10. Cellular cementum on surface of acellular cementum and again covered by acellular cementum (incremental lines). Lacunae of cellular cementum appear empty, indicating degeneration of cementocytes.

ment proper is confined to the most superficial or recently formed layer of cementum (Fig. 6-5). This would seem to indicate that the thickness of cementum does not enhance functional efficiency by increasing the strength of attachment of the individual fibers.

The location of acellular and cellular cementum is not definite. As a general rule, however, acellular cementum usually predominates on the coronal half of the root, whereas cellular cementum is more frequent on the apical half. Layers of acellular and cellular cementum may alternate in almost any pattern. Acellular cementum may occasionally be found on the surface of cellular cementum (Fig. 6-10). Cellular cementum is frequently formed on the surface of acellular cementum (Fig. 6-10), but

it may comprise the entire thickness of apical cementum (Fig. 6-12). It is always thickest around the apex and, by its growth, contributes to the length of the root (Fig. 6-13).

Extensive variations in the surface topography of cementum can be observed with the scanning electron microscope. Resting cemental surfaces, where mineralization is more or less complete, exhibit low, rounded projections corresponding to the centers of Sharpey's fibers (Fig. 6-14). Cemental surfaces with actively mineralizing fronts have numerous small openings that correspond to sites where individual Sharpey's fibers enter the tooth (Fig. 6-15). These openings represent unmineralized cores of the fibers. Numerous resorption bays and irregular ridges of cellular cemen-

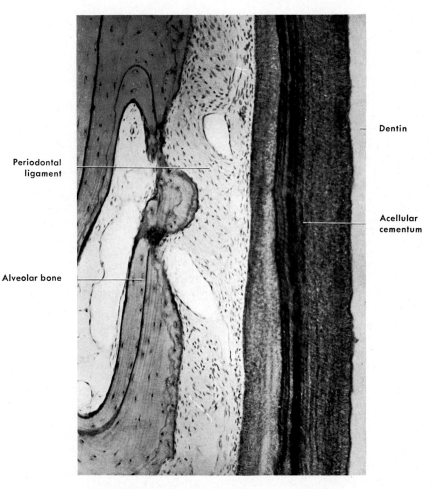

Periodontal
ligament

Alveolar bone

Dentin

Acellular
cementum

Fig. 6-11. Incremental lines in acellular cementum.

tum are also frequently observed on root surfaces (Fig. 6-16).

CEMENTODENTINAL JUNCTION

The dentin surface upon which cementum is deposited is relatively smooth in permanent teeth. The cementodentinal junction in deciduous teeth, however, is sometimes scalloped. The attachment of cementum to dentin in either case is quite firm, although the nature of this attachment is not fully understood.

The interface between cementum and dentin is clearly visible in decalcified and stained histologic sections using the light microscope (Figs. 6-10 and 6-11). In such preparations cementum usually stains more intensely than does dentin. When observed with the electron microscope, the cementodentinal junction is not as distinct as when observed with the light microscope. A narrow interface zone between the two tissues, however, can be detected with the electron microscope. In decalcified prepa-

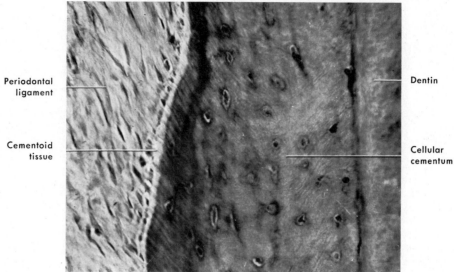

Periodontal ligament

Cementoid tissue

Dentin

Cellular cementum

Fig. 6-12. Cellular cementum forming entire thickness of apical cementum. (From Orban B: Dental histology and embryology, Philadelphia, 1929, P Blakiston's Son & Co.)

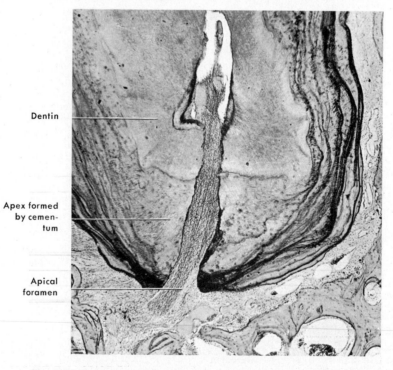

Dentin

Apex formed by cementum

Apical foramen

Fig. 6-13. Cementum thickest at apex, contributing to length of root.

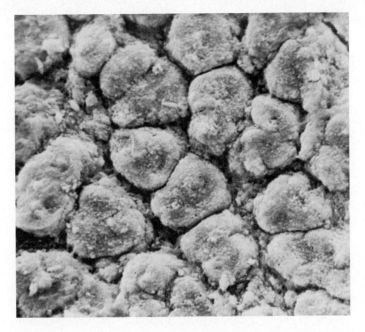

Fig. 6-14. Scanning electron micrograph of resting cemental surface of human premolar. Rounded projections correspond to insertion sites of Sharpey's fibers. (Anorganic preparation; ×3400.) (Courtesy A. Boyde, London.)

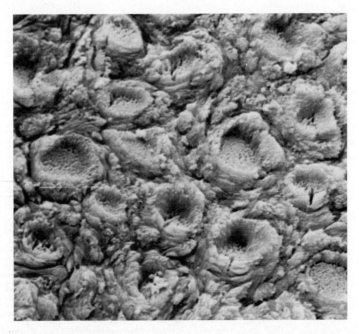

Fig. 6-15. Scanning electron micrograph of cemental surface of human molar with actively mineralizing front. Peripheral portions of Sharpey's fibers are more mineralized than their centers. (Anorganic preparation; approximately ×1500.) (From Jones SJ and Boyde A: Z Zellforsch 130:318, 1972.)

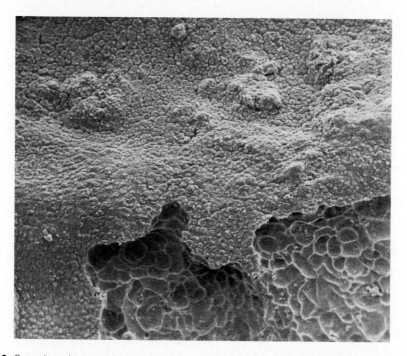

Fig. 6-16. Scanning electron micrograph of cemental surface of human molar showing numerous projections of Sharpey's fibers. Note large multiloculate resorption bay at bottom of field. (Anorganic preparation; ×250.) (From Jones SJ and Boyde A: Z Zellforsch 130:318, 1972.)

rations, cementum is more electron dense than dentin, and some of its collagen fibrils are arranged in relatively distinct bundles, whereas those of dentin are arranged somewhat haphazardly (Fig. 6-8). Since collagen fibrils of cementum and dentin intertwine at their interface in a very complex fashion, it is not possible to precisely determine which fibrils are of dentinal and which are of cemental origin.

Sometimes dentin is separated from cementum by a zone known as the intermediate cementum layer, which does not exhibit characteristic features of either dentin or cementum (Fig. 6-17). This layer is predominately seen in the apical two thirds of roots of molars and premolars and is only rarely observed in incisors or deciduous teeth. It is believed that this layer represents areas where cells of Hertwig's epithelial sheath become trapped in a rapidly deposited dentin or cementum matrix. Sometimes it is a continuous layer. Sometimes it is found only in isolated areas.

CEMENTOENAMEL JUNCTION

The relation between cementum and enamel at the cervical region of teeth is variable. In approximately 30% of all teeth, cementum meets the cervical end of enamel in a relatively sharp line (Fig. 6-18, A). In about 10% of the teeth, enamel and cementum do not meet. Presumably this occurs when enamel epithelium in the cervical portion of the root is delayed in its separation from dentin. In such cases there is no cementoenamel junction. Instead, a zone of the root is devoid of cementum and

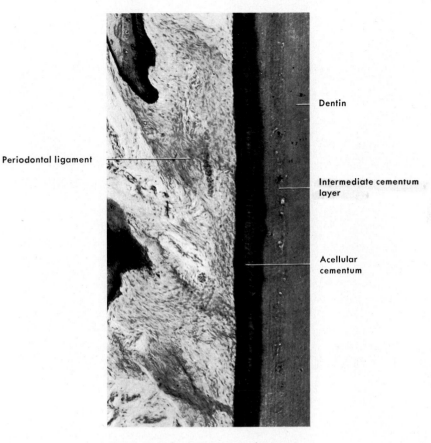

Periodontal ligament

Dentin

Intermediate cementum layer

Acellular cementum

Fig. 6-17. Intermediate layer of cementum.

is, for a time, covered by reduced enamel epithelium.

In approximately 60% of the teeth, cementum overlaps the cervical end of enamel for a short distance (Fig. 6-18, *B*). This occurs when the enamel epithelium degenerates at its cervical termination, permitting connective tissue to come in direct contact with the enamel surface. Electron microscopic evidence indicates that when connective tissue cells, probably cementoblasts, come in contact with enamel they produce a laminated, electron-dense, reticular material termed afibrillar cementum. Afibrillar cementum is so named because it

does not possess collagen fibrils with a 64 nm (640 Å) periodicity. If such afibrillar cementum remains in contact with connective tissue cells for a long enough time, fibrillar cementum with characteristic collagen fibrils may subsequently be deposited on its surface; thus the thickness of cementum that overlies enamel increases.

FUNCTION

The primary function of cementum is to furnish a medium for the attachment of collagen fibers that bind the tooth to alveolar bone. Since collagen fibers of the periodontal ligament cannot be incorporated into

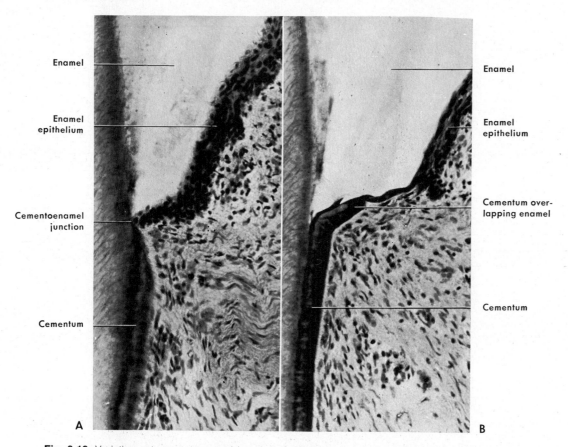

Enamel

Enamel epithelium

Cementoenamel junction

Cementum

Enamel

Enamel epithelium

Cementum overlapping enamel

Cementum

A · B

Fig. 6-18. Variations at cementoenamel junction. **A,** Cementum and enamel meet in sharp line. **B,** Cementum overlaps enamel.

dentin, a connective tissue attachment to the tooth is impossible without cementum. This is dramatically demonstrated in some cases of hypophosphatasia, a rare heredity disease in which loosening and premature loss of anterior deciduous teeth occurs. The exfoliated teeth are characterized by an almost total absence of cementum.

The continuous deposition of cementum is of considerable functional importance. In contrast to the alternating resorption and new formation of bone, cementum is not resorbed under normal conditions. As the most superficial layer of cementum ages, a new layer of cementum must be deposited to keep the attachment apparatus intact. The repeated apposition of cemental layers represents the aging of the tooth as an organ. In other words, a tooth is, functionally speaking, only as old as the last layer of cementum laid down on its root. The functional age of a tooth may be considerably less than its chronologic age.

Cementum serves as the major reparative tissue for root surfaces. Damage to roots such as fractures and resorptions can be repaired by the deposition of new cementum. Cementum may also be viewed as the tissue that makes functional adaptation of teeth possible. For example, deposition of cementum in an apical area can compensate for loss of tooth substance from occlusal wear.

HYPERCEMENTOSIS

Hypercementosis is an <u>abnormal thickening of cementum.</u> It may be diffuse or circumscribed. It may affect all teeth of the dentition, be confined to a single tooth, or even affect only parts of one tooth. If the overgrowth <u>improves the functional qualities of the cementum, it is termed a cementum hypertrophy.</u> If the overgrowth occurs <u>in nonfunctional teeth or if it is not corre-</u><u>lated with increased function, it is termed hyperplasia.</u>

In localized hypertrophy a spur or pronglike extension of cementum may be formed (Fig. 6-19). This condition frequently is found in teeth <u>that are exposed to great stress.</u> The pronglike extensions of cementum provide a larger surface area for the attaching fibers; thus a <u>firmer anchorage of the tooth to the surrounding alveolar bone</u> is assured.

Localized hypercementosis may sometimes be observed in areas in which enamel drops have developed on the dentin. The hyperplastic cementum covering the enamel drops (Fig. 6-20) occasionally is

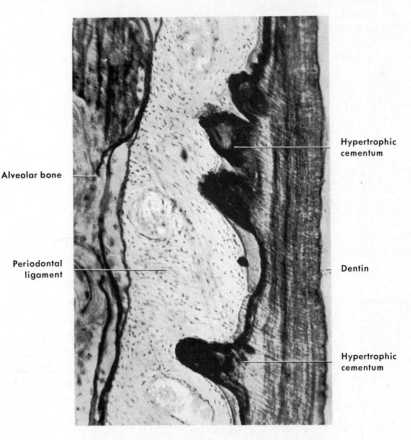

Fig. 6-19. Pronglike excementoses.

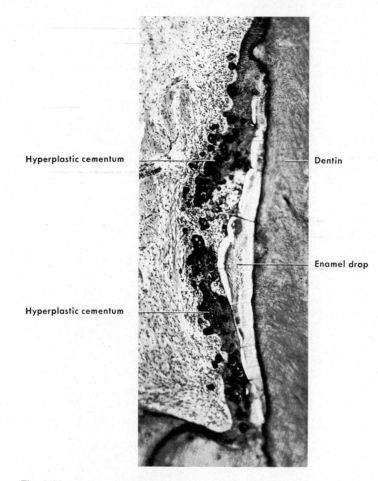

Hyperplastic cementum

Dentin

Enamel drop

Hyperplastic cementum

Fig. 6-20. Irregular hyperplasia of cementum on surface of enamel drop.

irregular and sometimes contains round bodies that may be calcified epithelial rests. The same type of embedded calcified round bodies frequently are found in localized areas of hyperplastic cementum (Fig. 6-21). Such knoblike projections are designated as excementoses. They too develop around degenerated epithelial rests.

Extensive hyperplasia of cementum is occasionally associated with chronic periapical inflammation. Here the hyperplasia is circumscribed and surrounds the root like a cuff.

A thickening of cementum is often observed on teeth that are not in function. The hyperplasia may extend around the entire root of the nonfunctioning teeth or may be localized in small areas. Hyperplasia of cementum in nonfunctioning teeth is characterized by a reduction in the number of Sharpey's fibers embedded in the root.

The cementum is thicker around the apex of all teeth and in the furcation of multirooted teeth than on other areas of the root. This thickening is found in embedded and in newly erupted teeth.

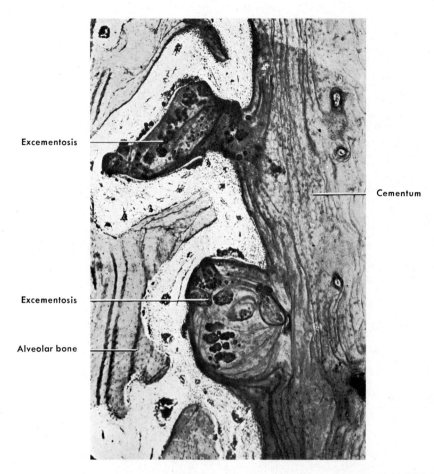

Excementosis

Cementum

Excementosis

Alveolar bone

Fig. 6-21. Excementoses in bifurcation of molar. (From Gottlieb B: Oesterr Z Stomatol 19:515, 1921.)

In some cases an irregular overgrowth of cementum can be found, with spikelike extensions and calcification of Sharpey's fibers and accompanied by numerous cementicles. This type of cemental hyperplasia can occasionally be observed on many teeth of the same dentition and is, at least in some cases, the sequela of injuries to the cementum (Fig. 6-22).

CLINICAL CONSIDERATIONS

Cementum is <u>more resistant to resorption than is bone,</u> and it is for this reason that orthodontic tooth movement is made possible. <u>When a tooth is moved by means of an orthodontic appliance, bone is resorbed on the side of the pressure, and new bone is formed on the side of tension</u>. On the side toward which the tooth is moved, pressure is equal on the surfaces of bone and cementum. Resorption of bone as well as of cementum may be anticipated. However, in careful orthodontic treatment, cementum resorption is minimal or absent, but bone resorption leads to tooth migration.

The difference in the resistance of bone

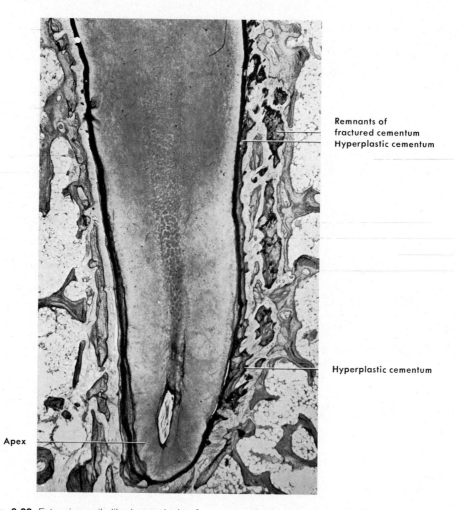

Remnants of
fractured cementum
Hyperplastic cementum

Hyperplastic cementum

Apex

Fig. 6-22. Extensive spikelike hyperplasia of cementum formed during healing of cemental tear.

and cementum to pressure may be caused by the fact that bone is richly vascularized, whereas cementum is avascular. Thus degenerative processes are much more easily effected by interference with circulation in bone, whereas cementum with its slow metabolism (as in other avascular tissues) is not damaged by a pressure equal to that exerted on bone.

Cementum resorption can occur after trauma or excessive occlusal forces. In se-

vere cases cementum resorption may continue into the dentin. After resorption has ceased, the damage usually is repaired, either by formation of acellular (Fig. 6-23, *A*) or cellular (Fig. 6-23, *B*) cementum or by alternate formation of both (Fig. 6-23, *C*). In most cases of repair there is a tendency to reestablish the former outline of the root surface. This is called *anatomic repair*. However, if only a thin layer of cementum is deposited on the surface of a deep re-

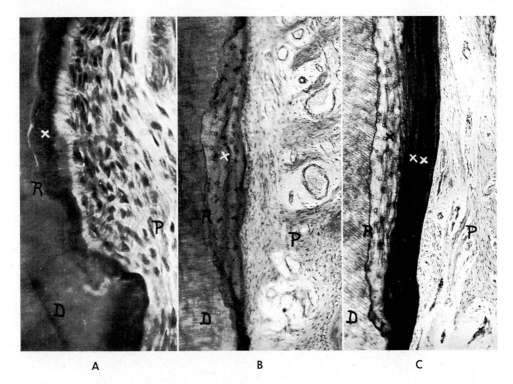

Fig. 6-23. Repair of resorbed cementum. **A,** Repair by acellular cementum, x. **B,** Repair by cellular cementum, x. **C,** Repair first by cellular, x, and later by acellular, xx, cementum, D, Dentin. R, Line of resorption. P, Periodontal ligament.

sorption, the root outline is not reconstructed, and a baylike recess remains. In such areas sometimes the periodontal space is restored to its normal width by formation of a bony projection so that a proper functional relationship will result. The outline of the alveolar bone in these cases follows that of the root surface (Fig. 6-24). In contrast to anatomic repair, this change is called *functional repair.*

If teeth are subjected to a severe blow, fragments of cementum may be severed from the dentin. The tear occurs frequently at the cementodentinal junction, but it may also be in the cementum or dentin.

Transverse fractures of the root may oc-

cur after trauma, and these may heal by formation of new cementum.

Frequently, hyperplasia of cementum is secondary to periapical inflammation or extensive occlusal stress. This is of practical significance because the extraction of such teeth may necessitate the removal of bone. This also applies to extensive excementoses, as shown in Fig. 6-21. They can anchor the tooth so tightly to the socket that the jaw or parts of it may be fractured in an attempt to extract the tooth. This possibility indicates the necessity for taking roentgenograms before any extraction. Small fragments of roots left in the jaw after extraction of teeth may be surrounded by cemen-

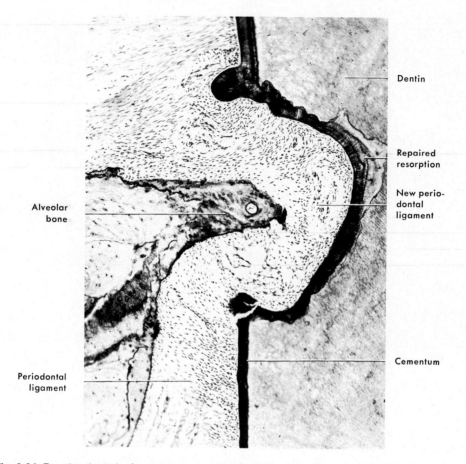

Dentin

Repaired resorption

New periodontal ligament

Cementum

Alveolar bone

Periodontal ligament

Fig. 6-24. Functional repair of cementum resorption by bone apposition. Normal width of periodontal ligament reestablished.

tum and remain in the jaw without causing any disturbance.

In periodontal pockets, plaque and its by-products can cause numerous alterations in the physical, chemical, and structural characteristics of cementum. The surface of pathologically exposed cementum becomes hypermineralized because of the incorporation of calcium, phosphorus, and fluoride from the oral environment. At the light-microscopic level no major structural changes occur in the surface of exposed ce-

mentum. However, at the ultrastructural level there is a loss or decrease in the cross-striations of collagen near the surface (Fig. 6-25). Endotoxin originating from plaque can be recovered from exposed cementum, but it is not known if the distribution of the cementum-bound endotoxin is limited to the cemental surface (adsorbed) or if it penetrates into deeper portions of the root (absorbed). Alterations in exposed cementum are of particular interest to the periodontal therapist since it is believed

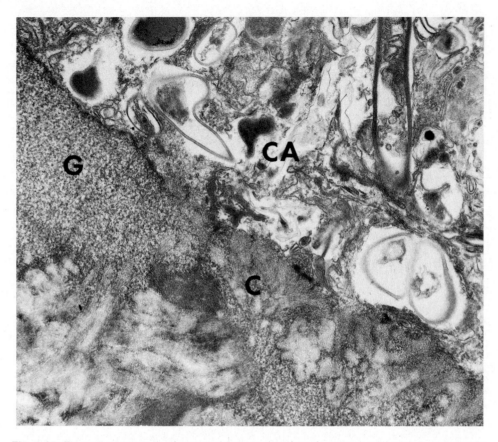

Fig. 6-25. Electron micrograph of exposed cemental surface from tooth with periodontal disease. Collagen fibrils at cemental surface *(C)* have lost their cross-striations or have been replaced by finely granular electron dense material *(G)*. Cell envelopes of bacteria can be observed in calculus *(CA)* on cemental surface. (Decalcified specimen; × 26,000.) (From Armitage GC: Periodont Abs 25:60, 1977.)

that they may interfere with healing during periodontal therapy. Consequently, in periodontal therapy, various procedures (mechanical and chemical) have been proposed that are intended to remove this altered cemental surface.

REFERENCES

Armitage GC: Alterations in exposed human cementum, Periodont Abs 25:60, 1977.

Beumer J, Trowbridge HO, Silverman S, Jr, et al.: Childhood hypophosphatasia and the premature loss of teeth. A clinical and laboratory study of seven cases, Oral Surg 35:631, 1973.

Blackwood HJJ: Intermediate cementum, Br Dent J 102:345, 1957.

Bruckner RJ, Rickles NH, and Porter DR: Hypophosphatasia with premature shedding of teeth and aplasia of cementum, Oral Surg 15:1351, 1962.

Denton GB: The discovery of cementum, J Dent Res 18:239, 1939.

Eastoe JE: Composition of the organic matrix of cementum, J Dent Res 54 (special issue) :L137, 1975 (abstract L547.)

El Mostehy MR and Stallard RE: Intermediate cementum, J Periodont Res 3:24, 1968.

Furseth R: A microradiographic and electron microscopic study of the cementum of human deciduous teeth, Acta Odontol Scand 25:613, 1967.

Furseth R: The fine structure of the cellular cementum of young human teeth, Arch Oral Biol 14:1147, 1969.

Gedalia I, Nathan H, Schapira J, et al.: Fluoride concentration of surface enamel, cementum, lamina dura and subperiosteal bone from the mandibular angle of Hebrews, J Dent Res 44:452, 1965.

Gottlieb B: Zementexostosen, Schmelztropfen und Epithelnester (Exostosis of cementum, enamel drops and epithelial rests), Osterr Z Stomatol 19:515, 1921.

Gottlieb B: Biology of the cementum, J Periodontol 13:13, 1942.

Jones SJ and Boyde A: A study of human root cementum surfaces as prepared for and examined in the scanning electron microscope, Z Zellforsch 130:318, 1972.

Kronfeld R: The biology of cementum, J Am Dent Assoc 25:1451, 1938.

Kronfeld R: Coronal cementum and coronal resorption, J Dent Res 17:151, 1938.

Lester KS: The incorporation of epithelial cells by cementum. J Ultrastruct Res 27:63, 1969.

Linden LA: Microscopic observations of fluid flow through cementum and dentine. An *in vitro* study on human teeth, Odontol Rev 19:367, 1968.

Listgarten MA: Phase-contrast and electron microscopic study of the junction between reduced enamel epithelium and enamel in unerupted human teeth, Arch Oral Biol 11:999, 1966.

Nihei I: A study on the hardness of human teeth, J Osaka Univ Dent Soc 4:1, 1959.

Olsen T and Johansen E: Inorganic composition of sound and carious human cementum. Preprinted abstracts. Fiftieth General Meeting of the International Association for Dental Research, Abstr no 174, 1972, p 91.

Orban B: Dental histology and embryology, ed 2, Philadelphia, 1929, P Blakiston's Son & Co.

Paynter KJ and Pudy G: A study of the structure, chemical nature, and development of cementum in the rat, Anat Rec 131:233, 1958.

Rautiola CA and Craig RG: The microhardness of cementum and underlying dentin of normal teeth and teeth exposed to periodontal disease, J Periodontol 32:113, 1961.

Rodriguez MS and Wilderman MN: Amino acid composition of the cementum matrix from human molar teeth. J Periodontol 43:438, 1972.

Schroeder HE and Listgarten MA: Fine structure of the developing epithelial attachment of human teeth. In Wolsky A, editor: Monographs in developmental biology, vol 2, Basel, 1971, S Karger, AG.

Selvig KA: Electron microscopy of Hertwig's epithelial root sheath and of early dentin and cementum formation in the mouse incisor. Acta Odontol Scand 21:175, 1963.

Selvig KA: An ultrastructural study of cementum formation, Acta Odontol Scand 22:105, 1964.

Selvig KA: The fine structure of human cementum, Acta Odontol Scand 23:423, 1965.

Selvig KA and Hals E: Periodontally diseased cementum studied by correlated microradiography, electron probe analysis and electron microscopy, J Periodont Res 12:419, 1977.

Van Kirk LE: Variations in structure of human enamel and dentin, J Am Dent Assoc 15:1270, 1928.

Zander HA and Hürzeler B: Continuous cementum apposition, J Dent Res 37:1035, 1958.

Zipkin I: The inorganic composition of bones and teeth. In Schraer H, editor: Biological calcification, New York, 1970, Appleton-Century-Crofts.

7
PERIODONTAL LIGAMENT

The periodontium is a connective tissue organ, covered by epithelium, that attaches the teeth to the bones of the jaws and provides a continually adapting apparatus for support of the teeth during function. The periodontium comprises four connective tissues, two mineralized and two fibrous. The two mineralized connective tissues are cementum and alveolar bone (see Chapters 6 and 8), and the two fibrous connective tissues are the periodontal ligament and the lamina propria of the gingiva (see Chapter 9). The periodontium is attached to the dentin of the root of the tooth by cementum and to the bone of the jaws by alveolar bone. The periodontal ligament occupies the periodontal space, which is located between the cementum and the periodontal surface of the alveolar bone, and

extends coronally to the most apical part of the lamina propria of the gingiva. By definition therefore the coronal part of the periodontal ligament is marked by the most superficial fibers, appearing to extend from cementum to alveolar bone. Collagen fibers of the periodontal ligament are embedded in cementum and alveolar bone so that the ligament provides soft-tissue continuity between the mineralized connective tissues of the periodontium.

The periodontal ligament is a fibrous connective tissue that is noticeably cellular (Fig. 7-1) and contains numerous blood vessels. All connective tissues, the periodontal ligament included, comprise cells as well as extracellular matrix consisting of fibers and ground substance. The majority of the fibers of the periodontal ligament are

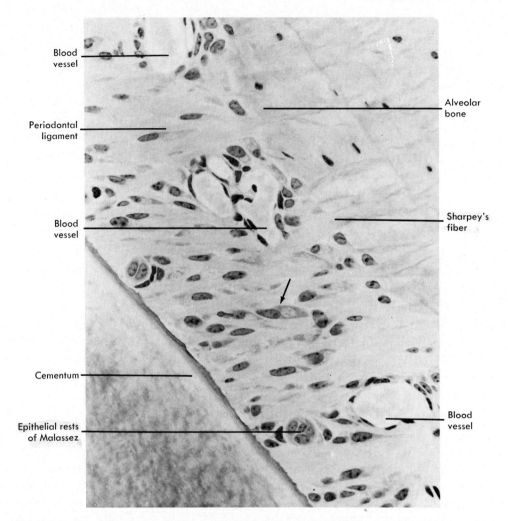

Fig. 7-1. Section, 1 μm thick, of mouse molar periodontal ligament. Tissue is cellular and vascular. The arrow indicates fibroblast that exhibits a negative image of the Golgi complex. (Hematoxylin and eosin; ×700.)

collagen, and the matrix is composed of a variety of macromolecules, the basic constituents of which are proteins and polysaccharides. It is important to remember that the extracellular matrix is produced and can be removed by the cells of the connective tissue.

The periodontal ligament has a number of functions, which include attachment and support, nutrition, synthesis and resorp-

tion, and proprioception. Over the years it has been described by a number of terms. Among them are desmodont, gomphosis, pericementum, dental periosteum, alveolodental ligament, and periodontal membrane. "Periodontal membrane" and "periodontal ligament" are the terms that are now most commonly used. Neither term describes the structure and its functions adequately. It is neither a typical membrane nor a typical ligament. However, because it is a complex soft connective tissue providing continuity between two mineralized connective tissues, the term "periodontal ligament" appears to be the more appropriate.

EVOLUTION

There is a fundamental difference between the attachment of reptilian and mammalian teeth. In the ancestral reptiles the teeth are ankylosed to the bone. In mammals they are suspended in their sockets by ligaments. The evolutionary step from reptile to mammal included a series of coordinated changes in the jaws. The central point of these changes is the radical "reconstruction" of the mandible. In reptiles the mandible consists of a series of bones united by sutures. Only the uppermost bone, the dentary, carries the ankylosed teeth. The mandibular articulation is formed by a separate bone of the mandible, the articulare, and a separate bone of the cranium, the quadratum. During the period of transition from advanced types of reptiles to the first mammals, the dentary attained larger proportions, whereas the other mandibular bones were reduced in size. Finally, only the dentary formed the mammalian mandible. The other bony components of the reptilian mandible were either lost or changed into two of the ossicles of the middle ear: the articulare survives as the malleus and the quadratum as the incus. Before this change could take place, the dentary, growing a condylar process, formed a "new" temporomandibular articulation that, for a time, functioned together with the old articulare-quadratum joint. Such "double-jointed" forms are now known.

The change from the many-boned reptilian to the single-boned mammalian mandible brought with it a radical change in the mode of growth. In the reptile the growth of the mandible is "sutural" in the same manner as the growth of the cranium. In the mammal the newly acquired cartilage of the condyle takes over as the most important growth site of the mandible. In the reptile growth of the mandibular body in height occurs in the mandibular sutures, whereas in the mammal it occurs by growth at the free margins of the alveolar process. In the reptile the mandibular (and maxillary) teeth "move" with the bones to which they are fused. In the mammal the teeth have to "move" as units independent of the bones, and this movement is made possible by the remodeling of the periodontium. The evolutionary change from the reptiles to mammals replaces the ankylosis of tooth and bone to a ligamentous suspension of the tooth. This change permits movement of mammalian teeth and the continual repositioning necessitated by jaw growth or tooth wear.

DEVELOPMENT

The dental organ (enamel organ) and, later in tooth development, Hertwig's epithelial root sheath are surrounded by a condensation of cells, the dental sac (see p. 31). A thin layer of these cells that apparently is continuous with the cells of the dental papilla lies adjacent to the dental organ. It has been suggested that the term *dental follicle* be reserved for this layer of cells and the term *perifollicular mesenchyme* for the cells that surround the dental follicle (Fig. 7-2). The cells of the dental follicle are probably derived from ancestral cells in the dental papilla. Dental follicle cells divide and differentiate into the dementoblasts that deposit cementum on the developing root, to the fibroblasts of the developing periodontal ligament, and possibly to the osteoblasts of the developing alveolar bone. The formation of the peri-

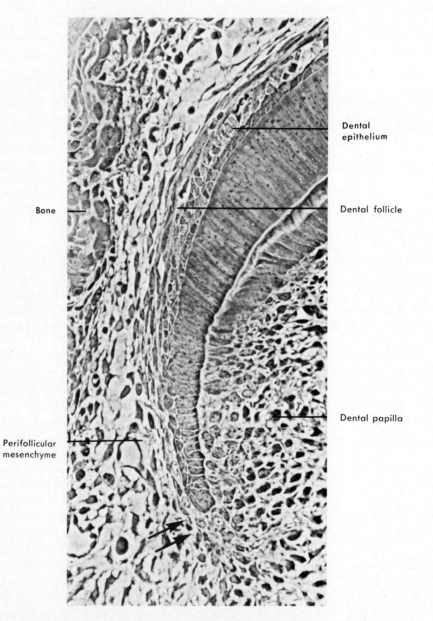

Bone

Dental
epithelium

Dental follicle

Dental papilla

Perifollicular
mesenchyme

Fig. 7-2. Montage phase-contrast photomicrograph of first molar tooth germ of 1-day-old mouse showing the dental follicle, which is continuous with the dental papilla around the cervical loop *(arrows).* (×450.) (From Freeman E and Ten Cate AR: J Periodontol 42:387, 1971.)

odontal ligament occurs after the cells of Hertwig's epithelial root sheath (see p. 41) have separated, forming the strands known as the *epithelial rests of Malassez* (see p. 42). This separation permits the cells of the dental follicle to migrate to the external surface of the newly formed root dentin. These migrant follicle cells then differentiate into cementoblasts and deposit cementum on the surface of the dentin. Other cells of the dental follicle differentiate into fibroblasts, which synthesize the fibers and ground substance of the periodontal ligament. The fibers of the periodontal ligament become embedded in newly developed cementum and alveolar bone and, as the tooth erupts, are oriented in characteristic fashion (see Chapter 11).

CELLS

The principal cells of the healthy, functioning periodontal ligament are concerned with the synthesis and resorption of alveolar bone and the fibrous connective tissue of the ligament and cementum. The cells of the periodontal ligament may be divided into three main categories:

Synthetic cells	Resorptive cells
Osteoblasts	Osteoclasts
Fibroblasts	Fibroblasts
Cementoblasts	Cementoclasts

The progenitors for the synthetic cells reside at least in part in the periodontal ligament, and the progenitors for osteoclasts and cementoclasts (but not fibroblasts) originate from hematopoietic cells.

There are, in addition, epithelial cells present in the ligament:

Epithelial rests of Malassez

And there are other types of cells derived from the hemopoietic line:

Mast cells
Macrophages

Synthetic cells

There are certain general cytologic criteria that distinguish all cells that are synthesizing proteins for secretion (e.g., extracellular substance of connective tissue), and these criteria can be applied equally to osteoblasts, cementoblasts, and fibroblasts. For a cell to produce protein, it must, among other activities, transcribe ribonucleic acid (RNA), synthesize ribosomes in the nucleolus and transport them to the cytoplasm, and increase its complement of rough endoplasmic reticulum (RER) and Golgi membranes for translation and transport of the protein. It must also have the means to produce an adequate supply of energy. Each of these functional activities is reflected morphologically when synthetically active tissues are viewed in the electron and light microscopes. Increased transcription of RNA and production of ribosomes is reflected by a large open-faced or vesicular nucleus containing prominent nucleoli. The development of large quantities of RER covered by ribosomes is readily recognized in the electron microscope and is reflected by hematoxyphilia of the cytoplasm when the cell is seen in the light microscope after staining by hematoxylin and eosin. The hematoxyphilia is the result of interaction of the RNA with the acid hematein in the stain. The Golgi saccules and vesicles are also readily seen in the electron microscope but are not stained by acid hematein and so, in the light microscope, they are seen in appropriate sections as a clear, unstained area in the otherwise hematoxyphilic cytoplasm. The increased requirement for energy is reflected in the electron microscope by the presence of relatively large numbers of mitochrondria. Accommodation of all these organelles in the cell requires a large amount of cytoplasm. Thus a cell that is actively secreting extracellular substance will be seen in the light microscope to exhibit a large, open-faced or vesicular nucleus with prominent nucleoli and to have abundant cytoplasm that tends to be hematoxyphilic, with, if the plane of section is favorable, a clear area representing the Golgi membranes (Fig. 7-1).

Cells with the morphology described above, if found at the periodontal surface of the alveolar bone, are active osteoblasts; if lying in the body of the soft connective tissue, they are active fibroblasts; and, if found at cementum, they are active cementoblasts. These cells all have, in addition to the features described above, the particular characteristics of osteoblasts, fibroblasts,

and cementoblasts. Detailed descriptions of the first two types of cells can be found in appropriate textbooks and of the third in the chapter on cementum (Chapter 6).

Synthetic cells in all stages of activity are present in the periodontal ligament, and this is reflected directly by the degree to which the characteristics described above are developed in each cell. Cells having a paucity of cytoplasm (i.e., cytoplasm that virtually cannot be distinguished in the light microscope) and having very few organelles and a close-faced nucleus are also found in the ligament.

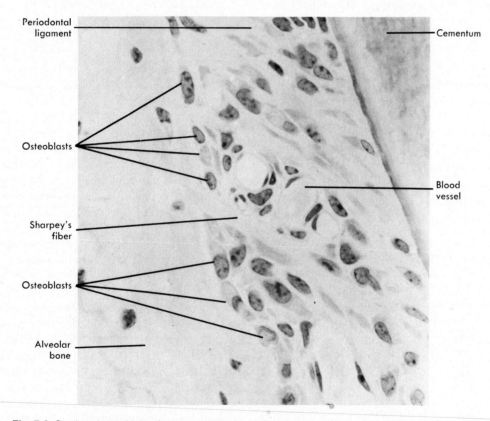

Fig. 7-3. Section, 1 μm thick, of mouse molar periodontal ligament. Note osteoblasts lining periodontal surface of alveolar bone, some of which exhibit a negative image of the Golgi complex. (Hematoxylin and eosin; ×1100.)

Osteoblasts. The osteoblasts covering the periodontal surface of the alveolar bone constitute a modified endosteum and not a periosteum. A periosteum can be recognized by the fact that it comprises at least two distinct layers, an inner cellular or cambium layer and an outer fibrous layer. A cellular layer, but not an outer fibrous layer, is present on the periodontal surface of the alveolar bone. The surface of the bone lining the dental socket must therefore be regarded as an interior surface of bone, akin to that lining medullary cavities, and not an external surface, which would be covered by periosteum. The surface of the bone is covered largely by osteoblasts in various stages of differentiation (Figs. 7-1, 7-3, and 7-4), as well as by occasional osteoclasts. Collagen fibers of the ligament that penetrate the alveolar bone intervene between the cells (Figs. 7-1, 7-3, and 7-5).

Fibroblasts. Fibroblasts in various stages of differentiation, and their progenitors, are found in the periodontal ligament, where they are surrounded by fibers and ground substance (Figs. 7-6 and 7-7). In longitudinal sections viewed by light microscopy, the cells of the ligament frequently appear to be oriented parallel to the oriented bundles of collagen fibers (Figs. 7-4 and 7-5).

Cementoblasts. The distribution on the tooth surface of variously differentiated cementoblasts (Fig. 7-8) is similar to the distribution of osteoblasts on the bone surface.

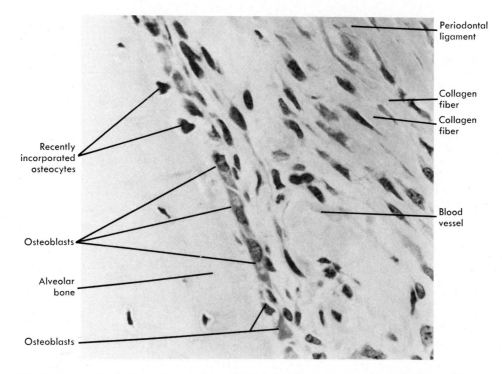

Fig. 7-4. Section, 1 μm thick, of mouse molar periodontal ligament. Note osteoblasts lining periodontal surface of alveolar bone, some of which exhibit a negative image of the Golgi complex. (Hematoxylin and eosin; ×1000.)

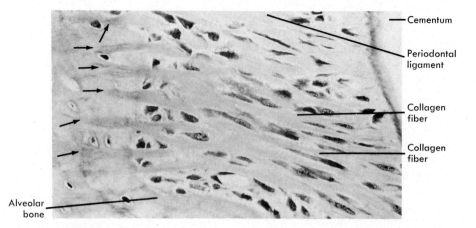

Fig. 7-5. Section, 1 μm thick, of mouse molar periodontal ligament. Collagen fibers from ligament that pass between osteoblasts to penetrate alveolar bone as Sharpey's fibers are shown by arrows. (Hematoxylin and eosin; ×1000.)

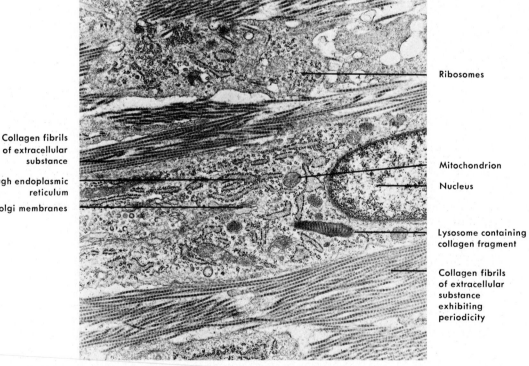

Fig. 7-6. Fibroblasts and collagen fibrils of mouse molar periodontal ligament. The lower cell exhibits numerous profiles of rough endoplasmic reticulum and Golgi membranes, and a collagen-containing lysosome. (×9250.) (Courtesy Dr. A.R. Ten Cate, Toronto.)

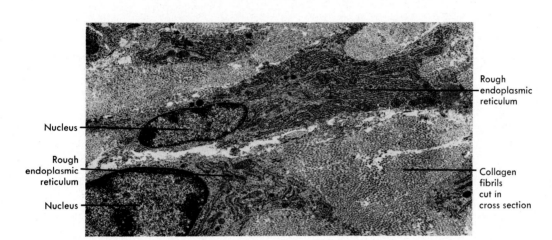

Fig. 7-7. Fibroblasts and collagen fibrils of mouse molar periodontal ligament. Upper cell cytoplasm exhibits relatively more rough endoplasmic reticulum than does that of lower cell. (×8000.)

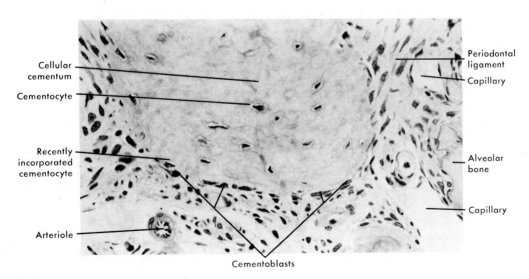

Fig. 7-8. Section, 1 μm thick, of mouse molar periodontal ligament. Note cementoblasts on surface of cellular cementum at apex of root. (Hematoxylin and eosin; ×650.)

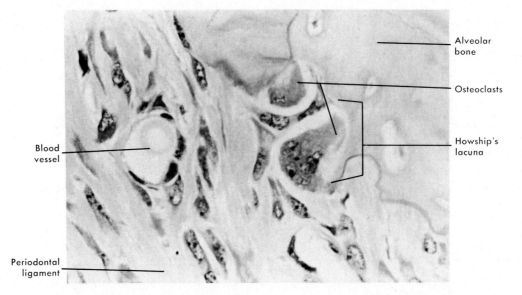

Blood
vessel

Periodontal
ligament

Alveolar
bone

Osteoclasts

Howship's
lacuna

Fig. 7-9. Section, 1 μm thick, illustrating osteoclasts located on periodontal surface of alveolar bone of mouse molar. (Hematoxylin and eosin; ×1600.)

Resorptive cells

Osteoclasts. Osteoclasts are cells that resorb bone and tend to be large and multinucleated (Fig. 7-9) but can also be small and mononuclear. Multinucleated osteoclasts are formed by fusion of precursor cells similar to circulating monocytes. These characteristic multinucleated cells usually exhibit an eosinophilic cytoplasm and are easily recognizable. When viewed in the light microscope, the cells may sometimes appear to occupy bays in bone (Howship's lacunae) or surround the end of a bone spicule. In the electron microscope their cytoplasm is seen to exhibit numerous mitochondria and lysosomes, abundant Golgi saccules, and free ribosomes but little RER. The part of the plasma membrane lying adjacent to bone that is being resorbed is raised in characteristic folds and is termed the *ruffled* or *striated border*. The ruffled border is separated from the rest of the plasma membrane by a zone of specialized membrane that is closely applied to the bone, the underlying cytoplasm of which tends to be devoid of organelles and has been called the *clear zone* (Fig. 7-10). The area of bone that is sealed off by the ruffled border is exposed to a highly acidic pH by virtue of the active pumping of protons by the osteoclast into this environment. The bone related to the ruffled border can be seen undergoing resorption. Resorption occurs in two stages: first, the mineral is removed from a narrow zone at the bone margin; then the recognizable exposed organic matrix is disintegrated. The osteoclast appears to accomplish both demineralization and disaggregation of the organic matrix, the latter possibly achieved by the secretion of appropriate enzymes. However, this question has not been settled. The ruffled border disappears in inactive osteoclasts. Light

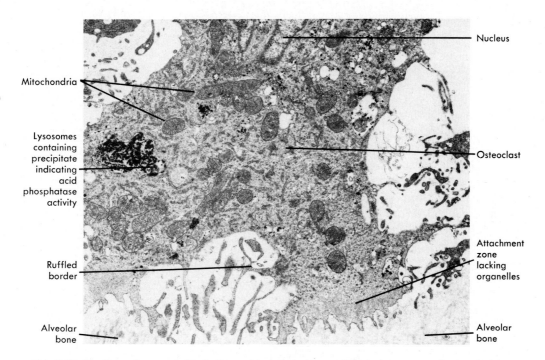

Nucleus

Mitochondria

Lysosomes
containing
precipitate
indicating
acid
phosphatase
activity

Osteoclast

Ruffled
border

Attachment
zone
lacking
organelles

Alveolar
bone

Alveolar
bone

Fig. 7-10. Electron micrograph illustrating acid phosphatase activity in lysosomes of osteoclast located on periodontal surface of alveolar bone of mouse molar. (×14,000.)

and electron microscopic histochemical tests can be used to show that osteoclasts are rich in acid phosphatase, which is contained in lysosomes (Fig. 7-10).

The presence of osteoclasts on the periodontal surface of the alveolar bone (Figs. 7-9 and 7-10) indicates that resorption was active or had recently ceased in that area at the time the tissue was removed. Osteoclasts are seen regularly in normal functioning periodontal ligament, in which the cells play a part in the removal and the deposition of bone that are responsible for its remodeling, a process that allows functional changes in the position of teeth that must be accommodated by the supporting tissues (see Chapter 11).

Fibroblasts. It has recently become evident that the collagen fibrils of mammalian

periodontal ligament can be resorbed under physiologic conditions by mononuclear fibroblasts. These cells exhibit lysosomes that contain fragments of collagen that appear to be undergoing digestion (Fig. 7-6). The activity of these fibroclastic cells does not appear necessarily to be restricted to destruction of collagen, because large portions of their cytoplasm may be filled with the organelles normally associated with protein synthesis. It must be made clear that there does not appear to be a unique cell that resorbs the extracellular substance of soft connective tissue but the fibroblast may be capable of both synthesis and resorption. Collagen-resorbing fibroblasts are found in normal functioning periodontal ligament, and their presence, like that of osteoclasts in relation to bone, indicates resorption of fibers occurring during physiologic turnover or remodeling of periodontal ligament.

Cementoclasts. Cementoclasts resemble osteoclasts and are occasionally found in normal functioning periodontal ligament. This observation is consistent with the knowledge that cementum is not remodeled in the fashion of alveolar bone and periodontal ligament but that it undergoes continual deposition during life. However, resorption of cementum can occur under certain circumstances, and in these instances mononuclear cementoclasts or multinucleated giant cells, often located in Howship's lacunae, are found on the surface of the cementum. The origin of cementoclasts is unknown, but it is conceivable that they arise in the same manner as osteoclasts.

Progenitor cells

All connective tissues, including periodontal ligament, contain progenitors for synthetic cells that have the capacity to undergo mitotic division. If they were not present, there would be no cells available to replace differentiated cells dying at the end of their life span (Fig. 7-11) or as a result of trauma. Although the process is not well understood, it is believed that after cell division, one of the daughter cells differentiates into a functional type of connective tissue cell (i.e., any one of the synthetic cell types described above) while the other remains an undifferentiated progenitor cell retaining the capacity to divide when stimulated appropriately. Progenitor cells tend to have a small, close-faced nucleus and very little cytoplasm and are

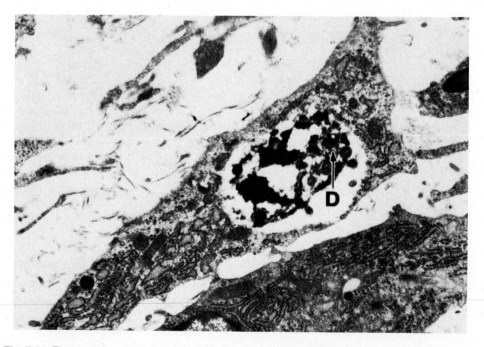

Fig. 7-11. Electron micrograph illustrating fibroblast in body of periodontal ligament that exhibits disintegrating cytoplasm and electron dense masses *(D)*. (×12,870.)

found in highest concentrations close to blood vessels.

Little is known about the progenitor cells of the ligament. For example, it is not known whether a single population of progenitor cells gives rise to all of the specialized synthetic cells in the ligament or if there are a number of populations, each of which gives rise to a different specialized cell. That progenitor cells are present is evident from the burst of mitoses that occur after application of pressure to a tooth as in orthodontic therapy or after wounding, maneuvers that stimulate proliferation and differentiation of cells of periodontal liga-

ment. The cells that divide in response to normal biologic requirements and to wounding of the periodontal ligament apparently are located predominantly in the vicinity of blood vessels but may also enter the periodontal ligament through penetrations from adjacent endosteal spaces (Fig. 7-12).

Relationship between cells

The cells of the periodontal ligament form a three-dimensional network, and, in appropriately oriented sections, their processes can be seen to surround the collagen fibers of the extracellular substance. Cells of periodontal ligament associated with bone, fibrous connective tissue, and cementum are not separated from one another, but adjacent cells generally are in contact with their neighbors, usually through their processes (Fig. 7-13). The site of some of the contacts between adjacent cells may be marked by modification of the structure of the contiguous plasma membranes (Fig. 7-14). The nature of these junctions has not yet been elucidated satisfactorily. Although many appear to be zonulae occludens, it is conceivable that they are in fact gap junctions. Gap junctions in other tissues occur between cells that have been found to be in direct communication with one another. It is likely that some form of communication must exist between the cells of the periodontal ligament; to facilitate the homeostatic mechanisms that are known to operate in the periodontal ligament.

Epithelial rests of Malassez

The periodontal ligament contains epithelial cells that are found close to the cementum (Fig. 7-15). These cells were first described by Malassez in 1884 and are the remnants of the epithelium of Hertwig's epithelial root sheath (see Chapter 2). At

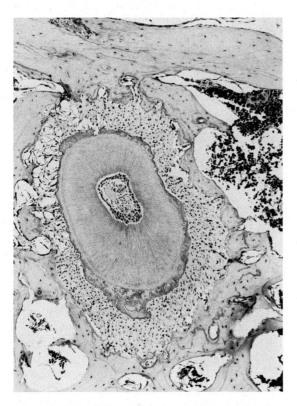

Fig. 7-12. Section, 1 μm thick illustrating continuity between endosteal spaces and periodontal ligament in rat mandibular molar. (×160.)

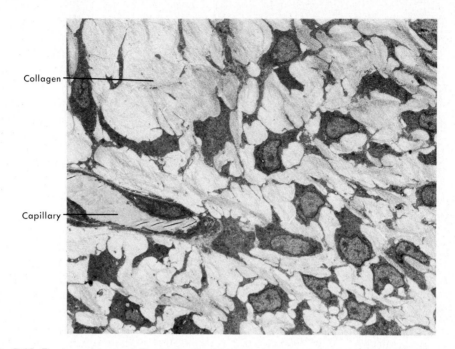

Collagen

Capillary

Fig. 7-13. Electron micrograph illustrating fibroblasts and mutual contacts made by their processes in periodontal ligament of mouse molar. (×3040.)

the time of cementum formation the continuous layer of epithelium that covers the surface of the newly formed dentin breaks into lacelike strands (Fig. 7-16). The epithelial rests persist as a network, strands, islands, or tubulelike structures near and parallel to the surface of the root (Figs. 7-15 and 7-17).

Only in sections almost parallel to the root can the true arrangment of these epithelial strands be seen. When the tooth is sectioned longitudinally or transversely, the strands of the network are cut in cross section or obliquely and, as a result, appear as isolated islands when viewed in the light microscope. The cause of disintegration of the epithelium and any inductive influence that it may have on the cells of the dental follicle has not been elucidated.

In rat and mouse molars, most but not all

of the epithelium of the developing root is incorporated into the cementum, and consequently the epithelial rests of Malassez are sparse.

Electron microscopic observations show that the epithelial rest cells exhibit tonofilaments (Fig. 7-18) and that they are attached to one another by desmosomes. The epithelial cell clusters are isolated from the connective tissue cells by a basal lamina similar to that occurring at the junction of epithelium and connective tissue elsewhere in the body. It is evident from their ultrastructure, response to histochemical tests, and behavior in cell, tissue, and organ culture that, although the epithelial cells appear in some mammals to decrease with age, they are not effete. However, their physiologic role, if any, in the functioning periodontal ligament is unknown.

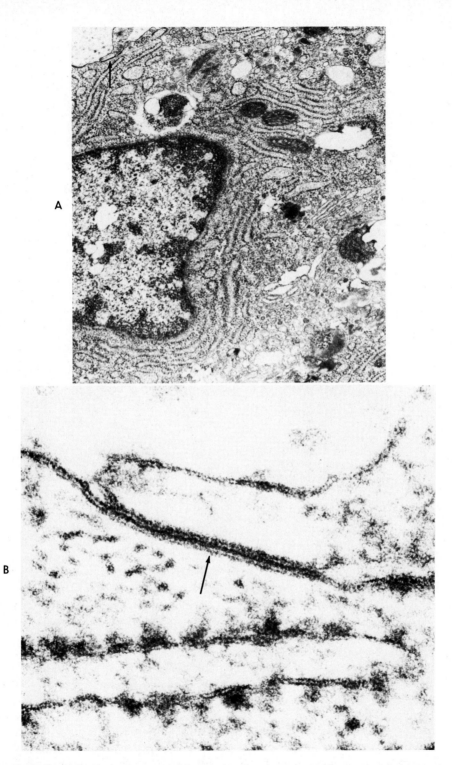

Fig. 7-14. Specialized structure, possibly gap junction *(arrow),* marking contact between plasma membranes of adjacent fibroblasts in periodontal ligament of mouse molar. (**A,** ×32,000; **B,** ×450,000.)

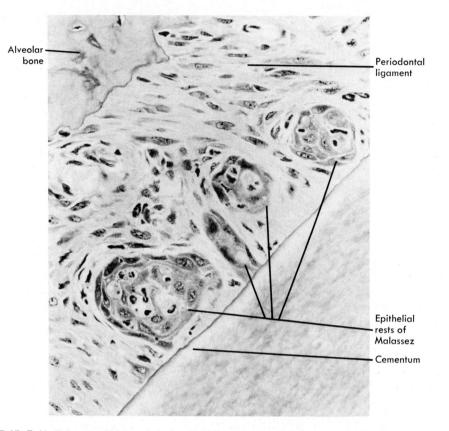

Alveolar bone

Periodontal ligament

Epithelial rests of Malassez

Cementum

Fig. 7-15. Epithelial rests of Malassez in 1 μm thick section of periodontal ligament of mouse molar. (Hematoxylin and eosin; ×640.)

The fact that methods have recently been described for culturing the rest cells in vitro suggests that it may soon be possible to obtain new information about their functional capabilities. When certain pathologic conditions are present, cells of the epithelial rests can undergo rapid proliferation and can produce a variety of cysts and tumors that are unique to the jaws.

Mast cells

The mast cell is a relatively small, round or oval cell having a diameter of about 12 to 15 μm. The cells are characterized by numerous cytoplasmic granules, which frequently obscure the small, round nucleus. The granules stain with basic dyes but are most readily demonstrated by virtue of their capacity to stain metachromatically with metachromatic dyes such as azure A. They are also positively stained by the periodic acid–Schiff reaction. The granules have been shown to contain heparin and histamine and, in some animals, serotonin. In some preparations, mast cells may be seen to have degranulated so that many or all of the granules are located outside the cell.

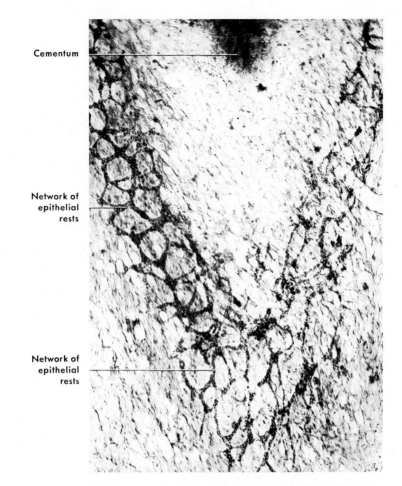

Fig. 7-16. Network of epithelial rests in periodontal ligament. (Tangential section almost parallel to root surface.)

Electron microscopy shows the mast cell cytoplasm contains free ribosomes, short profiles of granular endoplasmic reticulum, few round mitochondria, and a prominent Golgi apparatus. The granules average about 0.5 to 1 μm in diameter and are membrane bound.

The physiologic role of heparin in mast cells does not appear to be clear. Mast cell histamine plays a role in the inflammatory reaction, and mast cells have been shown to degranulate in response to antigen-anti-body formation on their surface. Occasional mast cells may be seen in the healthy periodontal ligament. The release of histamine into the extracellular environment causes proliferation of endothelial cells and mesenchymal cells. Consequently, mast cells may play an important role in regulating endothelial and fibroblast cell populations.

Macrophages

Macrophages are also found in the ligament (Fig. 7-19) and are predominantly lo-

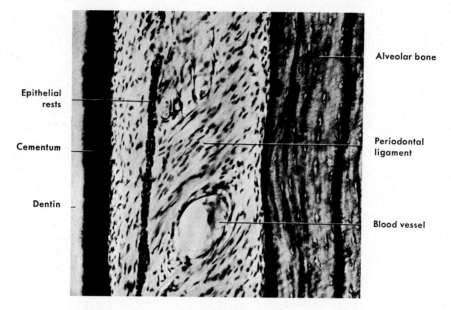

Epithelial
rests

Cementum

Dentin

Alveolar bone

Periodontal
ligament

Blood vessel

Fig. 7-17. Long strand of epithelium in periodontal ligament.

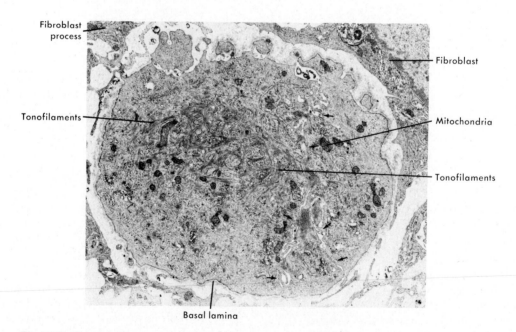

Fibroblast
process

Tonofilaments

Fibroblast

Mitochondria

Tonofilaments

Basal lamina

Fig. 7-18. Electron micrograph illustrating cluster of three epithelial rest cells in periodontal ligament of mouse molar. Contiguous surfaces of cells are marked by arrows. (×13,840.)

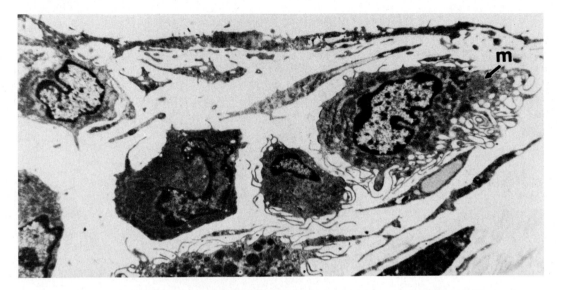

Fig. 7-19. Electron micrograph depicting macrophages *(m)* in rat periodontal ligament adjacent to blood vessel. Note reinform nucleus and microvilli. (×6006.)

cated adjacent to blood vessels. However, it is important to understand that the only certain criterion by which macrophages can be distinguished from fibroblasts in the light microscope is by the presence of phagocytosed material in their cytoplasm and, further, that differentiated cells in the periodontal ligament are capable of phagocytosis. The wandering type of macrophage, probably derived from blood monocytes, has a characteristic ultrastructure that permits it to be readily distinguished from fibroblasts. It has a nucleus, generally of regular contour, which may be horseshoe or kidney shaped and which exhibits a dense uneven layer of peripheral chromatin. Nucleoli are rarely seen. Macrophages are readily identified in the electron microscope, and it is apparent that the surface of the cell is generally raised in microvilli and the cytoplasm contains numerous free ribosomes. The rough endoplasmic reticulum is relatively sparse and is adorned with

widely spaced polysomes that are composed of only two to four ribosomes each. The Golgi apparatus is not well developed, but the cytoplasm contains numerous lysosomes in which identifiable material may be seen. In the periodontal ligament macrophages may play a dual role: (1) phagocytosing dead cells and (2) secreting growth factors that regulate the proliferation of adjacent fibroblasts.

EXTRACELLULAR SUBSTANCE

The extracellular substance of the periodontal ligament comprises the following:

Fibers	Ground substance
Collagen	Proteoglycans
Oxytalan	Glycoproteins

Fibers

The fibers in human periodontal ligament are made up of collagen and oxytalan. Elastic fibers are restricted almost entirely to the walls of the blood vessels. The majority of fibers in the periodontal ligament are collagen.

Collagen. Collagen is a specific, high-molecular-weight protein to which are attached a small number of sugars and a heterogeneous collection of small glycoproteins. There are at least 12 different types of collagen, all basically similar in chemical structure but with each exhibiting certain specific and unique chemical characteristics and each known to be the product of different genes. Periodontal ligament appears to be made up predominantly of type I and type III collagen. Collagen *macromolecules* are rodlike, being very long in relation to their diameter, and are arranged to form *fibrils*. These fibrils show a highly ordered periodic banding pattern that is definitive for collagen when viewed in longitudinal section in the electron microscope (Fig. 7-6), but because of their small diameter, they cannot be resolved by light microscopy. However, the fibrils are packed side by side to form bundles or *fibers*, which, when of diameter greater than 0.2 µm, can be seen at the highest magnification of the light microscope. Fibers are the smallest order of collagen that can be resolved by light microscopy. Collagen fibers are further gathered together to form larger bundles, and these are readily resolved by light microscopy. The collagen fibrils of periodontal ligament, when examined by transmission electron microscopy, are seen to be gathered together to form fibers. When examined in the light microscope, many of the collagen fibers are found to be gathered into bundles having clear orientation relative to the periodontal space, and these are termed *principal fibers.*

The principal fibers of the periodontal ligament (Figs. 7-20 to 7-22) are arranged in five particular groups, each group having a name, as follows:

1. *Alveolar crest group.* The fiber bundles of this group radiate from the crest of the alveolar process and attach themselves to the cervical part of the cementum.
2. *Horizontal group.* The bundles run at right angles to the long axis of the tooth from the cementum to the bone.
3. *Oblique group.* The bundles run obliquely. They are attached in the cementum somewhat apically from their attachment to the bone. These fiber bundles are most numerous and constitute the main attachment of the tooth.
4. *Apical group.* The bundles are irregularly arranged and radiate from the apical region of the root to the surrounding bone.
5. *Interradicular group.* From the crest of the interradicular septum, bundles extend to the furcation of multirooted teeth.

There are also fiber bundles in the lamina propria of the gingiva that have specific orientation, and some of them lie immediately coronal to the periodontal ligament (see Chapter 9). The most superficial fibers of the alveolar crest group of principal fibers mark the coronal extremity of the periodontal ligament.

Collagen fibers are embedded into cementum on one side of the periodontal space and into alveolar bone on the other. The embedded fibers are termed *Sharpey's fibers* (Figs. 7-1, 7-3, and 7-5). There is some evidence from small rodents and monkeys that Sharpey's fibers may traverse the bone of the alveolar process, particularly in the crestal region, to continue interdentally as principal fibers in the adjacent periodontal ligament or to mingle buccally and lingually with the fibers of the periosteum covering the alveolar process. Although not a common finding when viewed

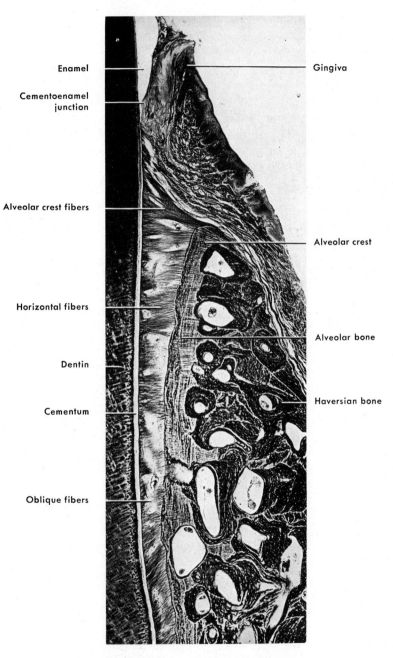

Enamel

Cementoenamel junction

Alveolar crest fibers

Horizontal fibers

Dentin

Cementum

Oblique fibers

Gingiva

Alveolar crest

Alveolar bone

Haversian bone

Fig. 7-20. Fibers of periodontal ligament.

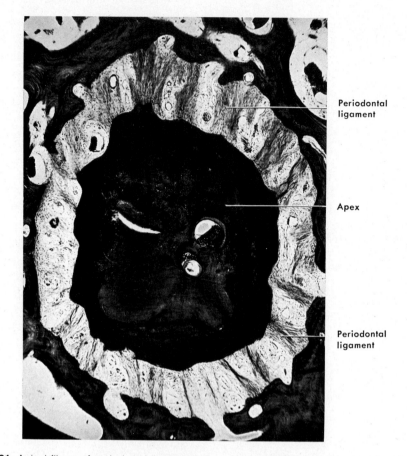

Periodontal
ligament

Apex

Periodontal
ligament

Fig. 7-21. Apical fibers of periodontal ligament. (From Orban B: Dental histology and embryology, Philadelphia, 1929, P Blakiston's Son & Co.)

through conventional light microscopy, transalveolar fibers are readily seen in the high-voltage electron microscope. Conceivably these fibers become entrapped in alveolar bone either during development of the interdental septum or by bone deposition at the alveolar crest. As a result of tooth drift and the resultant bone remodeling, the fibers may be severed, and some may be relinked to periodontal ligament fibers by an unbanded link protein. Transalveolar fibers may serve as a mechanism to connect adjacent teeth (Fig. 7-23).

The principal fibers frequently run a wavy course from cementum to bone. It may appear in some sections examined in the light microscope as though fibers arising from cementum and bone are joined in the midregion of the periodontal space, giving rise to a zone of distinct appearance, the so-called *intermediate plexus* (Fig. 7-22, *B*) (see also Chapter 11). It used to be believed that the intermediate plexus provides a site where rapid remodeling of fibers occurs, allowing adjustments in the ligament to be made to accommodate small

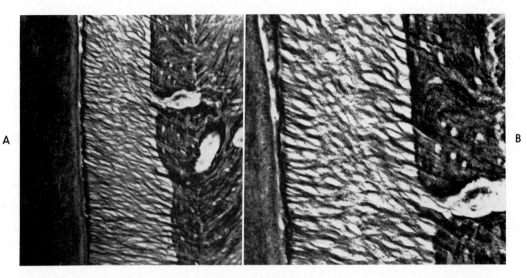

Fig. 7-22. A, Periodontal ligament of monkey premolar demonstrating principal fibers. **B,** Higher magnification of an area of **A.**Z one described as intermediate plexus is evident. (Silver impregnation, **A,** ×400; **B,** ×800.) (Courtesy Dr. I. Sciaky, Jerusalem.)

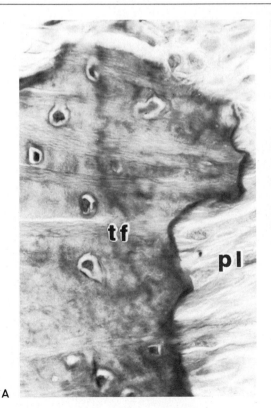

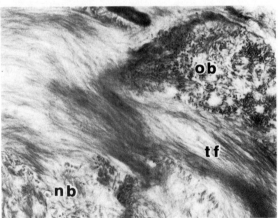

Fig. 7-23. A, Section through mouse alveolar bone illustrating transalveolar fibers *(tf)* that appear to extend from periodontal ligament *(pl)* into interdental septum and then into adjacent periodontal ligament. **B,** High voltage electron micrograph illustrating transalveolar fibers *(tf)* that appear to be continuous through both relatively old bones *(ob)* and newly synthesized *(nb)* in remodelling interdental septum. (**A,** ×1000; **B,** ×18,000.) (**A** from Johnson RB: J Periodont Res 19:512, 1984; **B** from Johnson RB: Anat Rec 217:339, 1987; courtesy of Laboratory for High-voltage Electron Microscopy, University of Colorado, Boulder, Colo.)

movements of the tooth. However, evidence derived from electron microscopy, radioautography, and surgical experiments on teeth of limited eruption provide no support for this belief. The so-called intermediate plexus is evidently an artifact arising out of the plane of section and may be attributable to the fact that the collagen fibers do not course only in one bundle but may move from one bundle to the other. This is most readily seen in horizontal sections of the ligament, where the fibers are found to be arranged in many small bundles on the tooth side but in a few large bundles on the bone side.

Oxytalan. Although elastic fibers are found in the periodontal ligaments of some animals, they are largely restricted to the walls of the blood vessels in humans. A fiber termed oxytalan, which may be an immature elastic fiber, is found in human periodontal ligament. Oxytalan fibers can be demonstrated in the light microscope in tissue stained by certain methods used to color elastic fibers, provided that the tissues are oxidized prior to staining. In the electron microscope, fibers believed to be oxytalan resemble developing elastic fibers.

The orientation of the oxytalan fibers is

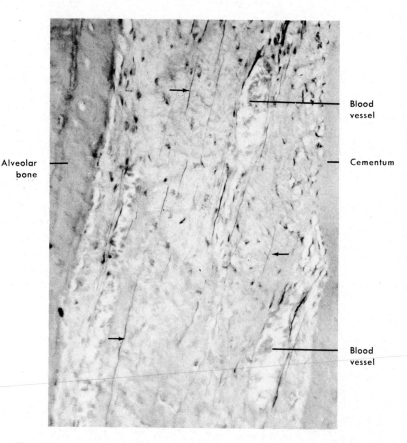

Fig. 7-24. Oxytalan fibers *(arrows)* in monkey periodontal ligament. (×245.)

quite different from that of the collagen fibers. Instead of running from bone to tooth, they tend to run in an axial direction (Fig. 7-24), one end being embedded in cementum or possibly bone and the other often in the wall of a blood vessel. In the vicinity of the apex they form a complex network. The function of the oxytalan fibers is unknown, but it has been suggested that they may play a part in supporting the blood vessels of the periodontal ligament.

Ground substance

The space between cells, fibers, blood vessels, and nerves in the periodontal space is occupied by ground substance. Indeed, the ground substance is present in every nook and cranny, including the interstices between fibers and between fibrils. It is important to understand that all anabolites reaching the cells from the microcirculation in the ligament and all catabolites passing in the opposite direction must pass through the ground substance. Its integrity is essential if the cells of the ligament are to function properly. The importance of the ground substance is frequently overlooked, possibly because it is a difficult substance to investigate and also because it is not demonstrated and therefore not recognizable in tissue prepared by routine methods for light and electron microscopy.

In essence, the ground substance is made up of two major groups of substances, proteoglycans and glycoproteins. Both groups are composed of proteins and polysaccharides but of different type and arrangement, and proteoglycans carry a much stronger negative charge than do the glycoproteins. The interested reader will find detailed descriptions of protein polysaccharides and glycoproteins in texts concerned with connective tissue biochemistry.

It was mentioned above that neither of these substances is demonstrated by routine histologic or electron-microscopic methods; they are demonstrated only by histochemical methods. A histochemical method is in essence a technique that attaches a material that can be recognized microscopically to specific chemical groups in the substance to be demonstrated (see Chapter 15). For light microscopy the specific substance is a dye that can be recognized by its color, and for electron microscopy, an electron-dense material. In the case of the proteoglycans, a number of methods that utilize their strong negative charges have been developed to demonstrate the location of these substances in both the light and electron microscopes. Examples of the chemicals used are Alcian blue 8GX and toluidine blue for light microscopy and ruthenium red for electron miscroscopy. Glycoproteins possess comparatively unique chemical groups (1, 2, glycols) that can be demonstrated in light microscopy by the periodic acid–Schiff method and in electron microscopy by the periodic acid–silver methenamine technique. These methods show quite clearly that ground substance is a significant constituent of the periodontal ligament (Fig. 7-25).

A particular glycoprotein, *fibronectin*, occurs in filamentous form in the periodontal ligament. It contains chemical groups that attach to the surface of the fibroblasts and to collagen, certain proteoglycans, and fibrin. Its orientation may be related to that of the microfilaments in the cytoplasm of contiguous fibroblasts.

Interstitial tissue

Some of the blood vessels, lymphatics, and nerves of the periodontal ligament are surrounded by loose connective tissue, and these areas can readily be recognized in the light microscope (Fig. 7-26). These ar-

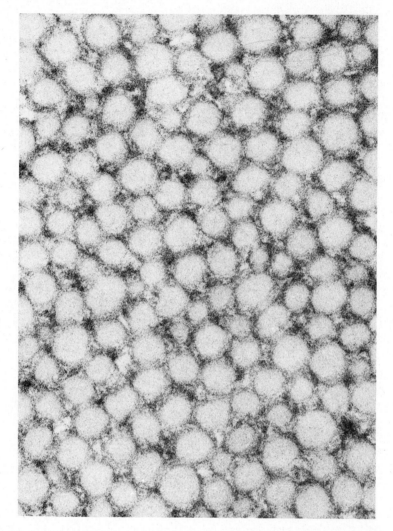

Fig. 7-25. Mouse periodontal ligament stained with ruthenium red to demonstrate proteoglycan of ground substance. Collagen are electron lucent, and ground substance is electron dense. (×162,000.)

eas have been termed *interstitial tissue,* but it is not known whether they have any particular biologic significance.

STRUCTURES PRESENT IN CONNECTIVE TISSUE

The following discrete structures are present in the connective tissue of the periodontal ligament:

Blood vessels   Nerves
Lymphatics   Cementicles

Blood vessels. The arterial vessels of the periodontal ligament are derived from three sources:

Branches in the periodontal ligament from apical vessels that supply the dental pulp.
Branches from intra-alveolar vessels. These

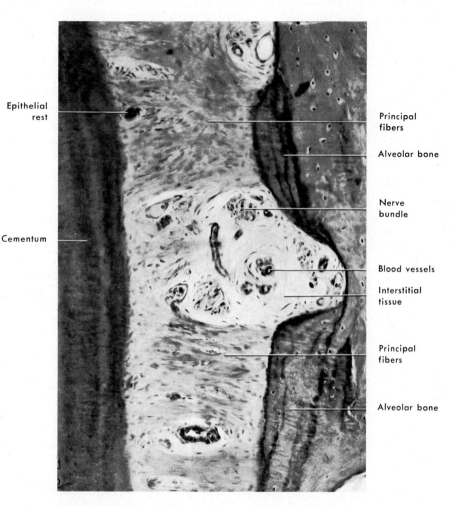

Epithelial rest

Cementum

Principal fibers

Alveolar bone

Nerve bundle

Blood vessels

Interstitial tissue

Principal fibers

Alveolar bone

Fig. 7-26. Interstitial spaces in periodontal ligament contain loose connective tissue, vessels, and nerves. (From Orban B: J Am Dent Assoc 16:405, 1929.)

branches run horizontally, penetrating the alveolar bone to enter the periodontal ligament (Fig. 7-27) (see Chapter 8).

Branches from gingival vessels. These enter the periodontal ligament from the coronal direction.

The arterioles and capillaries of the microcirculation ramify in the periodontal ligament, forming a rich network of arcades that is more evident in the half of the peri-odontal space adjacent to bone than that adjacent to cementum. There is a particularly rich vascular plexus at the apex and in the cervical part of the ligament. The venous vessels tend to run axially to drain to the apex. There are numerous arteriovenous anastomoses between the two sides of the microcirculation, as well as glomerulus-like structures, and these are possibly involved in the role that the circulation plays

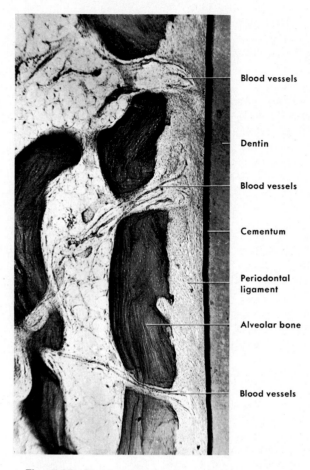

Blood vessels

Dentin

Blood vessels

Cementum

Periodontal
ligament

Alveolar bone

Blood vessels

Fig. 7-27. Blood vessels enter periodontal ligament through openings in alveolar bone. (From Orban B: Dental histology and embryology, Philadelphia, 1929, P Blakiston's Son & Co.)

in supporting the teeth during function.

Lymphatics. A network of lymphatic vessels, following the path of the blood vessels, provides the lymph drainage of the periodontal ligament. The flow is from the ligament toward and into the adjacent alveolar bone.

Nerves. Nerves, which usually are associated with blood vessels, pass through foramina in the alveolar bone, including the

apical foramen, to enter the periodontal ligament. In the region of the apex, they run toward the cervix, whereas along the length of the root they branch and run both coronally and apically. The nerve fibers are either of large diameter and myelinated or of small diameter, in which case they may or may not be myelinated. The small fibers appear to end in fine branches throughout the ligament and the large fibers in a variety of endings, for example, knoblike, spindlelike, and Meissner-like, but these seem to vary among the species. The large-diameter fibers appear to be concerned with discernment of pressure and the small-diameter ones with pain. Some of the unmyelinated smalldiameter fibers evidently are associated with blood vessels and presumably are autonomic.

Cementicles. Calcified bodies called cementicles are sometimes found in the periodontal ligament. These bodies are seen in older individuals, and they may remain free in the connective tissue, they may fuse into large calcified masses, or they may be joined with the cementum (Fig. 7-28). As the cementum thickens with advancing age, it may envelop these bodies. When they are adherent to the cementum, they form excementoses. The origin of these calcified bodies is not established. It is possible that degenerated epithelial cells form the nidus for their calcification.

FUNCTIONS

The periodontal ligament has the following functions:

Supportive	Nutritive
Sensory	Homeostatic

Supportive. When a tooth is moved in its socket as a result of forces acting on it during mastication or through application of an orthodontic force, part of the periodontal space will be narrowed and the periodontal

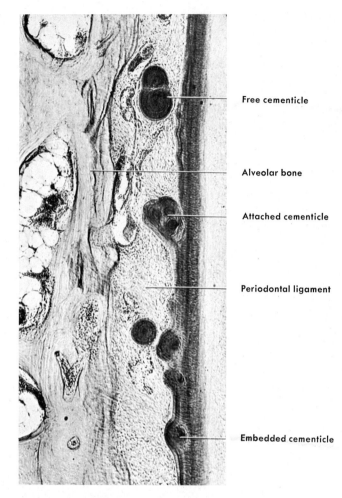

Free cementicle

Alveolar bone

Attached cementicle

Periodontal ligament

Embedded cementicle

Fig. 7-28. Cementicles in periodontal ligament.

ligament contained in these areas will be compressed. Other parts of the periodontal space will be widened. The compressed periodontal ligament provides support for the loaded tooth. The collagen fibers in the compressed ligament, in concert with water molecules and other molecules bound to collagen, act as a cushion for the displaced tooth. The pressure of blood in the numerous vessels also provides a hydraulic cushion for the support of the teeth. It has

often been suggested that the collagen fibers in the widened parts of the periodontal space are extended to their limit when a force is applied to a tooth and, being nonelastic, prevent the tooth from being moved too far. However, evidence to support this contention is lacking, and the role of the collagen fibers seems restricted largely to (1) attaching the cementum that is fused to the dentin of the root to alveolar bone and (2) acting as a cushion. The collagen fibers may be extended when a tooth is rotated excessively.

Sensory. The periodontal ligament, through its nerve supply, provides a most efficient proprioceptive mechanism, allowing the organism to detect the application of the most delicate forces to the teeth and very slight displacement of the teeth. Anyone who has bitten into soft food containing a small hard object such as stone or shot knows the importance of this mechanism in protecting both the supporting structures of the tooth and the substance of the crown from the effects of excessively vigorous masticatory force.

Nutritive. The ligament contains blood vessels, which provide anabolites and other substances required by the cells of the ligament, by the cementocytes, and presumably by the more superficial osteocytes of the alveolar bone. Experimental extirpation of the ligament results in necrosis of underlying cementocytes. The blood vessels are also concerned with removal of catabolites. Occlusion of blood vessels leads to necrosis of cells in the affected part of the ligament; this occurs when too heavy a force is applied to a tooth in orthodontic therapy.

Homeostatic. It is evident that the cells of the periodontal ligament have the capacity to resorb and synthesize the extracellular substance of the connective tissue of the ligament, alveolar bone, and cementum. It is also evident that these processes are not activated sporadically or haphazardly but function continuously, with varying intensity, throughout the life of the tooth. Alveolar bone appears to be resorbed and replaced (i.e., remodeled) at a rate higher than other bone tissue in the jaws. Furthermore the collagen of the periodontal ligament is turned over at a rate that may be the fastest of all connective tissues in the body, and the cells in the bone half of the

ligament may be more active than those on the cementum side. Visual evidence for the high turnover of *protein* in the periodontal ligament is provided by the numerous silver grains seen in radioautographs of the tissue removed from animals a few hours after they have received an injection of a radioactive precursor, for example, ^{3}H-proline (Fig. 7-29). On the other hand, deposition of cementum by cementoblasts appears to be a slow, continuous process, and resorption is not a regular occurrence.

The mechanisms whereby the cells responsible for these processes of synthesis and resorption are controlled are largely unknown. It is evident that the processes are exquisitely controlled because, under normal conditions of function, the various tissues of the periodontium maintain their integrity and relationship to one another. However, when these homeostatic mechanisms are upset, derangement of the periodontium occurs. If periodontal ligament, either in part or whole, is irreparably destroyed, bone will be deposited in the periodontal space, obliterating it, and this will result in ankylosis between bone and tooth. If the balance between synthesis and resorption is disturbed, the quality of the tissues will be changed. For example, if an experimental animal is deprived of substances essential for collagen synthesis such as vitamin C or protein, resorption of collagen will continue unabated, but its synthesis and replacement will be markedly reduced. This will result in progressive destruction and loss of extracellular substance of periodontal ligament, more advanced on the bone side of the ligament than on the cementum side. This eventually will lead to loss of attachment between bone and tooth and finally to loss of the tooth such as occurs in scurvy when vitamin C is absent from the diet.

From kinetic studies using labeled pre-

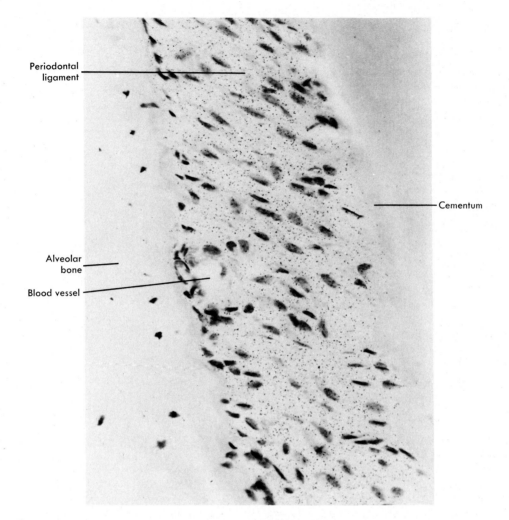

Periodontal
ligament

Cementum

Alveolar
bone

Blood vessel

Fig. 7-29. Light microscope radioautograph of periodontal ligament of molar of mouse that had received an intraperitoneal injection of ^{3}H-proline 24 hours before death. Black dots (silver grains) mark sites where isotope was incorporated into protein. (×650.)

cursors of DNA and radioautography, it appears that the connective tissue cells of the periodontal ligament are also turned over. That is, in all areas of the periodontal ligament, there is apparently a continual slow death of cells, which are replaced by new cells that are provided by cell division of progenitor cells in the ligament.

Another aspect of homeostasis relates to function. A periodontal ligament supporting a fully functional tooth exhibits all the structural features described above. However, with loss of function, much of the extracellular substance of the ligament is lost, possibly because of diminished synthesis of substances required to replace structural

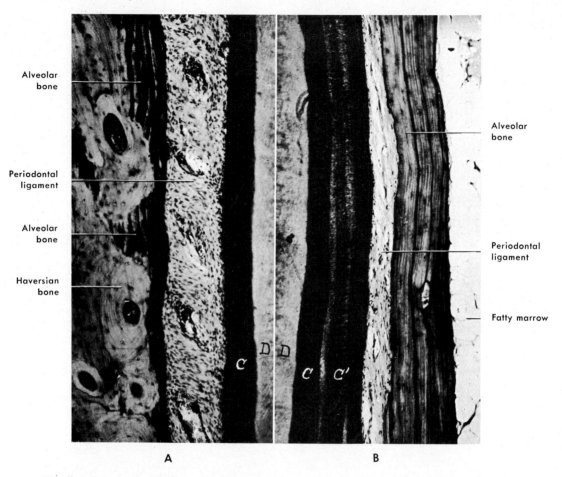

Fig. 7-30. Periodontal ligament of a functioning, **A**, and of a nonfunctioning, **B**, tooth. In the functioning tooth, the periodontal ligament is wide, and principal fibers are present. Cementum, *C*, is thin. In the nonfunctioning tooth, the periodontal space is narrow, and no principal fiber bundles are seen. Cementum is thick, *C* and *C'*. Alveolar bone is lamellated. *D*, Dentin.

molecules resorbed during normal turn-over, and the width of the periodontal space is subsequently decreased (Fig. 7-30). These changes are accompanied by increased deposition of cementum and a decrease in alveolar bone tissue mass per unit volume. The process is reversible if the tooth is returned to function, but the precise nature of the stimuli that control the changed activity of the cells is unknown.

CLINICAL CONSIDERATIONS

The primary role of the periodontal ligament is to support the tooth in the bony socket. Its thickness varies in different individuals, in different teeth in the same person, and in different locations on the same tooth, as is illustrated in Tables 3 and 4.

The measurements shown in Tables 3 and 4 indicate that it is not feasible to refer

Table 3. Thickness of periodontal ligament of 154 teeth from 14 human jaws*

	Average at alveolar crest (mm)	Average at midroot (mm)	Average at apex (mm)	Average for entire tooth (mm)
Ages 11-16 (83 teeth from 4 jaws)	0.23	0.17	0.24	0.21
Ages 32-50 (36 teeth from 5 jaws)	0.20	0.14	0.19	0.18
Ages 51-67 (35 teeth from 5 jaws)	0.17	0.12	0.16	0.15

From Coolidge ED: J Am Dent Assoc 24:1260, 1937.
*The table shows that the width of the periodontal ligament decreases with age and that it is wider at the crest and at the apex than at the midroot.

Table 4. Comparison of periodontal ligament in different locations around the same tooth (subject 11 years of age)*

	Mesial (mm)	Distal (mm)	Labial (mm)	Lingual (mm)
Upper right central incisor, mesial and labial drift	0.12	0.24	0.12	0.22
Upper left central incisor, no drift	0.21	0.19	0.24	0.24
Upper right lateral incisor, and labial drift	0.27	0.17	0.11	0.15

From Coolidge ED: J Am Dent Assoc 24:1260, 1937.
*The table shows the variation in width of the mesial, distal, labial, and lingual sides of the same tooth.

to an average figure as normal width of the periodontal ligament. Measurements of a large numer of ligaments range from 0.15 to 0.38 mm. The fact that the periodontal ligament is thinnest in the middle region of the root seems to indicate that the fulcrum of physiologic movement is in this region. The thickness of the periodontal ligament seems to be maintained by the functional movements of the tooth. It is thin in functionless and embedded teeth and wide in teeth that are under excessive occlusal stresses (Fig. 7-30).

For the practice of restorative dentistry the importance of these changes in structure is obvious. The supporting tissues of a tooth long out of function are poorly adapted to carry the load suddenly placed on the tooth by a restoration. This applies to bridge abutments, teeth opposing bridges or dentures, and teeth used as anchorage for removable bridges. This may account for the inability of a patient to use a restoration immediately after its placement. Some time must elapse before the supporting tissues become adapted again to the new functional demands. An adjustment period, likewise, must be permitted after orthodontic treatment.

Acute trauma to the periodontal ligament, accidental blows, or rapid mechanical separation may produce pathologic changes such as fractures or resorption of the cementum, tears of fiber bundles, hemorrhage, and necrosis. The adjacent alveolar bone is resorbed, the periodontal ligament is widened, and the tooth becomes loose. When trauma is eliminated, repair usually take place. Occlusal trauma is always restricted to the intra-alveolar tissues and does not cause changes of the gingiva such as recession or pocket formation or gingivitis.

Orthodontic tooth movement depends on resorption and formation of both bone and periodontal ligament. These activities can be stimulated by properly regulated pressure and tension. The stimuli are transmitted through the medium of the periodontal ligament. If the movement of teeth is within physiologic limits (which may vary with the individual), the initial compression of the periodontal ligament on the pressure side is compensated for by bone resorption, whereas on the tension side bone apposition is seen. Application of large forces results in necrosis of periodontal ligament and alveolar bone on the pressure side, and movement of the tooth will occur only after the necrotic bone has been resorbed by osteoclasts located on its endosteal surface.

The periodontal ligament in the periapical area of the tooth is often the site of a pathologic lesion. Inflammatory diseases of the pulp progress to the apical periodontal ligament and replace its fiber bundles with granulation tissue. This lesion, called a dental granuloma, may contain epithelial cells that undergo proliferation and produce a cyst. The dental granuloma and the apical cyst are the most common pathologic lesions of the jaws.

Safeguarding the integrity of the periodontal ligament (and the alveolar bone) is one of the most important challenges for the clinician. Gingivitis, or inflammation of the gingiva, is the most common dental disease of humans. If not controlled or treated, periodontitis may develop, and destruction may extend into the periodontal ligament and bone. Once destroyed by periodontitis, the periodontal ligament and the alveolar bone are very difficult to regenerate.

REFERENCES

Anderson DJ, Hannam AG, and Mathews B: Sensory mechanisms in mammalian teeth and their supporting structures, Physiol Rev 50:171, 1970.

Arnim SS and Hagerman DA: The connective tissue fibers of the marginal gingiva, J Am Dent Assoc 47:271, 1953.

Bernick S: Innervation of teeth and periodontium after enzymatic removal of collagenous elements, Oral Surg 10:323, 1957.

Bernick S, Levy BM, Dreizen S, and Grant DA: The intraosseous orientation of the alveolar component of Marmoset alveodental fibers, J Dent Res 56:1409, 1977.

Box KF: Evidence of lymphatics in the periodontium, J Can Dent Assoc 15:8, 1949.

Brunette DM, Kanoza RJ, Marmary Y, et al.: Interactions between epithelial and fibroblast-like cells in cultures derived from monkey periodontal ligament, J Cell Sci 27:127-140, 1977.

Brunette DM, Melcher AH, and Moe HK: Culture and origin of epithelium-like and fibroblast-like cells from porcine periodontal ligament explants and cell suspensions, Arch Oral Biol 21:393, 1976.

Bruszt P: Ueber die netzartige Anordnung des paradentalen Epithels (The network arrangement of the epithelium in the periodontal membrane), Z Stomatol 30:679, 1932.

Butler WT, Birkedal-Hansen H, Beegle WF, et al.: Proteins of the periodontium. Identification of collagens with the $[\alpha 1(I)]_{2\alpha 2}$ and $[\alpha_1(III)]_3$ structures in bovine periodontal ligament, J Biol Chem 250:8907, 1975.

Carmichael GG and Fullmer HM: The fine structure of the oxytalan fiber, J Cell Biol 28:33, 1966.

Cohn SA: Disuse atrophy of the periodontium in mice, Arch Oral Biol 10:909, 1965.

Cohn SA: A re-examination of Sharpey's fibres in alveolar bone of the mouse, Arch Oral Biol 17:255, 1972.

Cohn SA: A re-examination of Sharpey's fibres in alveolar bone of the marmoset (Saguinus fuscicollis), Arch Oral Biol 17:261, 1972.

Cohn SA: Transalveolar fibres in the human periodontium, Arch Oral Biol 20:257, 1975.

Connor NS, Aubin JE, and Melcher AH: The distribution of fibronectin in rat tooth and periodontal tissue: an immunofluorescence study using a monoclonal antibody, J Histochem Cytochem 32:565, 1984.

Coolidge ED: The thickness of the human periodontal membrane, J Am Dent Assoc 24:1260, 1937.

Deporter DA and Ten Cate AR: Fine structural localization of acid and alkaline phosphatase in collagen-containing vesicles of fibroblasts, J Anat 114:457, 1973.

Folke LEA and Stallard RE: Periodontal microcirculation as revealed by plastic microspheres, J Periodont Res 2:53, 1967.

Freeman E and Ten Cate AR: Development of the periodontium: an electron microscopic study, J Periodontol 42:387, 1971.

Fullmer HM: Connective tissue components of the periodontium. In Miles AEW, editor: Structural and chemical organization of the teeth, vol 2, New York, 1967, Academic Press, Inc.

Garant PR, Cho MI, and Cullen MR: Attachment of periodontal ligament fibroblasts to the extracellular-matrix in squirrel monkey, J Periodont Res 17:70,1982.

Garfunkel A and Sciaky I: Vascularization of the periodontal tissues in the adult laboratory rat, J Dent Res 50:880, 1971.

Goldman HM: The effects of dietary deprivation and of age on periodontal tissues of the rat and spider monkey, J Periodontol 25:87, 1954.

Goldman HM and Gianelly AA: Histology of tooth movement, Dent Clin North Am 16:439, 1972.

Gould TRL, Melcher AH, and Brunette DM: Location of progenitor cells in periodontal ligament of mouse molar stimulated by wounding, Anat Rec 188:133, 1977.

Griffin CJ: Unmyelinated nerve endings in the periodontal membrane of human teeth, Arch Oral Biol 13:1207, 1968.

Ham AW: Histology, ed. 7, Philadelphia, 1974, JB Lippincott Co.

Holtrop ME, Raisz LG, and Simmons HA: The effects of parathormone, colchicine and calcitonin on the ultrastructure and the activity of osteoclasts in organ culture, J Cell Biol 60:346, 1974.

Ishimitsu K: Beitrag zur Kenntnis der Morphologie and Entwicklungsgeschichte der Glomeruli periodontii (Contribution to the knowledge of morphology and development of the periodontal glomeruli), Yokohama Med Bull 11:415, 1960.

Johnson RB: A classification of Sharpey's fibers within the alveolar bone of the mouse: a high-voltage electron microscopic study, Anat Rec 217:339, 1987.

Kindlova M and Matena V: Blood vessels of the rat molar, J Dent Res 41:650, 1962.

Kvam E: Cellular dynamics on the pressure side of the rat periodontium following experimental tooth movement, Scand J Dent Res 80:369-383, 1972.

Leblond C.P, Messier B, and Kopriwa B: Thymidine-^{3}H as a tool for the investigation of the renewal of cell populations, Lab Invest 8:296, 1959.

Leibovich SJ and Ross R: The role of the macrophage in wound repair. A study with hydrocortisone and antimacrophage serum. Am J Pathol 78:71, 1975.

Malassez ML: Sur l'existence de masses epitheliales dans le ligament alveolodentaire (On the existence of epithelial masses in the periodontal membrane), Comp Rend Soc Biol 36:241, 1884.

Malkani K, Luxembourger M-M, and Rebel A: Cytoplasmic modifications at the contact zone of osteoclasts and calcified tissue in the diaphyseal growing plate of foetal guinea-pig tibia, Calcif Tissue Res 11:258, 1973.

McCulloch CAG, Barghava V, and Melcher AH: Cell death and the regulation of cell populations in the periodontal ligament, Cell Tissue Res 255:129, 1989.

McCulloch CAG and Melcher AH: Cell density and cell generation in the periodontal ligament of mice, Am J Anat 167:43, 1983.

Melcher AH: Repair of wounds in the periodontium of the rat. Influence of periodontal ligament on osteogenesis, Arch Oral Biol 15:1183, 1970.

Melcher AH and Correia MA: Remodeling of periodontal ligament in erupting molars of mature rats, J Periodont Res 6:118, 1971.

Picton DCA: The effects of external forces in the periodontium. In Melcher AH and Bowen WH, editors: Biology of the periodontium, New York, 1969, Academic Press, Inc.

Revel JP and Karnovsky MJ: Hexagonal array of subunits in intercellular junctions of the mouse heart and liver, J Cell Biol 33:C7, 1967.

Roberts WE, Chase DC, and Jee WSS: Counts of labelled mitoses in the orthodontically-stimulated periodontal ligament in the rat, Arch Oral Biol 19:665, 1974.

Rygh P: Ultrastructural cellular reactions in pressure zones of rat molar periodontium incident to orthodontic tooth movement, Acta Odontol Scand 30:575, 1972.

Sakamoto S, Goldhaber P, and Glimcher MJ: The further purification and characterization of mouse bone collagenase, Calcif Tissue Res 10:142, 1972.

Sodek J: A new approach to assessing collagen turnover by using a microassay. A highly efficient and rapid turnover of collagen in rat periodontal tissues. Biochem J 160:243, 1976.

Sodek J: A comparison of the rates of synthesis and turnover of collagen and non-collagen proteins in adult rate periodontal tissues and skin using a microassay, Arch Oral Biol 22:655, 1977.

Stallard RE: The utilization of ^{3}H-proline by the connective tissue elements of the periodontium, Periodontics 1:185, 1963.

Svoboda ELA, Brunette DM, and Melcher AH: *In vitro* phagocytosis of exogenous collagen by fibroblasts from the periodontal ligament: an electronmicroscopic study, J Anat 128:301, 1979.

Ten Cate AR and Mills C: The development of the periodontium: the origin of alveolar bone, Anat Rec 173:69, 1972.

Ten Cate AR, Mills C, and Solomon G: The development of the periodontium. A transplantation and autoradiographic study, Anat Rec 170:365, 1971.

Vaes G: Excretion of acid and of lysosomal hydrolytic enzymes during bone resorption induced in tissue culture by parathyroid extract, Exp Cell Res 39:470, 1965.

Valderhaug JP and Nylen MU: Function of epithelial rests as suggested by their ultrastructure, J Periodont Res 1:69, 1966.

Waerhaug J: Effect of C-avitaminosis on the supporting structures of the teeth, J Periodontol 29:87, 1958.

Walker DG: Bone resorption restored in osteopetrotic mice by transplants of normal bone marrow and spleen cells, Science 190:784, 1975.

Yajima T and Rose GC: Phagocytosis of collagen by human gingival fibroblasts in vitro, J Dent Res 56:1271, 1977.

Zwarych PD and Quigley MB: The intermediate plexus of the periodontal ligament: history and further observations, J Dent Res 44:383, 1965.

8

MAXILLA AND MANDIBLE (ALVEOLAR PROCESS)

DEVELOPMENT OF MAXILLA AND MANDIBLE

In the beginning of the second month of fetal life the skull consists of three parts:

1. The chondrocranium, which is cartilaginous, is made up of the base of the skull with the otic and nasal capsules.
2. The desmocranium, which is membranous, forms the lateral walls and roof of the braincase.
3. The appendicular or visceral part of the skull, which is cartilaginous, consists of the skeletal rods of the branchial arches.

The bones of the skull develop either by endochondral ossification, replacing the cartilage, or by intramembranous ossification in the mesenchyme. Intramembranous bone may develop in proximity to cartilaginous parts of the skull or directly in the membranous capsule of the brain called desmocranium.

The endochondral bones are the bones of the base of the skull: ethmoid bone; inferior concha (turbinate bone); body, lesser wings, basal part of the greater wings, and the lateral plate of the pterygoid process of the sphenoid bone; petrosal part of the temporal bone; and basilar, lateral, and lower part of the squamous portion of the occipital bone. The following bones develop in the desmocranium: frontal bones; parietal bones; squamous and tympanic parts of the temporal bone; parts of the greater wings and the medial plate of the pterygoid process of the sphenoid bone; and the upper part of the squamous portion of the occipital bone. All the bones of the upper face develop by intramembranous ossification, most of them close to the cartilage of the nasal capsule. The mandible develops as intramembranous bone, lateral to the cartilage of the mandibular arch. This cartilage, Meckel's cartilage, is in its proximal parts the primordium for two of the auditory ossicles: the incus (anvil) and the malleus (hammer). The third auditory ossicle, the stapes (stirrup), develops from the proximal part of the skeleton in the second branchial arch, which also gives rise to the styloid process, the stylohyoid ligament, and part of the hyoid bone. The latter is completed by the derivatives of the third arch. The fourth and fifth arches form the skeleton of the larynx.

Maxilla. The human maxilla is homologous to two bones, the maxilla proper and the premaxilla. The latter, in most animals a separate bone, carries the incisors and forms the anterior part of the hard palate and the rim of the piriform aperture. The ossification centers of the premaxilla and maxilla may be separate for a very short time, or only one center of ossification, common to both the premaxilla and max-

illa, appears. That humans therefore may not have an independent premaxilla, even in the first developmental stages, does not change the fact that they possess the homologue of a premaxilla. The composition of the human maxilla from premaxilla and maxilla is indicated by the incisive fissure, which is clearly visible in young skulls. It is seen on the palate where it extends from the incisive foramen to the alveolus of the canine.

Mandible. The mandible makes its ap-

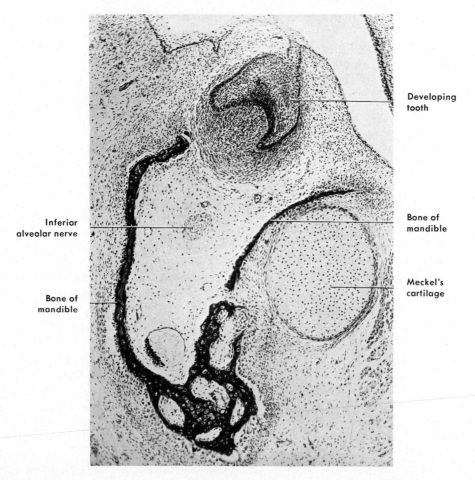

Fig. 8-1. Development of mandible as intramembranous bone lateral to Meckel's cartilage (human embryo 45 mm in length).

pearance as a bilateral structure in the sixth week of fetal life as a thin plate of bone lateral to, and at some distance from, Meckel's cartilage (Fig. 8-1). The latter is a cylindric rod of cartilage. Its proximal end (close to the base of the skull) gives rise to the malleus and the incus and therefore is continuous with and lies in contact with these bones, respectively. Its distal end at the midline is bent upward and is in contact with the cartilage of the other side. The greater part of Meckel's cartilage disappears without contributing to the formation of the bone of the mandible. Only a small part of the cartilage, some distance from the midline, is the site of endochondral ossification. Here the cartilage calcifies and is destroyed by chrondoclasts, being replaced by connective tissue and then by bone. Throughout fetal life the mandible is a paired bone. Right and left mandibles are joined in the midline by fibrocartilage in the mandibular symphysis. The cartilage at the symphysis is not derived from Meckel's cartilage but differentiates from the connective tissue in the midline. In it, small irregular bones known as the mental ossicles develop and at the end of the first year fuse with the mandibular body. At the same time the two halves of the mandible unite by ossification of the symphyseal fibrocartilage (Fig. 8-2).

DEVELOPMENT OF ALVEOLAR PROCESS

Near the end of the second month of fetal life the maxilla as well as the mandible forms a groove that is open toward the surface of the oral cavity (Fig. 8-1). The tooth germs are contained in this groove, which also includes the alveolar nerves and vessels. Gradually bony septa develop between the adjacent tooth germs, and much later the primitive mandibular canal is separated from the dental crypts by a horizontal plate of bone.

An alveolar process in the strict sense of the word develops only during the eruption of the teeth. It is important to realize that during growth part of the alveolar process is gradually incorporated into the maxillary or mandibular body while it grows at a fairly rapid rate at its free borders. During the period of rapid growth a tissue may develop at the alveolar crest that combines characteristics of cartilage and bone. It is called chondroid bone (Fig. 8-3). The alveolar process forms with the development and the eruption of teeth, and, conversely, it gradually diminishes in height after the loss of teeth.

STRUCTURE OF ALVEOLAR PROCESS

The alveolar process may be defined as that part of the maxilla and the mandible that forms and supports the sockets of the teeth (Fig. 8-4). Anatomically, no distinct boundary exists between the body of the maxilla or the mandible and their respective alveolar processes. In some places the alveolar process is fused with, and partly masked by, bone that is not functionally related to the teeth. In the anterior part of the maxilla the palatine process fuses with the oral plate of the alveolar process. In the posterior part of the mandible the oblique line is superimposed laterally on the bone of the alveolar process (Fig. 8-4, *D* and *E*).

As a result of its adaptation to function, two parts of the alveolar process can be distinguished. The first consists of a thin lamella of bone that surrounds the root of the tooth and gives attachment to principal fibers of the periodontal ligament. This is the *alveolar bone proper.* The second part is the bone that surrounds the alveolar bone proper and gives support to the socket. This has been called *supporting alveolar bone*. The latter, in turn, consists of two parts: (1) cortical plates, which consist of compact bone and form the outer and in-

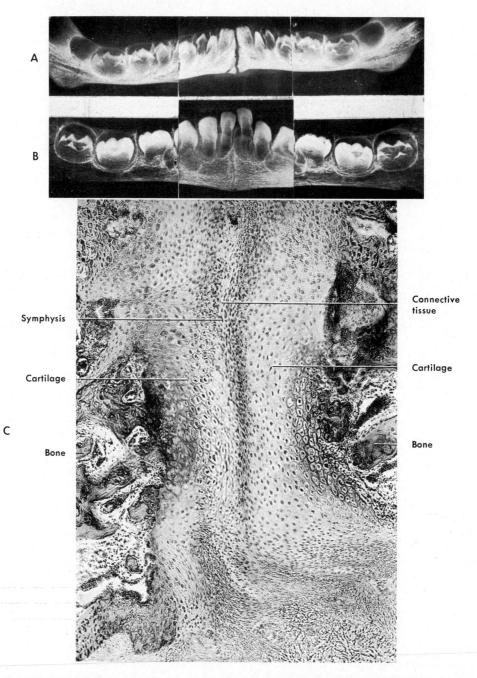

Fig. 8-2. Development of mandibular symphysis. **A,** Newborn infant. Symphysis wide open. Mental ossicle (roentgenogram). **B,** Child 9 months of age. Symphysis partly closed. Mental ossicles fused to mandible (roentgenogram). **C,** Frontal section through mandubular symphysis of newborn infant. Connective tissue in midline connects plates of cartilage on either side. Cartilage is later replaced by bone.

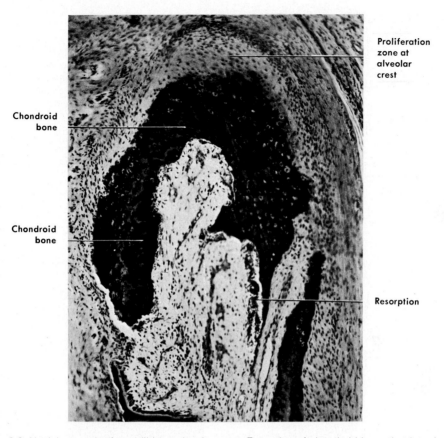

Proliferation zone at alveolar crest

Chondroid bone

Chondroid bone

Resorption

Fig. 8-3. Verticle growth of mandible at alveolar crest. Formation of chondroid bone that later is replaced by typical bone.

ner plates of the alveolar processes, and (2) the spongy bone, which fills the area between these plates and the alveolar bone proper (Figs. 8-4 and 8-5).

The cortical plates, continuous with the compact layers of the maxillary and mandibular body, are generally much thinner in the maxilla than in the mandible. They are thickest in the premolar and molar regions of the lower jaw, especially on the buccal side. In the maxilla the outer cortical plate is perforated by many small openings through which blood and lymph vessels pass. In the lower jaw the cortical bone of the alveolar process is dense. In the region of the anterior teeth of both jaws the supporting bone usually is very thin. No spongy bone is found here, and the cortical plate is fused with the alveolar bone proper (Fig. 8-4, *B* and *C*). In such areas, notably in the premolar and molar regions of the maxilla, defects of the outer alveolar wall are fairly common. Such defects, where periodontal tissues and covering mucosa fuse, do not impair the firm attachment and function of the tooth.

The shape of the outlines of the crest of the alveolar septa in the roentgenogram is

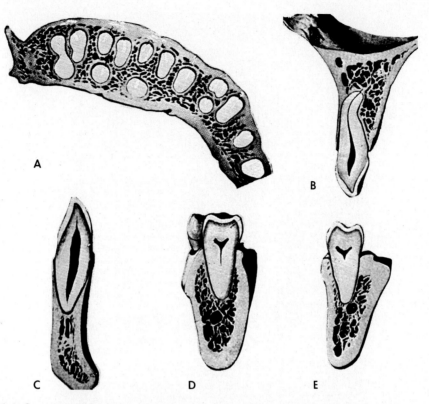

Fig. 8-4. Gross relations of alveolar processes. **A,** Horizontal section through upper alveolar process. **B,** Labiolingual section through upper lateral incisor. **C,** Labiolingual section through lower canine. **D,** Labiolingual section through lower second molar. **E,** Labiolingual section through lower third molar. (From Sicher H and Tandler J: Anatomie für Zahnärzte [Anatomy for dentists], Vienna, 1928, Julius Springer Verlag.)

dependent on the position of the adjacent teeth. In a healthy mouth the distance between the cementoenamel junction and the free border of the alveolar bone proper is fairly constant. If the neighboring teeth are inclined, therefore, the alveolar crest is oblique. In the majority of individuals the inclination is most pronounced in the premolar and molar regions, with the teeth being tipped mesially. Then the cementoenamel junction of the mesial tooth is situated in a more occlusal plane than that of the distal tooth, and the alveolar crest therefore slopes distally (Fig. 8-6).

The interdental and interradicular septa contain the perforating canals of Zuckerkandl and Hirschfeld (nutrient canals), which house the interdental and interradicular arteries, veins, lymph vessels, and nerves (Fig. 8-7).

Histologically, the cortical plates consist of longitudinal lamellae and haversian sys-

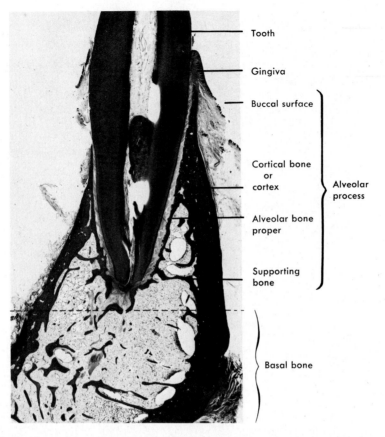

Tooth

Gingiva

Buccal surface

Cortical bone
or
cortex

Alveolar bone
proper

Supporting
bone

Alveolar
process

Basal bone

Fig. 8-5. Section through mandible showing relationship of tooth to alveolar process and basal bone. (From Bhaskar SN: Synopsis of oral histology, St Louis, 1962, The CV Mosby Co.)

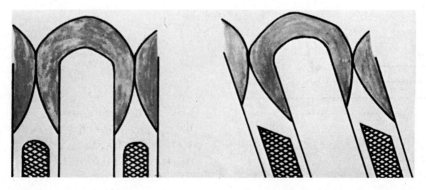

Fig. 8-6. Diagram of relation between cementoenamel junction of adjacent teeth and shape of crests of alveolar septa. (From Ritchey B and Orban B: J Periodontol 24:75, 1953.)

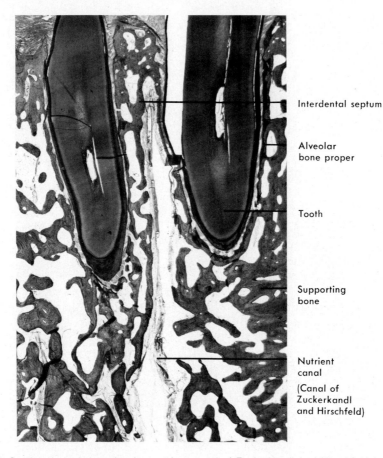

Interdental septum

Alveolar
bone proper

Tooth

Supporting
bone

Nutrient
canal

(Canal of
Zuckerkandl
and Hirschfeld)

Fig. 8-7. Section through jaw showing nutrient canal of Zuckerkandl and Hirschfeld in interdental bony septum. (From Bhaskar SN: Synopsis of oral histology, St Louis, 1962, The CV Mosby Co.)

tems (Fig. 8-8). In the lower jaw, circumferential or basic lamellae reach from the body of the mandible into the cortical plates.

The study of roentgenograms permits the classification of the spongiosa of the alveolar process into two main types. In type I the interdental and interradicular trabeculae are regular and horizontal in a ladderlike arrangement (Fig. 8-9, A to C). Type II shows irregularly arranged, numerous, delicate interdental and interradicular trabeculae (Fig. 8-9, D). Both types show a varia-

tion in thickness of trabeculae and size of marrow spaces. The architecture of type I is seen most often in the mandible and fits well into the general idea of a trajectory pattern of spongy bone. Type II, although evidently functionally satisfactory, lacks a distinct trajectory pattern, which seems to be compensated for by the greater number of trabeculae in any given area. This arrangement is more common in the maxilla. From the apical part of the socket of lower molars, trabeculae are sometimes seen radiating in a slightly distal direction. These

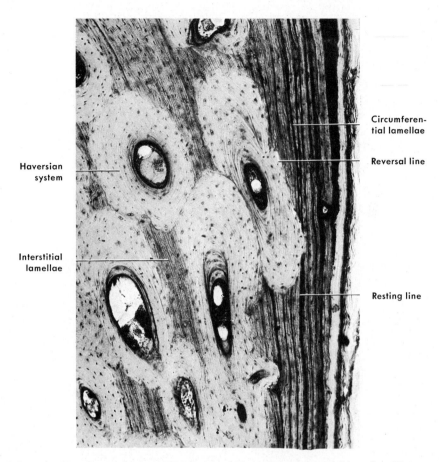

Haversian system

Interstitial lamellae

Circumferential lamellae

Reversal line

Resting line

Fig. 8-8. Appositional growth of mandible by formation of circumferential lamellae. These are replaced by haversian bone; remnants of circumferential lamellae in the depth persisting as interstitial lamellae.

trabeculae are less prominent in the upper jaw because of the proximity of the nasal cavity and the maxillary sinus. The marrow spaces in the alveolar process may contain hematopoietic marrow, but usually they contain fatty marrow. In the condylar process, in the angle of the mandible, in the maxillary tuberosity, and in other isolated foci, hematopoietic cellular marrow is found.

The alveolar bone proper, which forms the inner wall of the socket (Fig. 8-10), is perforated by many openings that carry branches of the interalveolar nerves and blood vessels into the periodontal ligament (see Chapter 7), and it is therefore called the _cribriform plate_. The alveolar bone proper consists partly of _lamellated_ and partly of _bundle bone_. Some lamellae of the lamellated bone are arranged roughly parallel to the surface of the adjacent marrow spaces, whereas others form haversian systems. Bundle bone is that bone in which the principal fibers of the periodontal liga-

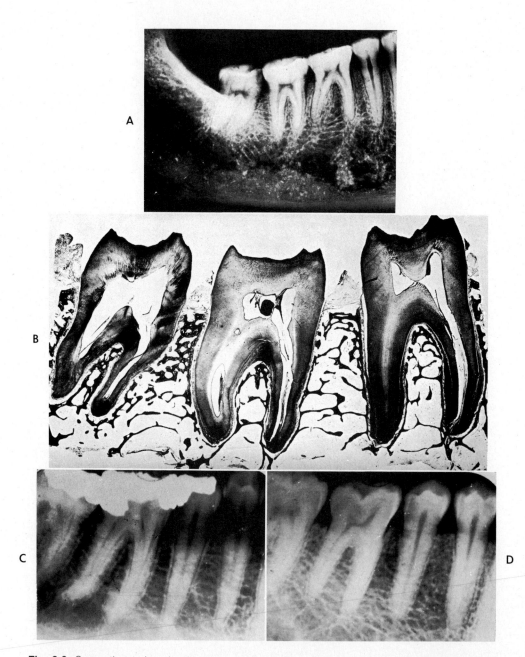

Fig. 8-9. Supporting trabeculae between alveoli. **A,** Roentgenogram of mandible. **B,** Mesiodistal section through mandibular molars showing alveolar bone proper and supporting bone. **C,** Type I alveolar spongiosa. Note regular horizontal trabeculae. **D,** Type II alveolar spongiosa. Note irregularly arranged trabeculae. (Courtesy Dr. N. Brescia, Chicago.)

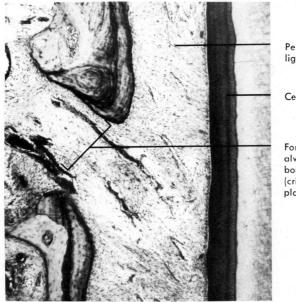

Fig. 8-10. Histologic section showing foramen in alveolar bone proper (cribriform plate). (From Bhaskar SN: Synopsis of oral histology, St Louis, 1962, The CV Mosby Co.)

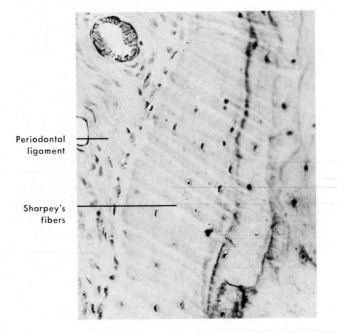

Fig. 8-11. Histologic section showing Sharpey's fibers in alveolar bone proper. (From Bhaskar SN: Synopsis of oral histology, St Louis, 1962, The CV Mosby Co.)

ment are anchored. The term "bundle bone" was chosen because the bundles of the principal fibers continue into the bone as Sharpey's fibers (Fig. 8-11). The bundle bone is characterized by the scarcity of the fibrils in the intercellular substance. These fibrils, moreover, are all arranged at right angles to Sharpey's fibers. The bundle bone contains fewer fibrils than does lamellated bone, and therefore it appears dark in routine hematoxylin and eosin stained sections and much lighter in prepa- rations stained with silver than does lamel- lated bone (Fig. 8-12). In some areas the al- veolar bone proper consists mainly of bun- dle bone. Since bundle bone contains more calcium salts per unit area than other types of bone tissue, such areas are seen in roent- genograms as dense radiopacities.

PHYSIOLOGIC CHANGES IN ALVEOLAR PROCESS

Bone consists of about 65% inorganic and 35% organic material. The inorganic mate-

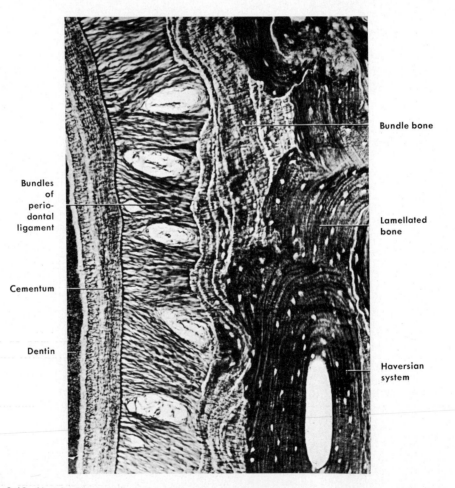

Bundle bone

Bundles of perio- dontal ligament

Lamellated bone

Cementum

Dentin

Haversian system

Fig. 8-12. Alveolar bone proper consisting of bundle bone and haversian bone on distal alveolar wall. A reversal line separates the two (silver impregnation).

rial is hydroxyapatite, whereas the organic material is primarily type I collagen, which lies in a ground sustance of glycoproteins and proteoglycans. The glycoproteins are proteins with a small amount of monosaccharide, disaccharide, polysaccharide, or oligosaccharide, and the proteoglycans are sulfated and nonsulfated glycosaminoglycans (high-molecular-weight carbohydrates) with a small amount of proteins. The approximate composition of bone is as follows:

Inorganic = 65%
Organic = 35%
  Collagen = 88%-89%
  Noncollagen = 11%-12%
    Glycoproteins = 6.5%-10%
    Proteoglycans = 0.8%
    Sialoproteins = 0.35%
    Lipids = 0.4%

The inorganic material almost exclusively consists of calcium and inorganic orthophosphate in the form of hydroxyapatite crystals. These crystals are deposited on and between the molecules of collagen (which form the collagen fibrils) as well as in the noncollagen, organic material that makes up the ground substance of bone. The exact mechanism by which hydroxyapatite crystals are deposited in the bone matrix produced by osteoblasts is still unknown. However, certain enzymes, alkaline phosphatase, ATPase, and pyrophosphatase, have been shown to participate in this process.

The internal structure of bone is adapted to mechanical stresses. It changes continuously during growth and alteration of functional stresses. In the jaws, structural changes are correlated to the growth, eruption, movements, wear, and loss of teeth. All these processes are made possible only by a coordination of destructive and formative activities. Specialized cells, the osteoclasts, eliminate overage bony tissue or

bone that is no longer adapted to mechanical forces, whereas osteoblasts produce new bone. Osteoblasts secrete the type I collagen as well as the noncollagenous matrix of bone. Their ultrastructure is characteristic of any actively secreting cell, that is, a prominent Golgi apparatus, rough endoplasmic reticulum, mitochondria, nucleoli, and many secretory vesicles and vacuoles. Osteoblasts differentiate from progenitor or precursor cells of the connective tissue at the site of bone formation. The mechanisms that determine bone formation at any given site are unknown. They must, however, be varied and in part must be determined on a genetic and functional basis. Although there are many theories and opinions in this regard, specific details have not yet been elucidated. As the osteoblasts secrete the organic matrix of bone, it is at first devoid of mineral salts, and at this stage it stains pink in routine hematoxylin and eosin stains and is called *osteoid tissue.* As this material is produced, some of the osteoblasts become embedded in it and form the *osteocytes.* In areas of bone formation, mineralization always lags behind the production of bone matrix, and therefore in such areas a superficial layer of osteoid tissue is always seen. In routine sections mineralized bone is basophilic and can be easily distinguished from the osteoid tissue.

Osteoclasts are, as a rule, multinucleated giant cells (Fig. 8-13, *left*). The number of nuclei in one cell may rise to a dozen or more. However, occasionally uninucleated osteoclasts are found. The cell body is irregularly oval or club shaped and may show many branching processes. In general, osteoclasts are found in baylike depressions in the bone called *Howship's lacunae.* Osteoclasts have prominent mitochondria, lysosomes, vacuoles, and little rough endoplasmic reticulum. Their many nuclei have condensed chromatin and a

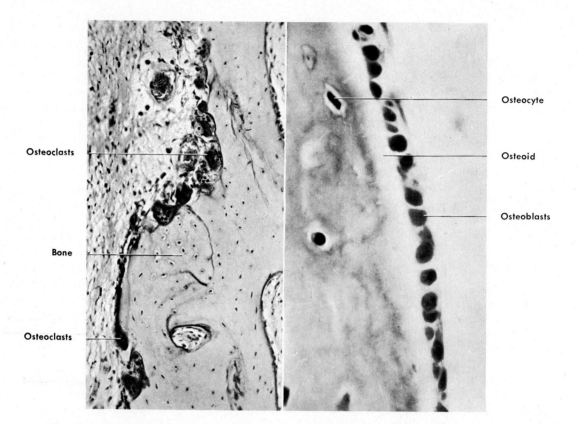

Osteoclasts

Bone

Osteoclasts

Osteocyte

Osteoid

Osteoblasts

Fig. 8-13. Resorption and apposition of bone. *Left,* Osteoclasts in Howship's lacunae. *Right,* Osteoblasts along bone trabecula. Layer of osteoid tissue is a sign of bone formation.

single nucleolus. The part of the cell in contact with the bone shows a convoluted surface, the _ruffled border_, which is the site of great activity. Here, pieces of bone are broken off and released into the extracellular spaces. The ruffled border is surrounded by a *clear zone* that has no organelles but only fine granular cytoplasm with microfilaments. Osteoclasts are probably derived from the circulating blood cells (monocytes), but they may differentiate from the mesenchymal cells in situ. Whereas the major position of bone resorption occurs through the mediation of osteoclasts, on rare occasions bone resorption by

osteocytes has been described (osteocytic osteolysis). This, however, is only of academic interest.

It has been suggested that bone resorption at any site is a chemotactic phenomenon; that is, it is initiated by the release of some soluble factor that attracts monocytes to the target site. In the bone resorption phenomenon, however, the role of genetic and functional influences cannot be underestimated. It might be that aging osteocytes, in their degeneration and death, liberate the substances that cause the differentiation of the osteoclasts.

During bone resorption, three processes

occur in more or less rapid succession: (1) decalcification, (2) degradation of matrix, and (3) transport of soluble products to the extracellular fluid or the blood vascular system. Since calcified matrix is resistant to proteases of all kinds, bone must first be decalcified; this is achieved at the ruffled border of the osteoclasts by secretion of organic acids (citric and lactic acid), which chelate bone, and by H^+, which increases the solubility of hydroxyapatite. After this decalcification process, pieces of matrix are released by the activity of cathepsin B_1 (lysosomal acid protease) and collagenase enzymes. (Collagenase is secreted as a proenzyme that is activated by specific neutral proteases.) Collagenolytic activity takes place outside the osteoclast and occurs at a specific site on the tropocollagen (collagen) molecule. This site is one third the distance from the caboxyl end of the molecule. The broken fragments of collagen are further decalcified, and breakdown of collagen by proteases other than collagenase continues. Collagenolysis occurs outside the osteoclast, and only calcium phosphate can be identified within these cells. After the degradation of the matrix, the breakdown products of bone must be transported to the extracellular fluids and to the blood vascular system, but the details of this mechanism are yet unknown.

INTERNAL RECONSTRUCTION OF BONE

The bone in the alveolar process is identical to bone elsewhere in the body and is in a constant state of flux. During the growth of the maxilla and the mandible, bone is deposited on the outer surfaces of the cortical plates. In the mandible, with its thick, compact cortical plates, bone is deposited in the shape of basic or circumferential lamellae (Fig. 8-8). When the lamellae reach a certain thickness, they are replaced from the inside by haversian bone. This reconstruction is correlated to the functional and nutritional demands of the bone. In the haversian canals, closest to the surface, osteoclasts differentiate and resorb the haversian lamellae and part of the circumferential lamellae. The resorbed bone is replaced by proliferating loose connective tissue. This area of resorption is sometimes called the *cutting cone* or the *resorption tunnel*. After a time the resorption ceases and new bone is apposed onto the old. The scalloped outline of Howship's lacunae that turn their convexity toward the old bone remains visible as a darkly stained cementing line, a *reversal line* (Fig. 8-14). This is in contrast to those cementing lines that correspond to a rest period in an otherwise continuous process of bone apposition. They are called *resting lines* (Fig. 8-8). Resting and reversal lines are found between layers of bone of varying age.

Wherever a muscle, tendon, or ligament is attached to the surface of bone, Sharpey's fibers can be seen penetrating the basic lamellae. During replacement of the latter by haversian systems, fragments of bone containing Sharpey's fibers remain in the deeper layers. Thus the presence of these lamellae containing Sharpey's fibers indicates the former level of the surface.

Alterations in the structure of the alveolar bone are of great importance in connection with the physiologic eruptive movements of the teeth. These movements are directed mesio-occlusally. At the alveolar fundus the continual apposition of bone can be recognized by resting lines separating parallel layers of bundle bone. When the bundle bone has reached a certain thickness, it is resorbed partly from the marrow spaces and then replaced by lamellated bone or spongy trabeculae. The presence of bundle bone indicates the level at which the alveolar fundus was situated pre-

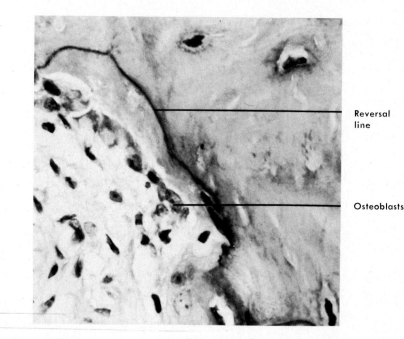

Reversal
line

Osteoblasts

Fig. 8-14. Reversal line in bone. (From Bhaskar SN: Synopsis of oral histology, St Louis, 1962, The CV Mosby Co.)

viously. During the mesial drift of a tooth, bone is apposed on the distal and resorbed on the mesial alveolar wall (Fig. 8-15). The distal wall is made up almost entirely of bundle bone. However, the osteoclasts in the adjacent marrow spaces remove part of the bundle bone when it reaches a certain thickness. In its place, lamellated bone is deposited (Fig. 8-12).

On the mesial alveolar wall of a drifting tooth, the sign of active resorption is the presence of Howship's lacunae containing osteoclasts (Fig. 8-15). Bundle bone, however, on this side is always present in some areas but forms merely a thin layer (Fig. 8-16). This is because the mesial drift of a tooth does not occur simply as a bodily movement. Thus resorption does not involve the entire mesial surface of the alveolus at one and the same time. Moreover,

periods of resorption alternate with periods of rest and repair. It is during these periods of repair that bundle bone is formed, and detached periodontal fibers are again secured. Islands of bundle bone are separated from the lamellated bone by reversal lines that turn their convexities toward the lamellated bone (Fig. 8-16).

During these changes, compact bone may be replaced by spongy bone or spongy bone may change into compact bone. This type of internal reconstruction of bone can be observed in physiologic mesial drift or in orthodontic mesial or distal movement of teeth. In these movements an interdental septum shows apposition on one surface and resorption on the other. If the alveolar bone proper is thickened by apposition of bundle bone, the interdental marrow spaces widen and advance in the direction

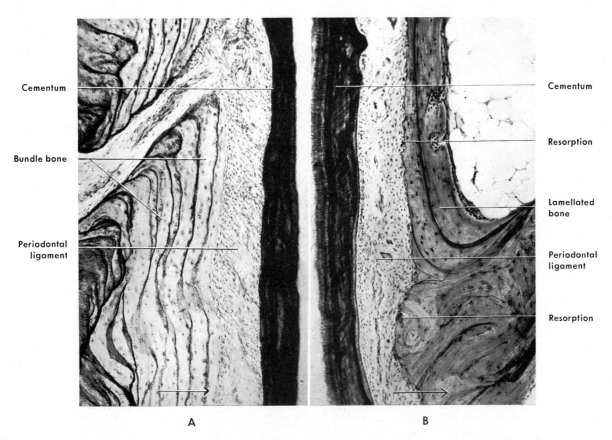

Fig. 8-15. Mesial drift indicated by arrow. **A,** Apposition of bundle bone on distal alveolar wall. **B,** Resorption of bone on mesial alveolar wall. (From Weinmann JP: Angle Orthod 11:83, 1941.)

of apposition. Conversely, if the plate of the alveolar bone proper is thinned by resorption, apposition of bone occurs on those surfaces that face the narrow spaces. The result is a reconstructive shift of the interdental septum.

CLINICAL CONSIDERATIONS

Bone, although one of the hardest tissues of the human body, is biologically a highly plastic tissue. Where bone is covered by a vascularized connective tissue, it is exceedingly sensitive to pressure, whereas tension acts generally as a stimulus to the pro-

duction of new bone. It is this biologic plasticity that enables the orthodontist to move teeth without disrupting their relations to the alveolar bone. Bone is resorbed on the side of pressure and apposed on the side of tension; thus the entire alveolus is allowed to shift with the tooth. It has been shown that on the pressure side there is an increase in the level of cyclic adenosine monophosphate (cAMP) in cells. This may play some role in bone resorption.

The adaptation of bone to function is quantitative as well as qualitative. Whereas increase in functional forces leads to forma-

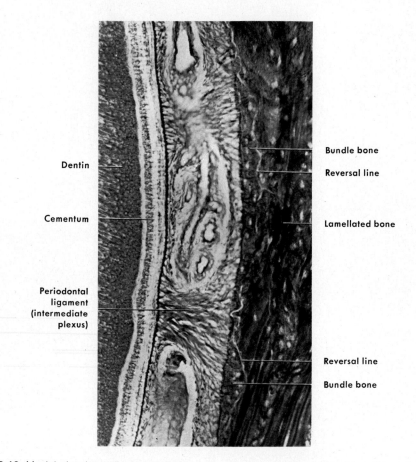

Dentin

Cementum

Periodontal
ligament
(intermediate
plexus)

Bundle bone

Reversal line

Lamellated bone

Reversal line

Bundle bone

Fig. 8-16. Mesial alveolar wall where alveolar bone proper consists mostly of lamellated bone and islands of bundle bone, which anchor principal fibers of periodontal ligament.

tion of new bone, decreased function leads to a decrease in the volume of bone. This can be observed in the supporting bone of teeth that have lost their antagonists. Here the spongy bone around the alveolus shows pronounced rarefaction: the bone trabeculae are less numerous and very thin (Fig. 8-17). The alveolar bone proper, however, is generally well preserved because it continues to receive some stimuli from the tension of the periodontal tissues.

During healing of fractures or extraction wounds an embryonic type of bone is formed, which only later is replaced by mature bone. The embryonic bone, also called immature or coarse fibrillar bone, is characterized, among other aspects, by the greater number, size, and irregular arrangement of the osteocytes than are found in mature bone (Fig. 8-18). The greater number of cells and the reduced volume of calcified intercellular substance render this immature bone more radiolucent than mature bone. This explains why bony callus cannot be seen in roentgenograms at a time when histologic examination of a fracture

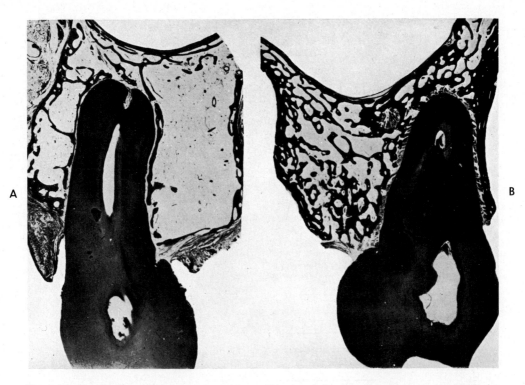

Fig. 8-17. Osteoporosis of alveolar process caused by inactivity of tooth that has no antagonist. La-biolingual sections through upper molars of same individual. **A,** Disappearance of bony trabeculae after loss of function. Plane of mesiobuccal root. Alveolar bone proper remains intact. **B,** Normal spongy bone in plane of mesiobuccal root of functioning tooth. (From Kellner E: Z Stomatol 18:59, 1920.)

reveals a well-developed union between the fragments and why a socket after an extraction wound appears to be empty at a time when it is almost filled with immature bone. The visibilty in radiographs lags 2 or 3 weeks behind actual formation of new bone.

The most frequent and harmful change in the alveolar process is that which is associated with periodontal disease. The bone resorption is almost universal, occurs more frequently in posterior teeth, is usually symmetrical, occurs in episodic spurts, is both of the horizontal and vertical type (i.e., occurs from the gingival and tooth side, respectively), and is intimately re-lated to bacterial plaque and pocket formation. Recent studies have revealed some of the mechanisms that contribute to this process. It has been shown, for example, the endotoxins produced by the gram-negative bacteria of the plaque lead to an increase in cAMP, which increases the osteoclastic activity. Furthermore, a peptide called *osteoclast activating factor* (OAF) has been demonstrated in the lymphocytes near the periodontal pocket. This substance is capable of increasing cAMP and osteoclastic activity and reducing osteoblastic activity at the target site. The insidious and progressive loss of alveolar bone in periodontal disease is difficult to control, and once lost,

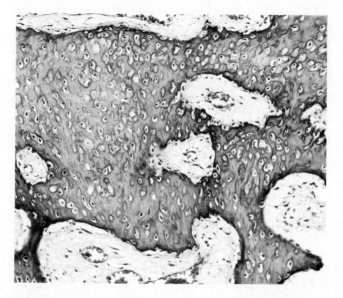

Fig. 8-18. Immature bone. Note many osteocytes and absence of lamellae or resting lines. (From Bhaskar SN: Synopsis of oral histology, St Louis, 1962, The CV Mosby Co.)

this bone is even more difficult to repair or regenerate. The therapeutic replacement or regeneration of just a few millimeters of bone tissue lost from the alveolar process in periodontal disease is the greatest challenge to the speciality of periodontics.

In the last few years synthetic materials have been introduced that are intended to replace bone tissue lost through disease or injury. These materials are of two types: the nonresorbable hydroxyapatite and the resorbable tricalcium phosphate. These synthetic inorganic products are currently being used for the augmentation of the alveolar ridges and for filling bone defects produced by periodontal disease. Although these materials are safe to use, they do not provide a basis for a new periodontal apparatus. However, their use stabilizes the compromised teeth, prolongs their life, and enhances their function. Results of their use in augmenting edentulous ridges have also been very successful.

Since the alveolar process of the maxilla and mandible develops and is maintained for the support of the teeth, when the teeth are lost, it undergoes gradual atrophy. In some instances the resorption may be so severe that the fabrication of a functional prosthesis may become difficult or even impossible. Studies in both humans and animals have shown that if during the extraction of teeth the root portion is retained in the alveolar process, this structure does not undergo a noticeable reduction in its height. Leaving the roots of the teeth within the jaws, however, requires time-consuming endodontic therapy.

REFERENCES

Bhaskar SN: Radiographic interpretation for the dentist, ed 3, St. Louis, 1979, The CV Mosby Co.

Bhaskar SN, Mohammed C, and Weinmann J: A morphological and histochemical study of osteoclasts, J Bone Joint Surg (Am) 38:1335, 1956.

Brodie AG: Some recent obsevations on the growth of the mandible, Angle Orthod 10:63, 1940.

Brodie AG: On the growth pattern of the human head from the third month to the eighth year of life, Am J Anat 68:209, 1941.

Council on Dental Materials, Instruments and Equipment, American Dental Association: Hydroxyapatite, beta tricalcium phosphate and autogenous and allogeneic bone for filling periodontal defects, alveolar ridge augmentation, and pulp capping, J Am Dent Assoc 108:822, 1984.

Glimcher MJ: Composition, structure and organization of bone and other mineralized tissues and the mechanism of calcification. In Greep RO and Aptwood EB, editors: The handbook of physiology. Section 7, vol 7, Washington, DC, 1976, American Physiological Society, pp 25-116.

Hall DA: Glycoproteins and proteoglycans. In The aging of connective tissue, New York, 1976, Academic Press, Inc.

Ham A and Leeson T: Histology, ed 4, Philadelphia, 1961, JB Lippincott Co.

Kaban LB and Glowacki J: Augmentation of rat mandibular ridge with demineralized bone implants, J Dent Res 63:998, 1984.

Marks SC and Schneider G: Evidence for a relationship between lymphoid cells and osteoclasts, Am J Anat 152:331, 1978.

Orban B: A contribution to the knowledge of the physiologic changes in the periodontal membrane, J Am Dent Assoc 16:405, 1929.

Ritchey B and Orban B: The crests of the interdental alveolar septa, J Periodontol 24:75, 1953.

Schaffer J: Die Verknöcherung des Unterkiefers (Ossification of the mandible), Arch Mikrosk Anat 32:266, 1888.

Sicher H and DuBrul EL: Oral anatomy, ed 6, St. Louis, 1975, The CV Mosby Co.

Urist MR: Biochemistry of calcification. In Bourne GH, editor: The biochemistry and physiology of bone, vol 4, ed 2, New York, 1976, Academic Press, Inc.

Weinmann JP: Das Knochenbild bei Störungen per physiologischen Wanderung der Zähne (Bone in disturbances of the physiologic mesial drift), Z Stomatol 24:397, 1926.

Weinmann JP: Bone changes related to eruption of the teeth, Angle Orthod 11:83, 1941.

Weinmann JP and Sicher H: Bone and bones; fundamentals of bone biology, ed 2, St. Louis, 1955, The CV Mosby Co.

9
ORAL MUCOUS MEMBRANE

The oral cavity is unique in structure. It contains the teeth. The salivary glands discharge their secretions into it. It contains the taste buds and can be used to perceive and sense in other ways. Thus it serves a variety of functions.

Food first enters the digestive tract through the oral cavity. Here the food is tasted, masticated, and mixed with saliva. Hard inedible particles are sensed and expectorated. Saliva secreted into the oral cavity lubricates the food and facilitates swallowing. Enzymes in the saliva initiate digestion.

Body cavities that communicate with the external surface are lined by mucous membranes, which are coated by serous and mucous secretions. The surface of the oral cavity is a mucous membrane. Its structure varies in an apparent adaptation to function in different regions of the oral cavity. Areas involved in the mastication of food, such as the gingiva and the hard palate, have a much different structure than does the floor of the mouth or the mucosa of the cheek.

Basing classification on these functional criteria, the oral mucosa may be divided into three major types:
1. Masticatory mucosa (gingiva and hard palate)
2. Lining or reflecting mucosa (lip, cheek, vestibular fornix, alveolar mucosa, floor of mouth and soft palate)
3. Specialized mucosa (dorsum of the tongue and taste buds)

The masticatory mucosa is bound to bone and <u>does not stretch.</u> It bears forces generated when food is chewed. The lining mucosa is not equally exposed to such forces. However, it covers the musculature and is distensible, adapting itself to the contraction and relaxation of <u>cheeks, lips, and tongue and to movements of the mandible produced by the muscles of mastication</u>. It makes up all the surfaces of the mouth except for the dorsum of the tongue and the masticatory mucosa. The specialized (sensory) mucosa is so-called because it bears the taste buds, which have a sensory function. These will be discussed below as will two areas with a slightly different structure—the dentogingival junction (the attachment of the gingiva to the tooth) and the red zone or vermilion border of the lips.

DEFINITIONS AND GENERAL CONSIDERATIONS

The structure of the oral mucous membrane resembles the skin in many ways. It is composed of two layers, epithelium and connective tissue (Fig. 9-1). The connective tissue component of oral mucosa is termed the *lamina propria*. The comparable part of skin is known as dermis or corium.

The two layers form an interface that is

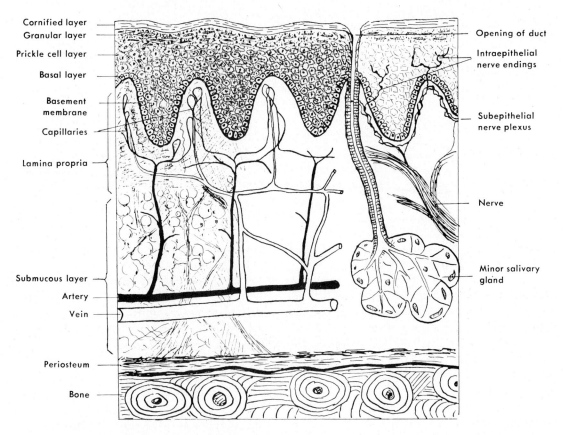

Fig. 9-1. Diagram of oral mucous membrane (epithelium, lamina propria, and submucosa).

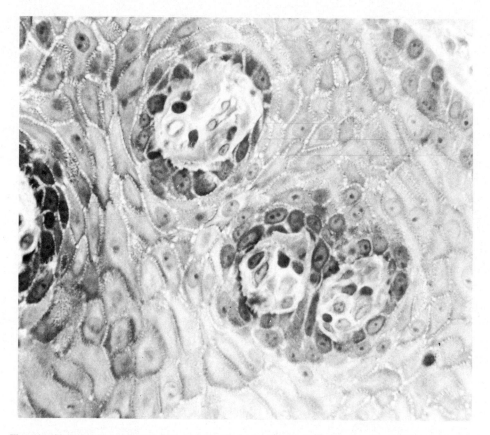

Fig. 9-2. Papillae of connective tissue protrude into epithelium. Blood vessels, fibroblasts, and collagen fibers are seen within them. Cells surrounding papillae are basal cells. The other cells are mainly spinous cells.

folded into corrugations. Papillae of connective tissue protrude toward the epithelium (Fig. 9-2) carrying blood vessels and nerves. Although some of the nerves actually pass into it, the epithelium does not contain blood vessels. The epithelium in turn is formed into ridges that protrude toward the lamina propria. These ridges interdigitate with the papillae and are called epithelial ridges. When the tissue is sectioned for microscopy, these ridges look like pegs as they alternate with the papillae, forming a serpentine interface. At one time, the epithelial ridges were mistakenly called epithelial pegs.

The two tissues are intimately connected. At their junction there are two different structures with very similar names, the basal lamina and the basement membrane. The *basal lamina* is evident at the electron microscopic level and is epithelial in origin (Fig. 9-3). The *basement membrane* is evident at the light microscopic level. It is found at the interface of epithelial and connective tissue within the connective tissue. It is a zone that is 1 to 4 μm

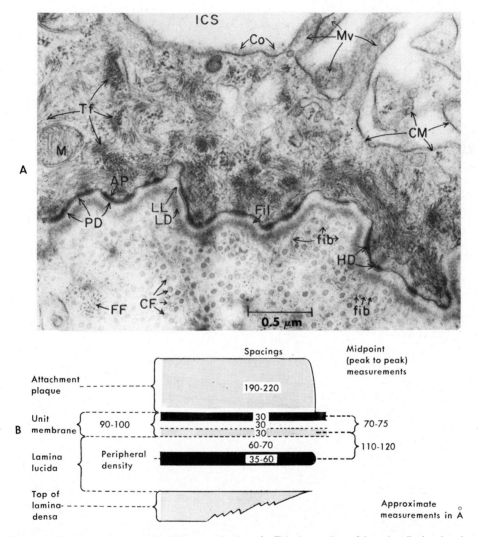

Fig. 9-3. Electron micrograph of human gingiva. **A,** This is portion of basal cell showing basal plasma membrane and also hemidesmosomes, *HD,* lamina lucida, *LL,* and lamina densa, *LD.* Collagen fibrils, *CF,* may be seen cut in cross section in connective tissue. There are also fine fibrils, *FF,* present as a grouping. Other special or anchoring fibrils, *fib,* may be seen inserting into connective tissue side of lamina densa. Area of intercellular space, *ICS,* is evident above epithelial cell. Microvilli, *Mv,* and coating, *Co,* on plasma membrane, *CM,* are present there. **B,** Approximate dimensions of hemidesmosome. (From Stern IB: Periodontics 3:224, 1965.)

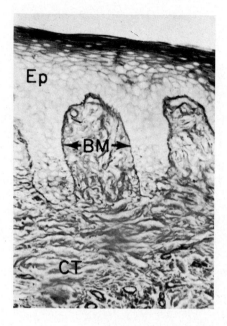

Fig. 9-4. Photomicrograph of human gingiva (PAS stain). PAS-positive basement membrane appears as dense line at epithelium—connective tissue junction. Note that blood vessels in lamina propria also have PAS-positive basement membrane. *BM,* Basement membrane; *CT,* connective tissue; *Ep,* epithelial cells. (× 160.) (From Stern IB: Periodontics 3:224, 1965.)

Fig. 9-5. Silver-stained section of human fetal tongue showing basement membrane as dense line separating epithelium above from connective tissue below. Extending for variable distance into connective tissue are dark-stained reticular fibers, which are found in greatest number immediately below basement membrane. This zone, known as reticular zone, is found whether or not papillae are present. Papillae delineate extent of papillary zone.

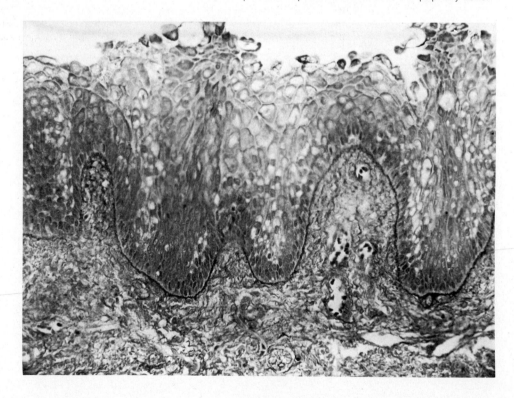

wide and is relatively cell free. This zone stains positively with the periodic acid–Schiff method, indicating that it contains neutral mucopolysaccharides (glycosaminoglycans) (Fig. 9-4). It also contains fine argyrophilic reticulin fibers (Fig. 9-5), as well as special anchoring fibrils (Fig. 9-6). In the skin the basement membrane zone has been shown to contain fibronectin and laminin (glycoproteins), heparin sulfate, proteoglycans, type IV collagen, as well as some special antigens (p. 269).

Lamina propria. The lamina propria may be described as a connective tissue of variable thickness that supports the epithelium. It is divided for descriptive reasons into two parts—papillary and reticular. The papillary portion is named for the papillae, the reticular portion for the reticular fibers. Since there is considerable variation in length and width of the papillae in different areas, the papillary portion is also of variable depth. A portion of the lamina propria subjacent to the basement membrane can be distinguished from the connective tissue because it has the property of taking up silver stain more strongly (argyrophilia) (Fig. 9-5). Fine immature collagen fibers that are argyrophilic and have a trellislike or latticelike arrangement are termed reticulin. This portion as well as the papillary portion contains reticular fibers. The two portions are not separate. They are a continuum, but the two terms are used to describe this region in different ways. The reticular zone is always present. The papillary zone may be absent in some areas such as the alveolar mucosa when the papillae are either very short or lacking.

The interlocking arrangement of the connective tissue papillae and the epithelial ridges and the even finer undulations and projections found at the base of each epithelial cell increases the area of contact between the lamina propria and epithelium (Fig. 9-7). This additional area facilitates exchange of material between the epithelium and the blood vessels in the connective tissue. In addition, cells with heavily arranged pedicles (serrations) may serve to strengthen the attachment to the connective tissue. Cells with flatter basal surfaces may be preparing to undergo cell division. The resultant cell will either remain in the proliferative pool in the basal layer or will become determined as a keratinocyte, cell destined to migrate to the tissue surface to become part of the stratum corneum.

The lamina propria may attach to the periosteum of the alveolar bone, or it may overlay the submucosa, which varies in different regions of the mouth such as the soft palate and floor of the mouth.

Submucosa. The submucosa consists of connective tissue of varying thickness and density. It attaches the mucous membrane to the underlying structures. Whether this attachment is loose or firm depends on the character of the submucosa. Glands, blood vessels, nerves, and also adipose tissue are present in this layer. It is in the submucosa that the larger arteries divide into smaller branches, which then enter the lamina propria. Here they again divide to form a subepithelial capillary network in the papillae. The veins originating from the capillary network course back along the path taken by the arteries. The blood vessels are accompanied by a rich network of lymph vessels. The sensory nerves of the mucous membrane tend to be more concentrated toward the anterior part of the mouth (rugae, tip of tongue, etc.). The nerve fibers are myelinated as they traverse the submucosa but lose their myelin sheath before splitting into their end arborizations. Sensory nerve endings of various types are found in the papillae (Fig. 9-8, *A*). Some of the fibers enter the epithelium, where they terminate between the epithelial cells as

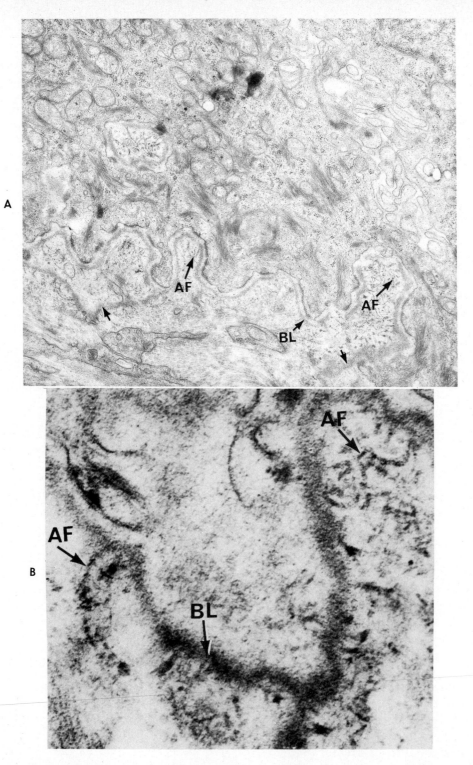

Fig. 9-6. A, Anchoring fibrils, *AF,* and basal lamina, *BL,* which are cut tangentially at places *(arrows).*
B, These fibrils branch, loop, and exhibit banding.

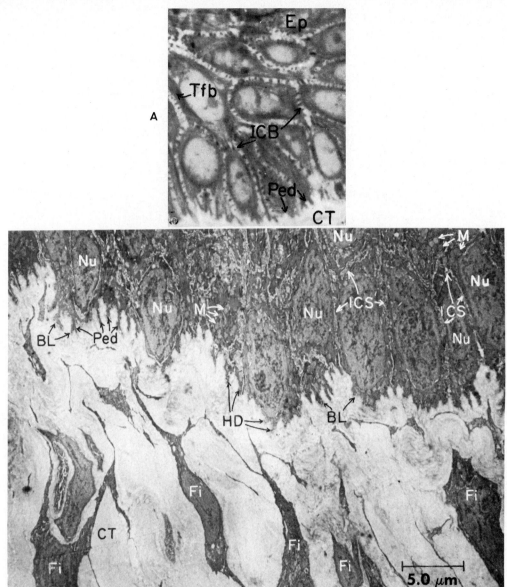

Fig. 9-7. A, Photomicrograph of human gingival epithelial cells, *Ep.* Pedicles, *Ped,* are present at base of basal cells and extend toward connective tissue, *CT.* Tonofibrils, *Tfb,* are evident both in cells and apparently coursing across intercellular bridges, *ICB.* **B,** Electron micrograph of rat gingiva. Several basal cells with apparent pedicles, *Ped,* extending toward connective tissue, *CT,* but separated from it by basal lamina, *BL,* which is barely visible. Fibroblasts, *Fi,* may be noted within connective tissue. Epithelial cells contain prominent nucleus, *Nu,* and are demarcated from adjacent cells by lighter appearance of intercellular spaces, *ICS.* Small, round, light areas in epithelial cells are mitochondria, *M.* Pedicles, *Ped,* in this electron micrograph are of a much smaller dimension than larger undulations of basal cell surface outlined by arrows at *HD.* These, in turn, are smaller than ridges shown in Fig. 9-7, *A.* (**A,** × 1400.) (From Stern IB: Periodontics 3:224, 1965.)

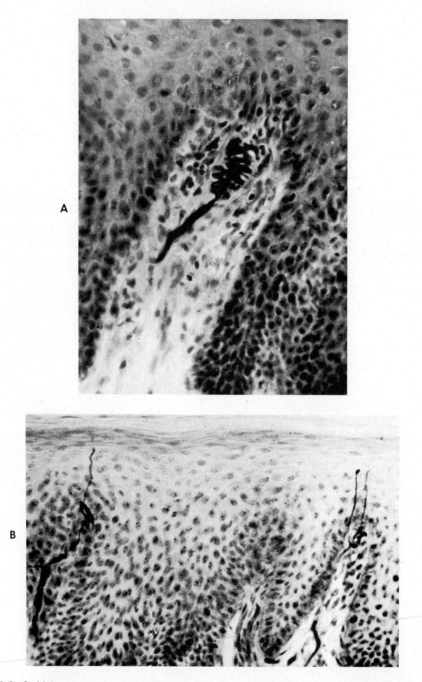

Fig. 9-8. A, Meissner tactile corpuscle in human gingiva (silver impregnation after Bielschowsky-Gros). **B,** Intraepithelial "ultraterminal" extensions and nerve endings in human gingiva (silver impregnation after Bielschowsky-Gros). (From Gairns FW and Aitchison JA: Dent Rec 70:180, 1950.)

free nerve endings (Fig. 9-8, *B*). The blood vessels are accompanied by nonmyelinated visceral nerve fibers that supply their smooth muscles. Other visceral fibers supply the glands.

In studying any mucous membrane, the following features should be considered: (1) type of covering epithelium, (2) structure of the lamina propria, its density and thickness, and the presence or lack of elasticity, (3) the form of junction between the epithelium and lamina propria, and (4) the membrane's fixation to the underlying structures, that is, the submucous layer. Considered as a separate and well-defined layer, submucosa may be present or absent. Looseness or density of its texture determines whether the mucous membrane is movably or immovably attached to the deeper layers. Presence or absence and location of adipose tissue or glands should also be noted.

Epithelium. The epithelium of the oral mucous membrane is of the stratified squamous variety. It may be keratinized, parakeratinized, or nonkeratinized, depending on location. In humans the epithelial tissues of the gingiva and the hard palate (masticatory mucosa) are keratinized (Fig. 9-9, *A*), although in many individuals the gingival epithelium is parakeratinized (Fig. 9-9, *C*). The cheek, faucial, and sublingual tissues are normally nonkeratinized (Fig. 9-9, *B*).

A common feature of all epithelial cells is that they contain keratin intermediate filaments as a component of their cytoskeleton. This is one of the distinguishing features of an epithelial cell, regardless of its function. The analogous components of connective tissue cells are called *vimentin;* in muscle cells they are called *desmin*, and in nerve cells *neural filaments*. These words are used with a biochemical orientation. All intermediate filaments resemble tonofilaments, are 7 to 11 nm in width, and can be reconstituted in vitro from the isolated filaments.

Keratinizing oral epithelium has four cell layers: basal, spinous, granular, and cornified. These are also referred to in Latin as *stratum basale, stratum spinosum, stratum granulosum*, and *stratum corneum*. These layers take their names from their morphologic appearance. A single cell is, at different times, a part of each layer. After mitosis, it may remain in the basal layer and divide again or it may become determined, during which time it migrates and is pushed upward. During its migration as a keratinocyte it becomes committed to biochemical and morphologic changes (differentiation), which culminate in the formation of a keratinized squama, a dead cell filled with densely packed protein contained within a toughened cell membrane. After reaching the surface it desquamates. This whole process from the onset of determination is called keratinization. A determined keratinocyte can no longer divide. For the tissue to remain in a steady state, undifferentiated cells must remain in the basal layer and form one differentiated cell for each cell that desquamates.

The basal layer is made up of cells that synthesize DNA and undergo mitosis, thus providing new cells (Fig. 9-10). New cells are generated in the basal layer. However, some mitotic figures may be seen in spinous cells just beyond the basal layer. These cells have become determined as they leave the basal layer. The basal cells and the parabasal spinous cells are referred to as the stratum germinativum, but only the basal cells can divide.

It has been proposed that the basal cells are made up of two populations. One population is serrated and heavily packed with tonofilaments, which are adaptations for attachment, and the other is nonserrated and

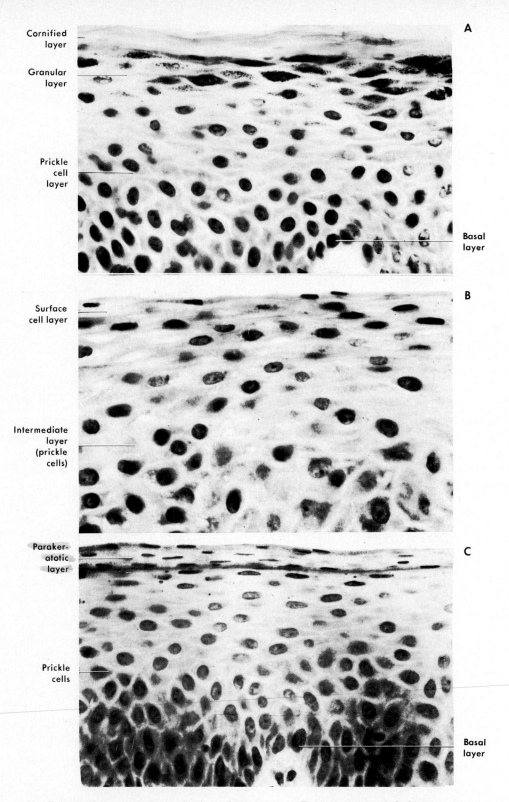

Cornified layer

Granular layer

Prickle cell layer

Basal layer

A

Surface cell layer

Intermediate layer (prickle cells)

B

Parakeratotic layer

Prickle cells

Basal layer

C

Fig. 9-9. Variations of gingival epithelium. **A,** Keratinized. **B,** Nonkeratinized. **C,** Parakeratinized.

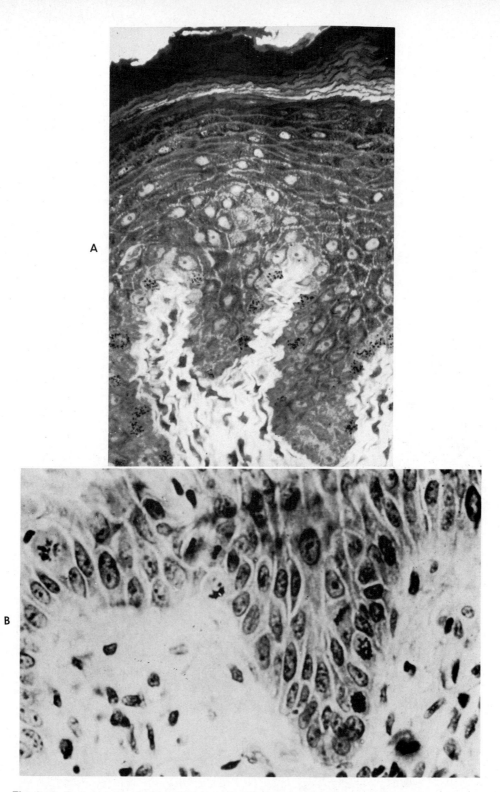

Fig. 9-10. A, Arrangement of labeling in oral epithelium 30 minutes after administration of tritiated thymidine. Grains are localized over nuclei in stratum basale. **B,** Oral epithelium showing many mitotic figures. (**A** from Anderson GS and Stern IB: Periodontics 4:115, 1966.)

is composed of slowly cycling stem cells. The stem cells give rise to a population of cells amplified for cell division, the proliferative compartment.

The serrated basal cells are a single layer of cuboid or high cuboid cells that have protoplasmic processes (pedicles) projecting from their basal surfaces toward the connective tissue (Fig. 9-7). Specialized structures called *hemidesmosomes,* which abut on the basal lamina (Fig. 9-3), are found on the basal surface. They consist of a single attachment plaque, the adjacent plasma membrane, and an associated extracellular structure that appears to attach the epithelium to the connective tissue. The basal lamina is made up of a clear zone (*lamina lucida*) just below the epithelial cells and a dark zone (*lamina densa*) beyond the lamina lucida and adjacent to the connective tissue (Fig. 9-3; also see p. 325). The lamina lucida thus far has been shown to contain laminin and bullous pemphigoid antigen. Laminin is a large, triple-chain molecule (Mr = 10^6). It and type IV collagen promote epithelial cell growth and guide epithelial cell movement through chemotaxis.

Basement membranes promote differentiation. They also promote peripheral nerve regeneration and growth, and they tend to prevent metastases. The lamina densa contains type IV collagen and an antigen bound by the antibody KF-1. Below the lamina densa is a fibrillar zone (sublamina densa fibrils) that is not of epithelial origin.

The lateral borders of adjacent basal cells are closely apposed and connected by desmosomes (Fig. 9-11, *B*). These are specializations of the cell surface, consisting of adjacent cell membranes and a pair of denser regions (attachment plaques) as well as intervening extracellular structures (Fig. 9-12). The basal cells contain tonofilaments, which course toward, and in some way are

attached to, the attachment plaques. There are other types of cell junctions such as tight, close, and gap junctions present. There are also ribosomes and elements of rough-surfaced endoplasmic reticulum, indicative of protein-synthesizing activity. Basal cells synthesize some of the proteins of the basal lamina. They also synthesize proteins, which form the intermediate filaments of the basal cells.

The *spinous cells* (stratum spinosum) are irregularly polyhedral and larger than the basal cells. On the basis of light microscopy, it appears that the cells are joined by "intercellular bridges" (Fig. 9-11, *A*). Tonofibrils seem to course from cell to cell across these bridges. Electron microscopic studies have shown that the "intercellular bridges" are desmosomes and the tonofibrils are bundles of tonofilaments (Fig. 9-13). The tonofilaments turn or loop adjacent to the attachment plaques and do not cross over into adjacent cells. It is suspected that an agglutinating material joins them to the attachment plaques. The desmosome attachment plaques contain the polypeptides desmoplakin I and II. Monoclonal antibodies to these polypeptides can be used to detect carcinomas (an epithelial tumor) by immunofluorescent microscopy. The intercellular spaces contain glycoprotein, glycosaminoglycans, and fibronectin.

Fig. 9-11. A, High magnification light micrograph showing epithelial cells with nuclei, *N;* intercellular spaces, *ICS;* tonofibrils, *T;* and intercellular bridges, *IB.* Speckled areas are intercellular bridges (desmosomes) cut tangentially or "en face." **B,** Electron micrograph of prickle cells of human gingiva. Portions of epithelial cells, *E,* are evident, separated by intercellular space, *ICS.* Several nuclei, *N,* are evident. Tonofilaments, *Tf,* are present in cytoplasm and extend toward desmosomes, *D,* located at periphery of cells. (**B** from Grant DA, Stern IB, and Listgarten MA: Periodontics in the tradition of Orban and Gottlieb, ed 6, St Louis, 1988, The CV Mosby Co.)

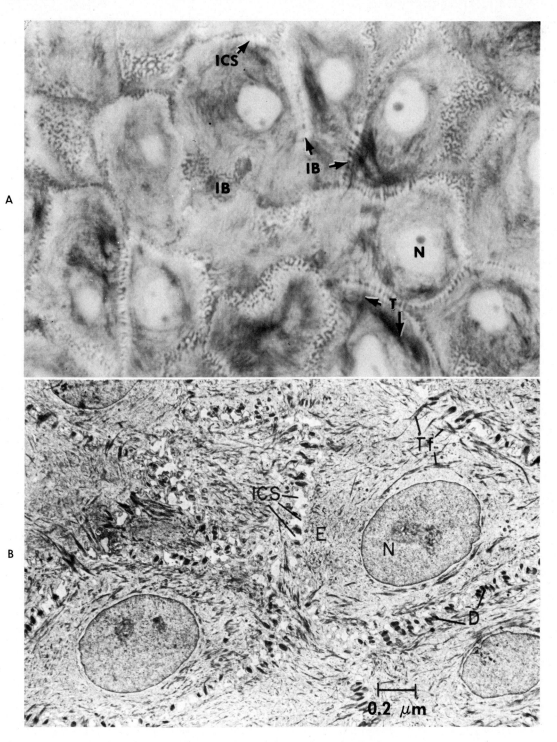

Fig. 9-11. For legend see opposite page.

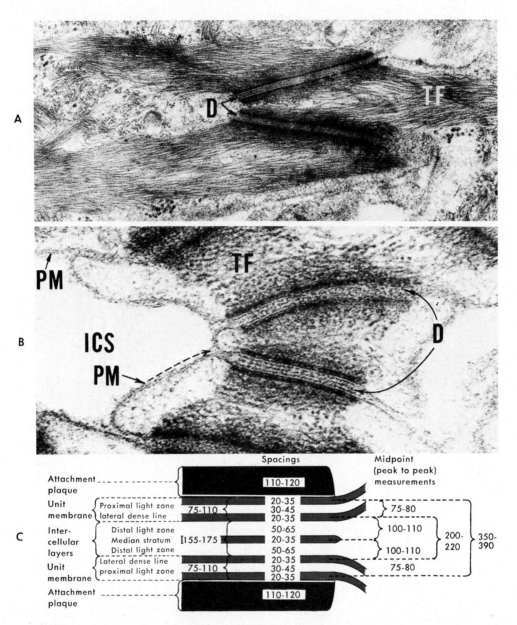

Fig. 9-12. A, Tonofilaments, *Tf,* extending to series of desmosomes, *D.* Tonofilaments are sectioned in long axis (human gingiva). **B,** Higher magnification of two desmosomes, *D,* showing substructure. Tonofilaments are cross sectioned. Intercellular space, *ICS,* is bounded by adjacent cell membranes, *PM,* whose unit membrane is clearly evident *(dashed arrow).* Unit membranes form part of substructure of desmosome. **C,** Diagrammatic cross-sectioned representation of desmosome and dimensions (in Ångström units) of various components. (From Stern IB: Periodontics 3:224, 1965.)

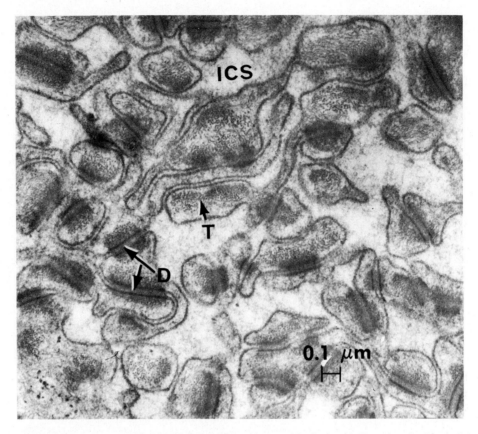

Fig. 9-13. Electron micrograph of prickle cell layer of human gingival epithelium showing intercellular bridges and tonofibrils. Here desmosomes are cut tangentially or "en face" as shown in light micrograph (Fig. 9-11, *A*). Note relatively close adaptation of cell processes ending in desmosomes, *D*. These processes contain tonofilaments, *T*, cut on end, which appear as fine dots. Relatively large intercellular space, *ICS*, contains cell-coating material.

The tonofilament network and the desmosomes appear to make up a tensile supporting system for the epithelium. The percentage of cell membrane occupied by hemidesmosomes is higher in basal cells of gingiva and palate than in alveolar mucosa, buccal mucosa, and tongue. The intercellular spaces of the spinous cells in keratinizing epithelia are large or distended; thus the desmosomes are made more prominent, and these cells are given a prickly appearance. The spinous (prickle) cells resemble a cockleburr or sticker that has each spine ending at a desmosome. Of the four layers, the spinous cells are the most active in protein synthesis. These cells synthesize additional proteins that differ from those made in the basal cells. This change indicates their biochemical commitment to keratinization. In terms of number and length the desmosomes of the spinous layer occupy more of the membrane in the tongue, gingiva, and palate than in either alveolar or buccal mucosa.

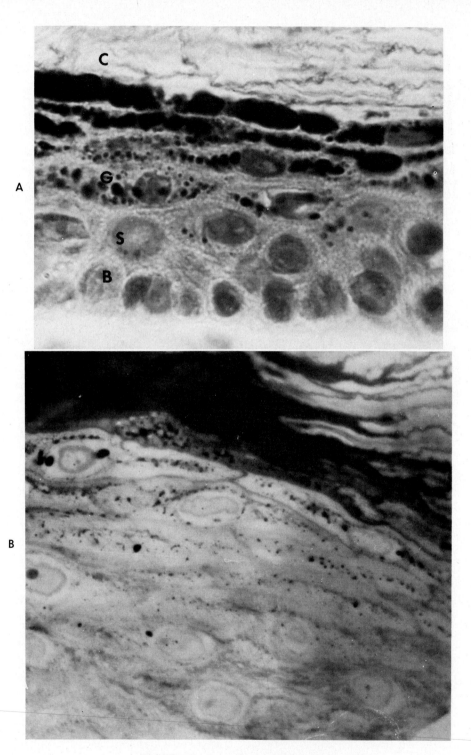

Fig. 9-14. For legend see opposite page.

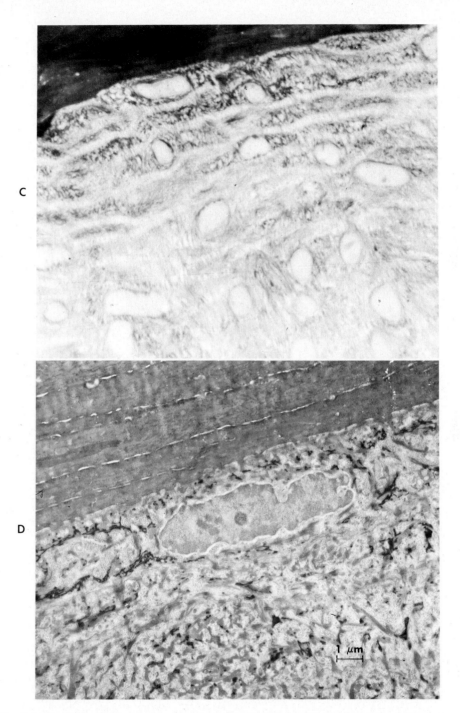

Fig. 9-14. A, Light micrograph of newborn rat skin showing basal cells, *B,* spinous cells, *S,* granular cells with numerous dense granules, *G,* and cornified (keratinized) components. **B** and **C,** Keratohyalin is formed as discrete spherical granules in some tissues or is formed as angular amorphous material in other tissues. **D** and **E,** Angular form is associated with tonofilaments primarily *(arrow);*

Continued.

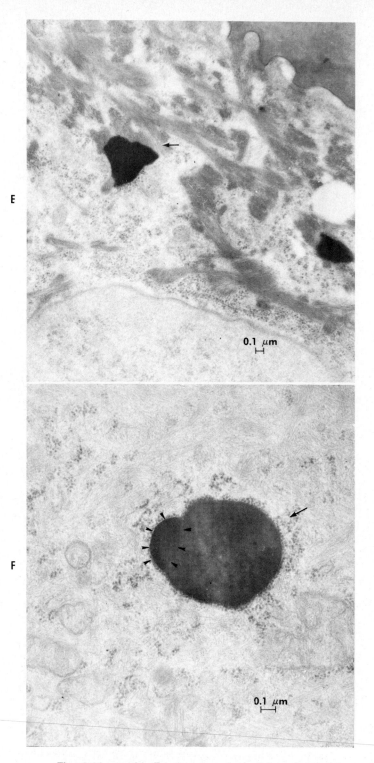

Fig. 9-14, cont'd. F, whereas spherical form is surrounded by ribosomes *(arrow)* and may contain more than one material *(small arrows).*

The next layer *(stratum granulosum)* contains flatter and wider cells. These cells are larger than the spinous cells. This layer is named for the basophilic keratohyalin granules (blue staining with hematoxylin and eosin) (Fig. 9-14, *A* to *C*) that it contains. The nuclei show signs of degeneration and pyknosis. This layer still synthesizes protein, but reports of synthesis rates at this level differ. However, as the cell approaches the stratum corneum, the rate diminishes. Tonofilaments are more dense in quantity and are often seen associated with keratohyalin granules (Fig. 9-14, *D* to *F*). Sometimes dense networks of tonofilaments and keratohyalin granules are evident. Keratohyalin granules contain at least two types of proteins, one that (solubilized by solutions containing high concentrations of salt) is rich in the amino acid histidine. It functions in the stratum corneum as a keratin filament matrix protein (see below).

In the stratum granulosum the cell surfaces become more regular and more closely applied to adjacent cell surfaces. At the same time the lamellar granule, a small organelle (also known as keratinosome, Odland body, or membrane-coating granule) forms in the upper spinous and granular cell layers. It has an internal lamellated structure (Fig. 9-15, *A* and *B*). Lamellar granules discharge their contents into the intercellular space forming an intercellular lamellar material, which contributes to the permeability barrier (Fig. 9-15, *C*). This barrier forms at the junction of granular and cornified cell layers. The intercellular space of this region has a lamellar structure similar to that of the lamellar granule (Fig. 9-15, *C*) and contains glycolipid. At approximately the same time during differentiation, the inner unit of the cell membrane thickens, forming the "cornified cell envelope." Several proteins contribute to this

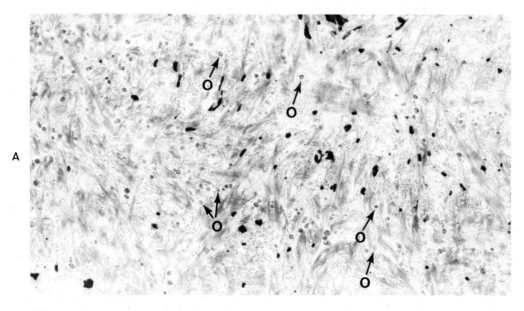

Fig. 9-15. A, Lamellar granules, *O,* are found close to cell membrane *(arrows)* and desmosomes in granular cells. *Continued.*

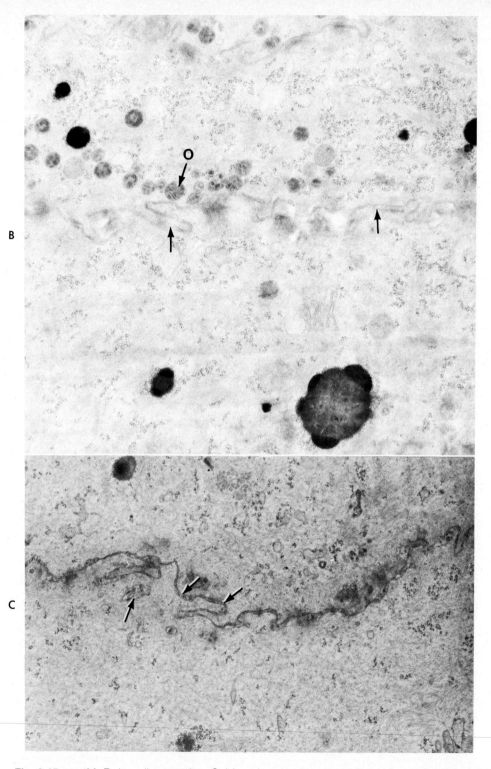

Fig. 9-15, cont'd. B, Lamellar granules, *O,* lying close to plasma membrane *(arrows)* and in cells containing ribosome-associated keratohyalin granules. Note that some of keratohyalin granules have two densities and perhaps two components. Lamellar granules contain an internal lamellar structure. **C,** Lamellar structure in intercellular space *(arrows)*. It is presumed that these lamellae are derived from lamellar granules that are no longer present.

structure, among which is involucrin (keratolinin), which is present at the upper half of the stratum spinosum. Thereafter the thickened membrane contains sulfur-rich proteins stabilized by covalent crosslinks. It forms a highly resistant structure.

In nonkeratinizing oral epithelium a small organelle similar to the lamellar granule forms. It differs in that its contents are granular rather than lamellar, but it may serve a similar function.

The *stratum corneum* is made up of keratinized squamae, which are larger and flatter than the granular cells. Here all of the nuclei and other organelles such as ribosomes and mitochondria have disappeared (Fig. 9-14, *D*).* The layer is acidophilic (red staining with hematoxylin and eosin) and is histologically amorphous. The keratohyalin granules have disappeared. Ultrastructurally the cells of the cornified layer are composed of densely packed filaments developed from the tonofilaments, altered, and coated by the basic protein of the keratohyalin granule, filaggrin.

The cells of the stratum corneum are densely packed with filaments in this nonfibrous interfilamentous matrix protein, filaggrin (named for its function in filament aggregation). When the purified solubilized matrix protein obtained from the epithelium is combined with solubilized keratin filaments in vitro, aggregates of matrix and highly oriented filaments form instantaneously (Fig. 9-16). Their ultrastructural appearance is similar to that of the contents of the stratum corneum. The active matrix protein, filaggrin, is derived from a precursor in the keratohyalin granules. Studies of the interaction of matrix and filaments have been performed with filaggrin and keratin

filaments obtained from epidermis; however, the same proteins can also be demonstrated in keratinizing oral epithelium. The keratinized cell becomes compact and dehydrated and covers a greater surface area than does the basal cell from which it developed. It does not synthesize protein. It is closely applied to adjacent squamae. The cell surface and desmosomes are altered, and the plasma membrane is denser and thicker than in the cells of deeper layers.

Epithelial cells that ultimately keratinize are called *keratocytes* or *keratinocytes*. Keratinocytes increase in volume in each successive layer from basal to granular. The cornified cells, however, are smaller in volume than the granular cells. The cells of each successive layer cover a larger area than do the cells of the layers immediately below.

Nonkeratinizing epithelia differ from keratinizing epithelia primarily because they do not produce a cornified surface layer, but there are other differences as well. The layers in nonkeratinizing epithelium are referred to as basal, intermediate, and superficial (*stratum basale, stratum intermedium, stratum superficiale*) (Fig. 9-9, *B*). The basal cells of both types are similar. The cells of the stratum intermedium are larger than cells of the stratum spinosum. The intercellular space is not obvious or distended and hence the cells do not have a prickly appearance. Nevertheless, the cells of the stratum intermedium often are referred to as spinous or prickle cells, even though morphologically they are not spinous and biochemically they do not keratinize. These cells do contain some intermediate keratin filaments, but they differ biochemically from those in keratinizing epithelia and are sparsely distributed within the cells. The cells of the stratum intermedium are attached by desmosomes and other junctions, and their cell surfaces

---

*In states such as dandruff the rates of cell division and desquamation increase and nuclei may persist in the desquamating cells.

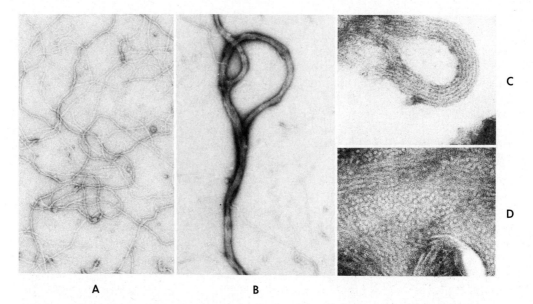

Fig. 9-16. A, Rat epidermal keratin subunits formed after solubilization in 8M urea. **B,** Aggregates of epidermal keratin filaments and filaggrin after mixing the proteins in a 0.25:1 ratio and allowing mixture to stand for 5 minutes. **C,** Aggregates formed as in **B,** fixed and embedded for transmission electron microscopy. Filaments 7 to 11 nm wide appear in longitudinal section separated at a uniform distance by darker staining material. **D,** Cross section of inner portion of rat stratum corneum showing keratin pattern of electron-lucent filament 7 to 11 nm wide embedded in an osmiophilic interfilamentous matrix. (**A** and **B** negatively stained with 1% uranyl acetate; ×62, 700. **C** and **D,** ×105,000.) (**A** to **C** from Dale BA, Holbrook KA, and Steinert PM: Nature 276:129, 1978. **D** courtesy B.A. Dale, K.A. Holbrook, and P.M. Steinert.)

are more closely applied than are spinous cells. There is no stratum granulosum (although incomplete or vestigial granules may form), nor is there a stratum corneum. Nucleated cells exist at the surface (Fig. 9-17). These cells ultimately desquamate, as do the cornified squamae. In general, nonkeratinizing oral mucosa have higher rates of mitoses than do the keratinizing oral mucosa.

In *orthokeratinization,* keratinized squamae form as has been described. In *parakeratinization,* the cells retain pyknotic and condensed nuclei and other partially lysed cell organelles until they desquamate. There are signs of condensation of the su-

perficial cells, which appear almost as if they were keratinizing. Tissues that are not keratinized at one stage of development may keratinize at another (Fig. 9-15). Similarly, tissues may be modulated from keratinized-parakeratinized and nonkeratinized variants in pathologic states. Although the terms "keratinized" and "parakeratinized" may be used interchangeably with the terms "parakeratosis" and "keratosis," the former terms refer to physiologic and the latter terms refer to pathologic stages. When keratinization occurs in a normally nonkeratinized tissue, it is referred to as keratosis. When normally keratinizing tissue such as the epidermis becomes parak-

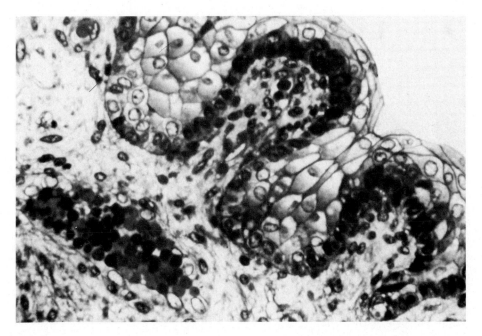

Fig. 9-17. Section of human fetal tongue showing three cell strata of nonkeratinized epithelium.

eratinized, it is referred to as parakeratosis.

The oral epithelium, in addition, contains melanocytes, Langerhans cells, Merkel cells, and various white blood cells (see p. 297).

Keratinocytes and lymphocytes interact. Keratinocytes can activate lymphocytes through the production of interleukin-1, but they may also inhibit lymphocyte proliferation. Stimulated lymphocytes produce gamma-interferon, which can stimulate keratinocytes to express HLA-DR antigen.

SUBDIVISIONS OF ORAL MUCOSA

For descriptive purposes the oral mucosa may be divided into the following areas:

    Keratinized areas
        Masticatory mucosa
        Vermilion border of lip
    Nonkeratinized areas
        Lining mucosa
        Specialized mucosa

Keratinized areas
Masticatory mucosa (gingiva and hard palate)

The masticatory mucosa is keratinized and is made up of the gingiva and the hard palate. They have similarities in thickness and keratinization of epithelium; in thickness, density, and firmness of lamina propria; and in being immovably attached. However, there are differences in their submucosa.

Hard palate. The mucous membrane of the hard palate is tightly fixed to the underlying periosteum and therefore immovable. Like the gingiva it is pink. The epithelium is uniform in form with a rather well-keratinized surface. The cells of the stratum corneum exhibit stacking, and in the rat there are complementary grooves and ridges between the apposing surfaces of the cells. The pedicles (see p. 265), the increase in number and length of desmosomes, the density of the tonofilaments, and the complementary grooves and ridges all appear to be adaptations of keratinizing epithelium to resist forces and to bind the epithelium to the connective tissue. The lamina propria, a layer of dense connective tissue, is thicker in the anterior than in the posterior parts of the palate and has numerous long papillae. Various regions in the hard palate differ because of the varying structure of the submucous layer. The following zones can be distinguished (Fig. 9-18):

1. Gingival region, adjacent to the teeth
2. Palatine raphe, also known as the median area, extending from the incisive or palatine papilla posteriorly
3. Anterolateral area or fatty zone between the raphe and gingiva
4. Posterolateral area or glandular zone between the raphe and gingiva

Except for narrow and specific zones, the palate has a distinct submucous layer. The zones that do not have a submucous layer occur peripherally where the palatine tissue is identical with the gingiva and along the midline for the entire length of the hard palate (the palatine raphe) (Fig. 9-18). The marginal area shows the same structure as the other regions of the gingiva. Only the lamina propria and periosteum are present below the epithelium (Fig. 9-19). Similarly, a submucosa is not found below the palatine raphe, or median area (Fig. 9-20). The lamina propria blends with the periosteum. If a palatine torus is present, the mucous membrane is thinner. The otherwise narrow raphe is widened and spreads over the entire torus.

The submucous layer occurs in wide regions extending between the palatine gingiva and palatine raphe. Despite this extensive submucosa, the mucous membrane is

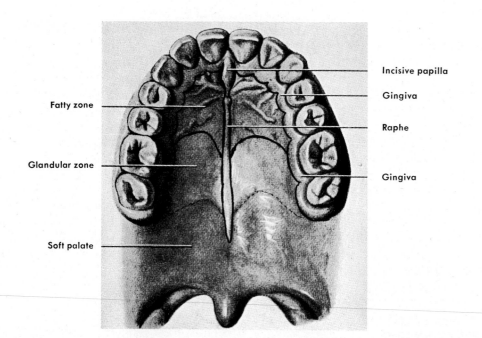

Fig. 9-18. Surface view of hard and soft palates. The different zones of palatine mucosa are outlined.

Fatty zone

Glandular zone

Soft palate

Incisive papilla

Gingiva

Raphe

Gingiva

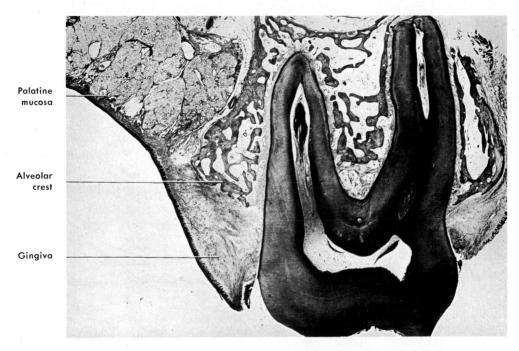

Palatine
mucosa

Alveolar
crest

Gingiva

Fig. 9-19. Structural differences between gingiva and palatine mucosa. Region of first molar.

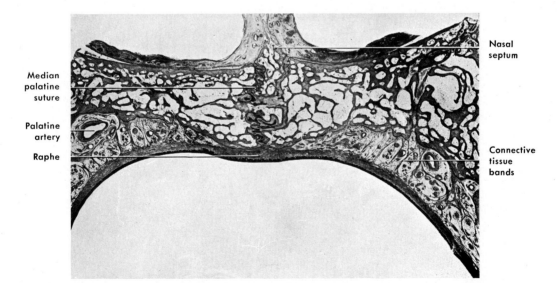

Nasal
septum

Median
palatine
suture

Palatine
artery

Raphe

Connective
tissue
bands

Fig. 9-20. Transverse section through hard palate. Palatine raphe. Fibrous bands connecting mucosa and periosteum in lateral areas. Palatine vessels. (From Pendleton EC: J Am Dent Assoc 21:488, 1934.)

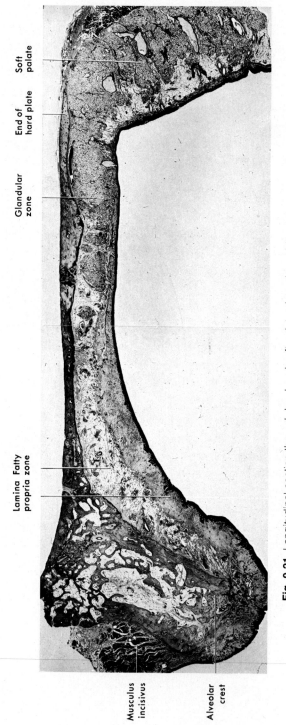
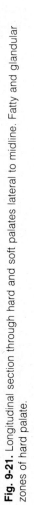

Fig. 9-21. Longitudinal section through hard and soft palates lateral to midline. Fatty and glandular zones of hard palate.

immovably attached to the periosteum of the maxillary and palatine bones. This attachment is formed by dense bands and trabeculae of fibrous connective tissue that join the lamina propria of the mucosa membrane to the periosteum. The submucous space is thus subdivided into irregular intercommunicating compartments of various sizes. These are filled with adipose tissue in the anterior part and with glands in the posterior part of the hard palate. The presence of fat or glands in the submucous layer acting as a cushion is comparable to the subcutaneous tissue of the palm of the hand and the sole of the foot.

When the submucosa of hard palate and that of gingiva are compared, there are pronounced differences. The dense connective tissue that makes up the lamina propria of gingiva is bound to the periosteum of the alveolar process or to the cervical region of the tooth. A submucous layer, as

such, cannot generally be recognized. In the lateral areas of the hard palate (Fig. 9-20), in both fatty and glandular zones, the lamina propria is fixed to the periosteum by bands of dense fibrous connective tissue. These bands are arranged at right angles to the surface and divide the submucous layer into irregularly shaped spaces. The distance between lamina propria and periosteum is smaller in the anterior than in the posterior parts. In the anterior zone the connective tissue contains fat (Fig. 9-21), whereas in the posterior part it contains mucous glands (Fig. 9-21). The glandular layers of the hard palate and of the soft palate are continuous.

At the junction of the alveolar process and the horizontal plate of the hard palate the anterior palatine vessels and nerves course, surrounded by loose connective tissue. This wedge-shaped area (Fig. 9-22) is large in the posterior part of the palate and

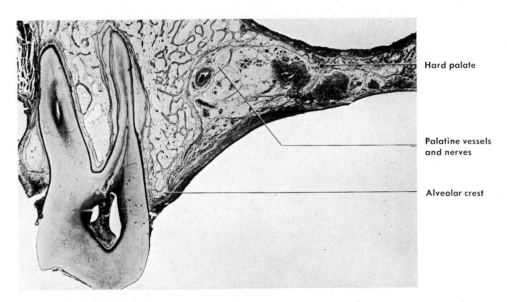

Hard palate

Palatine vessels and nerves

Alveolar crest

Fig. 9-22. Transverse section through posterior part of hard palate, region of second molar. Loose connective tissue in groove between alveolar process and hard palate around palatine vessels and nerves.

smaller in the anterior part. It is important for oral surgeons and periodontists to know the distribution of these vessels.

Incisive papilla. The oral incisive (palatine) papilla is formed of dense connective tissue. It contains the oral parts of the vestigial nasopalatine ducts. They are blind ducts of varying length lined by simple or pseudostratified columnar epithelium, rich in goblet cells. Small mucous glands open into the lumen of the ducts. These ducts sometimes become cystic in humans. Frequently the ducts are surrounded by small, irregular islands of hyaline cartilage, which are the vestigial extensions of the parasep-

tal cartilages. In most mammals the nasopalatine ducts are patent and, together with Jacobson's organ, are considered as auxiliary olfactory sense organs. Jacobson's organ (the vomeronasal organ) is a small ellipsoid (cigar-shaped) structure lined with olfactory epithelium that extends from the nose to the oral cavity. In humans, Jacobson's organ is apparent in the twelfth to fifteenth fetal week, after which it undergoes involution. In humans cartilage is sometimes found in the anterior parts of the papilla. In this location it bears no relation to the nasopalatine ducts (Fig. 9-23).

Palatine rugae (transverse palatine

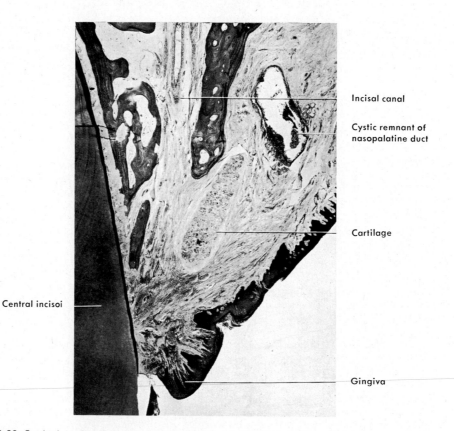

Fig. 9-23. Sagittal section through palatine papilla and anterior palatine canal. Note cartilage in papilla.

ridges). The palatine rugae, irregular and often asymmetric in humans, are ridges of mucous membrane extending laterally from the incisive papilla and the anterior part of the raphe. Their core is made of a dense connective tissue layer with fine interwoven fibers.

Epithelial pearls. In the midline, especially in the region of the incisive papilla, epithelial pearls may be found in the lamina propria. They consist of concentrically arranged epithelial cells that are frequently keratinized. They are remnants of the epithelium formed in the line of fusion between the palatine processes (see Chapter 1).

Gingiva. The gingiva extends from the dentogingival junction to the alveolar mucosa. It is subject to the friction and pressure of mastication. The morphology of both epithelium and connective tissues indicates the adaptation to these forces. The stratified squamous epithelium may be keratinized or nonkeratinized but most often is parakeratinized. The underlying lamina propria is dense. The collagen fibers of the lamina propria may either insert into the alveolar bone and the cementum or blend with the periosteum.

The gingiva is limited on the outer surface of both jaws by the mucogingival junction, which separates it from the alveolar mucosa (Fig. 9-24). The alveolar mucosa is red and contains numerous small vessels coursing close to the surface. On the inner surface of the lower jaw a line of demarcation is found between the gingiva and the mucosa on the floor of the mouth. On the palate the distinction between the gingiva and the peripheral palatal mucosa is not so sharp.*

The gingiva can be divided into the *free gingiva,* the "attached" *gingiva*† (Fig. 9-25), and the *interdental papilla.* The dividing line between the free gingiva and the gingiva is the *free gingival groove,* which runs parallel to the margin of the gingiva at a distance of 0.5 to 1.5 mm. The free gingival groove, not always visible microscopically, appears in histologic sections (Fig. 9-26, *A*) as a shallow V-shaped notch at a heavy epithelial ridge. The free gingival groove develops at the level of, or somewhat apical to, the bottom of the gingival sulcus. In some cases the free gingival groove is not so well defined as in others, and then the division between the free gingiva and the gingiva is not clear. The free gingival groove and the epithelial ridge are probably caused by functional impacts on the free gingiva. In the absence of a sulcus there is no free gingiva.

The gingiva is characterized by a surface that appears stippled (Fig. 9-26, *B*). Portions at the epithelium appear to be elevated, and between the elevations there are shallow depressions, the net result of which is stippling. The depressions corre-

*These surfaces are frequently referred to as buccal or labial, lingual or palatal. The oral cavity can be divided into two parts: the vestibulum oris (vestibule) and the cavum oris proprium (oral cavity proper). The term "vestibular" is used to describe those surfaces that face the vestibule; thus the need of differentiating between buccal and labial is eliminated. This tends to simplify descriptions and coincides with proper anatomic usage. The vestibular cavity is bounded anterolaterally by the mucous membranes of the lips and cheeks and internally by the teeth and gingiva. Vestibular would therefore apply to any tooth surface facing the vestibular cavity. Similarly the term "oral" describes the palatal and lingual. The oral cavity proper is bounded anterolaterally by the teeth and gingiva, superiorly by the soft and hard palate, inferiorly by the tongue and mucous membranes of the floor of the mouth, and posteriorly by the pillars of the fauces, the opening into the oral pharynx.

†At the International Conference on Research in the Biology of Periodontal Disease, Chicago, June 12-15, 1977, it was voted to drop the use of "attached" and simply refer to gingiva.

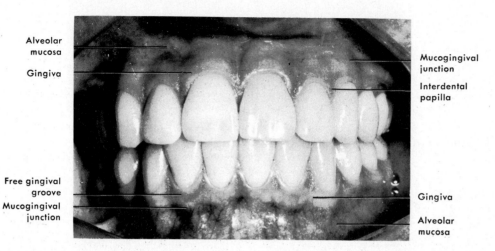

Alveolar mucosa

Gingiva

Free gingival groove

Mucogingival junction

Mucogingival junction

Interdental papilla

Gingiva

Alveolar mucosa

Fig. 9-24. Vestibular surface of gingiva of young adult. (Courtesy Dr. A. Ogilvie, Vancouver, British Columbia.)

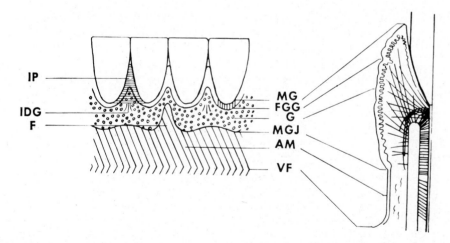

IP

IDG

F

MG

FGG

G

MGJ

AM

VF

Fig. 9-25. Diagrammatic illustration of surface characteristics of the clinically normal gingiva. *IP,* Interdental papilla; *IDG,* interdental groove; *F,* frenum; *MG,* marginal gingiva; *FGG,* free gingival groove; *G,* gingiva; *MGJ,* mucogingival junction; *AM,* alveolar mucosa; *VF,* vestibular fornix. (From Grant DA, Stern IB, and Listgarten MA: Periodontics in the tradition of Orban and Gottlieb, ed 6, St Louis, 1988, The CV Mosby Co.)

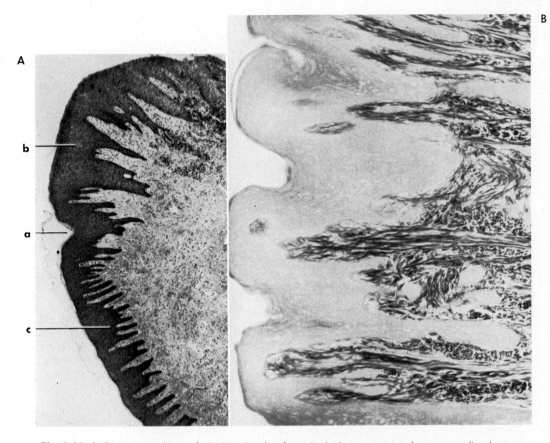

Fig. 9-26. A, Biopsy specimen of gingiva showing free gingival groove, *a,* and corresponding heavy epithelial ridge; *b,* free gingiva; *c,* gingiva. **B,** Gingival specimen showing stippling. Note relation of connective tissue fiber bundles to stippled surface (Mallory stain). (From Grant DA, Stern IB, and Listgarten MA: Periodontics in the tradition of Orban and Gottlieb, ed 6, St Louis, 1988, The CV Mosby Co.)

spond to the center of heavier epithelial ridges. There may be protuberances of the epithelium as well as stippling. They probably are functional adaptations to mechanical impacts. The disappearance of stippling is an indication of edema, an expression of an involvement of the gingiva in a progressing gingivitis.

Although the degree of stippling (Fig. 9-24) and the texture of the collagenous fibers vary with different individuals, there are also differences according to age and sex. In younger females the connective tissue is more finely textured than in the male. However, with increasing age the collagenous fiber bundles become more coarse in both sexes. Males tend to have more heavily stippled gingivae than do females. Like the human epidermis, the cells of the oral epithelium show another sex difference. In females the majority of the nuclei contain a large chromatin particle adjacent to the nuclear membrane.

The gingiva appears slightly depressed

between adjacent teeth, corresponding to the depression on the alveolar process between eminences of the sockets. In these depressions the gingiva sometimes forms slight vertical folds called interdental grooves.

The interdental papilla is that part of the gingiva that fills the space between two adjacent teeth. When viewed from the oral or vestibular aspect, the surface of the interdental papilla is triangular. In a three-dimensional view the interdental papilla of the posterior teeth is tent shaped, whereas it is pyramidal between the anterior teeth. When the interdental papilla is tent shaped, the oral and the vestibular corners are high, whereas the central part is like a valley. The central concave area fits below the contact point, and this depressed part of the interdental papilla is called the *col.* The col is covered by thin nonkeratinized epithelium, and it has been suggested that the col (the nonkeratinized epithelium) is more vulnerable to periodontal disease.

The lamina propria of the gingiva consists of a dense connective tissue that does not contain large vessels. Small numbers of lymphocytes, plasma cells, and macrophages are present in the connective tissue of normal gingiva (Fig. 9-27) subjacent to the sulcus and are involved in defense and re-

pair. The papillae of the connective tissue are characteristically long, slender, and numerous. The presence of these high papillae makes for ease in the histologic differentiation of gingiva and alveolar mucosa, in which the papillae are quite low (Fig. 9-28). The tissue of the lamina propria contains only few elastic fibers, and for the most part they are confined to the walls of the blood vessels. Other elastic fibers known as oxytalan fibers (because of special staining qualities) are also present. On the other hand, the alveolar mucosa and the submucosa contain numerous elastic fibers. These fibers are thickest in the submucosa.

The gingival fibers of the periodontal ligament enter into the lamina propria, attaching the gingiva firmly to the teeth (see Chapter 7). The gingiva is also immovably and firmly attached to the periosteum of the alveolar bone. Because of this arrangement it is often referred to as mucoperiosteum. Here a dense connective tissue, consisting of coarse collagen bundles (Fig. 9-29, *A*), extends from the bone to the lamina propria. In contrast, the submucosa underlying the alveolar mucous membrane is loosely textured (Fig. 9-29, *B*). The fiber bundles of the lamina propria of the alveolar mucosa are thin and regularly interwoven.

The gingiva contains dense fibers of collagen, sometimes referred to as the gingival ligament, which are divided into the following major groups.

1. *Dentogingival.* Extends from the cervical cementum into the lamina propria of the gingiva. The fibers of the gingival ligament constitute the most numerous group of gingival fibers.
2. *Alveologingival.* The fibers arise from the alveolar crest and extend into the lamina propria.
3. *Circular.* A small group of fibers that

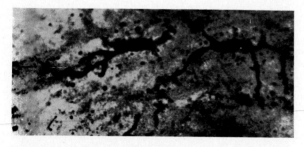

Fig. 9-27. Macrophages in normal gingiva. (Rio Hortega stain; ×1000.) (From Aprile EC de: Arch Hist Normal Pat 3:473, 1947.)

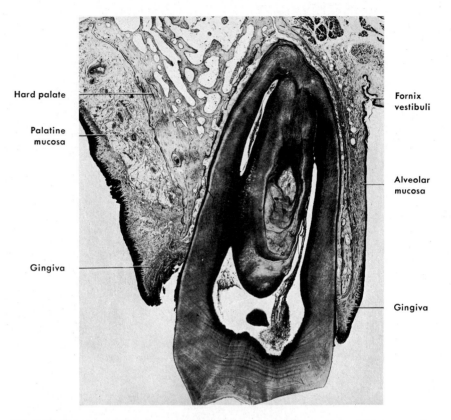

Hard palate

Palatine mucosa

Gingiva

Fornix vestibuli

Alveolar mucosa

Gingiva

Fig. 9-28. Structural differences between gingiva and alveolar mucosa. Upper premolar.

circle the tooth and interlace with the other fibers.

4. *Dentoperiosteal.* These fibers can be followed from the cementum into the periosteum of the alveolar crest and of the vestibular and oral surfaces of the alveolar bone.

There are also accessory fibers that extend interproximally between adjacent teeth and are also referred to as transseptal fibers. These fibers make up the *interdental ligament.*

The gingiva is normally pink but may sometimes have a grayish tint. The color depends in part on the surface (keratinized or not) and thickness and in part on pig-

mentation. The surface may be translucent or transparent, permitting the color of the underlying tissues to be seen. The reddish or pinkish tint is attributable to the color given the underlying tissue by the blood vessels and the circulating blood.

The following are three types of epithelial surface layers that result from differences in differentiation (Fig. 9-9).

1. *Keratinization,* in which the superficial cells form scales of keratin and lose their nuclei. A stratum granulosum is present.

2. *Parakeratinization,* in which the superficial cells retain pyknotic nuclei and show some signs of being kerati-

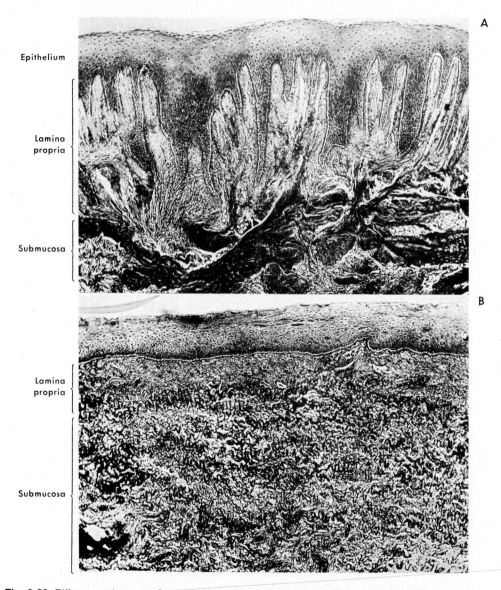

Fig. 9-29. Differences between **A,** gingiva, and **B,** alveolar mucosa. Silver impregnation of collagenous fibers. Note coarse bundles of fibers in gingiva and finer fibers in alveolar mucosa.

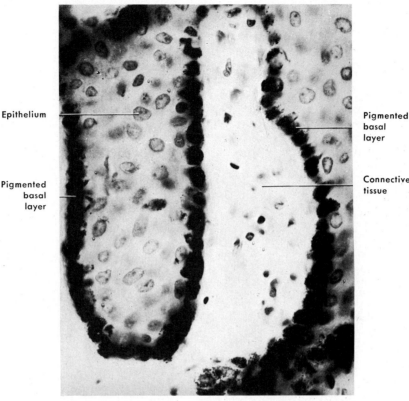

Epithelium

Pigmented
basal
layer

Pigmented
basal
layer

Connective
tissue

Fig. 9-30. Basal cells of gingiva showing pigmentation.

nized; however, the stratum granulosum is generally absent.

3. *Nonkeratinization,* in which the surface cells are nucleated and show no signs of keratinization.

The gingiva is parakeratinized in 75%, keratinized in 15%, and nonkeratinized in 10% of the population. It has been suggested that inflammation, which is seen in almost all gingival specimens, interferes with keratinization. The more highly keratinized the tissue, the whiter and less translucent is the tissue.

The presence of melanin pigment in the epithelium may give it a brown to black coloration. Pigmentation is most abundant at the base of the interdental papilla. It can be increased considerably in a number of pathologic states. Melanin is stored by the basal cells in the form of melanosomes, but these cells do not produce the pigment (Fig. 9-30). Melanin is elaborated by specific cells, *melanocytes,* residing in the basal layer and is transferred to the basal cells. The melanocytes are derived from the embryologic neural crest and migrate into the epithelium (Fig. 9-31). Oral pigmentation can be studied by use of either the dopa reaction or silver-staining techniques. In the dopa reaction the cells containing tyrosinase enzyme appear dark. Therefore the melanin-producing cells,

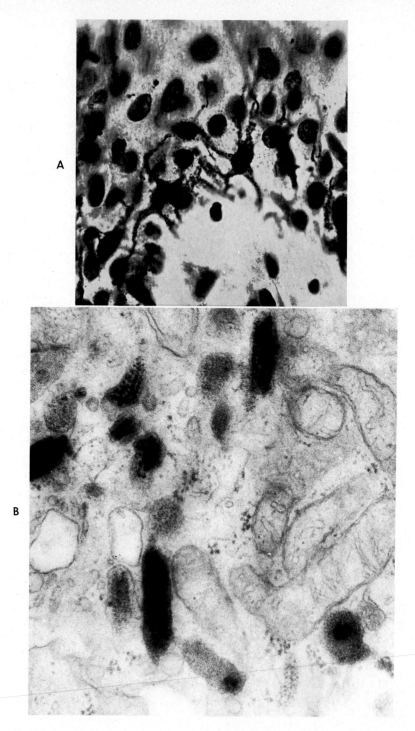

Fig. 9-31. A, Dendritic cells (melanocytes) in basal layer of epithelium. Biopsy of normal gingiva. **B,** Ultrastructural photographs of melanosomes from human gingiva showing substructural form. It is believed that tyrosinase associated with these structures is responsible for melanization and when melanosomes become fully melanized they are transferred to keratinocytes. (×1000.) (**A** from Aprile EC de: Arch Hist Normal Pat 3:473, 1947.)

which contain tyrosinase (dopa oxidase), are demonstrated. Silver stains also dye the melanin pigment. The dopa reaction is likewise found in certain connective tissue cells of the lamina propria that contain melanin (melanophages). These cells obtain the pigment from the melanocytes. Melanocytes appear as clear cells in hematoxylin sections. Silver stains reveal a spider-like (dendritic) appearance. Thus melanocytes are referred to as clear cells or dendritic cells. The number of melanocytes per square millimeter is quite constant for any particular region, and no difference in their numbers is found in the mucosa of blacks and whites.

The Langerhans cell is another clear cell or dendritic cell found in the upper layers of the skin and the mucosal epithelium restricted to zones of orthokeratinization. There is a correlation in the occurrence of a stratum granulosum and Langerhans' cells. This cell is free of melanin and does not give a dopa reaction. It stains with gold chloride, ATPase, and immunofluorescent markers. Neither the Langerhans cell nor the melanocyte forms desmosomal attachments to the epithelial cells. The Langerhans cell is a cell of hematopoietic origin.It has vimentin-type intermediate filaments (see p. 269). Langerhans cells are involved in the immune response. In the presence of antigenic challenge by bacterial plaque Langenhans cells migrate into the gingiva. They contain Ia antigens, which they present to primed T cells (thymocytes). They may function, as do macrophages, by picking up antigen and presenting it to lymphocytes, either locally or at lymph nodes. Langerhans cells with HLA-DR and T6 antigens also interact with lymphocytes but do so differently from keratinocytes (see p. 282). Langerhans cells present the antigen to specific helper T cells. The interleukin-1 secreted by the keratinocytes induces the T cells to produce interleukin-2, which binds to responsive T cells, causing them to proliferate. Another factor with common bochemical and biophysical properties to interleukin-1 is epidermal cell-derived thyrocyte-activating factor (ETAF), which apparently is produced by a subset of keratinocytes.

Another population of dendritic cells (Thy-1$^+$ dendritic epidermal cells) resides in murine epidermis and express a Thy-1 antigen. These cells have a bone marrow origin and may interact with suppressor T-cell populations. They have not yet been demonstrated in human epidermis.

The importance of these observations is that the skin and presumably the oral mucosa have an epithelial immunologic function and through this function the epithelium of the skin and oral mucosa interacts with the entire lymphoid system in concert with the Langerhans cells to help mount an immune response.

Another cell found among the basal cells, the *Merkel cell*, has nerve tissue immediately subjacent and is presumed to be a specialized neural pressure-sensitive receptor cell. It is believed to be slow acting, to have neurosecretory activity, and to be a migrant from the neural crest. Thus the oral epithelium not only contains the normal population of keratinocytes arranged in strata according to degree of differentiation, it also contains as residents three types of cells, the *melanocytes* (derived from the neural crest), the *Langerhans* cells (originating in the bone marrow), and the *Merkel cells.* The Merkel cell is neurally related but lacking neural filaments.

Other cells, such as lymphocytes and polymorphonuclear leukocytes, are also found at various levels of the epithelium. These cells are transients and can pass through the epithelium to the surface.

Blood and nerve supply. The blood supply of the gingiva is derived chiefly from the branches of the alveolar arteries that pass upward through the interdental septa. The interdental alveolar arteries perforate the alveolar crest in the interdental space and end in the interdental papilla, supplying it and the adjacent areas of the buccal and lingual gingiva. In the gingiva these branches anastomose with superficial branches of arteries that supply the oral and vestibular mucosa and marginal gingiva, for instance, with branches of the lingual, buccal, mental, and palatine arteries. The numerous lymph vessels of the gingiva lead to submental and submandibular lymph nodes.

The gingiva is well innervated. Different types of nerve endings can be observed, such as the Meissner or Krause corpuscles, end bulbs, loops, or fine fibers that enter the epithelium as "ultraterminal" fibers (Fig. 9-8).

Vermilion border of lip

The transitional zone between the skin of the lip and the mucous membrane of the lip is the red zone, or the vermilion border. It is found only in humans (Fig. 9-32). The skin on the outer surface of the lip is covered by a moderately thick, keratinized epithelium with a rather thick stratum corneum. The papillae of the connective tis-

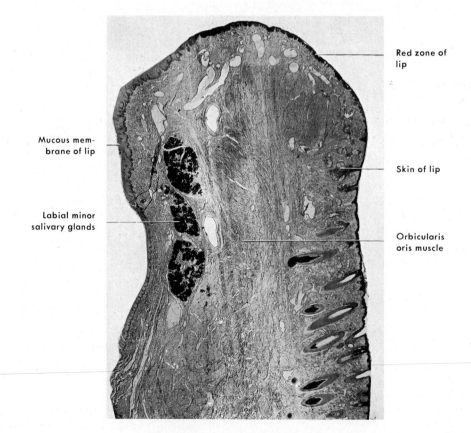

Mucous membrane of lip

Labial minor salivary glands

Red zone of lip

Skin of lip

Orbicularis oris muscle

Fig. 9-32. Section through the lip.

sue are few and short. Many sebaceous glands are found in connection with the hair follicles. Sweat glands occur between them.

The boundary between the red zone and the mucous membrane of the inner surface of the lip occurs where the keratinization of the transitional zone ends. The epithelium of the mucous membrane of the lip is not keratinized.

The transitional region is characterized by numerous, densely arranged, long papillae of the lamina propria, reaching deep into the epithelium and carrying large capillary loops close to the surface. Thus blood is visible through the thin parts of the translucent epithelium and gives the red color to the lips. Because this transitional zone contains only occasional sebaceous glands, it is subject to drying and therefore requires moistening by the tongue.

Nonkeratinized areas
Lining mucosa

Lining mucosa is found on the lip, cheek, vestibular fornix, and alveolar mucosa. All the zones of the lining mucosa are characterized by a relatively thick nonkeratinized epithelium and a thin lamina propria. Different zones of lining mucosa vary from one another in the structure of their submucosa. Where the lining mucosa reflects from the movable lips, cheeks, and tongue to the alveolar bone, the submucosa is loosely textured. The reflectory mucosa found in the fornix vestibuli and in the sublingual sulcus at the floor of the oral cavity has a submucosa that is loose and of considerable volume. The mucous membrane is movably attached to the deep structures and does not restrict the movement of lips and cheeks and the tongue.

Where lining mucosa covers muscle, as on the lips, cheeks, and underside of the tongue, the mucosa is fixed to the epimy-sium or fascia. In these regions the mucosa is also highly elastic. These two characteristics permit the mucosa to maintain a relatively smooth surface during muscular movement. Thus heavy folding, which could lead to injury during chewing if such folds were caught between the teeth, does not occur.

The mucosa of the soft palate is intermediate between this type of lining mucosa and the reflecting mucosa.

Lip and cheek. The epithelium of the mucosa of the lips (Fig. 9-32) and of the cheek (Fig. 9-33) is stratified squamous nonkeratinized epithelium. The lamina propria of the labial and buccal mucosa consists of dense connective tissue and has short, irregular papillae.

The submucous layer connects the lamina propria to the thin fascia of the muscles and consists of strands of densely grouped collagen fibers. There is loose connective tissue containing fat and small mixed glands between these strands. The strands of dense connective tissue limit the mobility of the mucous membrane, holding it to the musculature and preventing its elevation into folds. This prevents the mucous membrane of the lips and cheeks from lodging between the biting surfaces of the teeth during mastication. The mixed minor salivary glands of the lips are situated in the submucosa, whereas in the cheek the glands are larger and are usually found between the bundles of the buccinator muscle and sometimes on its outer surface. The cheek, lateral to the corner of the mouth, may contain isolated sebaceous glands called Fordyce spots (Fig. 9-34). These may occur lateral to the corner of the mouth and are often seen opposite the molars.

A comparison of masticatory and buccal mucosa shows that in the keratinized tissue the epithelium is thinner. It has a granular

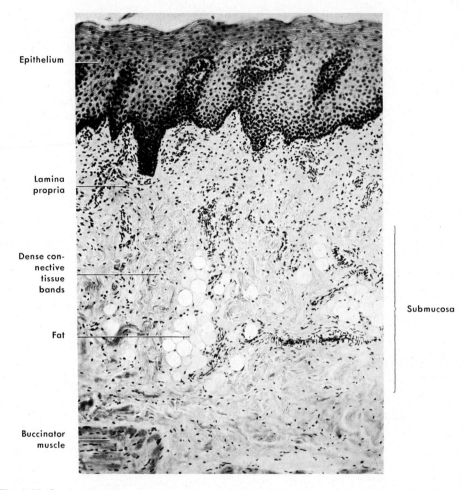

Epithelium

Lamina propria

Dense connective tissue bands

Fat

Buccinator muscle

Submucosa

Fig. 9-33. Section through mucous membrane of cheek. Note bands of dense connective tissue attaching lamina propria to fascia of buccinator muscle.

layer, the basal cells are larger, but the average cell size is smaller, and the cells have an angular shape. Furthermore, it is characterized by having many tonofibrils, wider intercellular spaces, and "prickles" that form "intercellular bridges." The cells of both tissues are joined by desmosomes. The appearance of the two differs by the heightened prominence of the "prickles" in the keratinized tissues, brought about by the increased width of the intercellular space and the greater density of the tonofibrils. Even the lamina propria of the two differ. In masticatory mucosa the basement membrane contains more reticular fibers, and its papillae are high and more closely spaced.

Vestibular fornix and alveolar mucosa. The mucosa of the lips and cheeks reflects from the vestibular fornix to the alveolar mucosa covering the bone. The mucous membrane of the cheeks and lips is attached firmly to

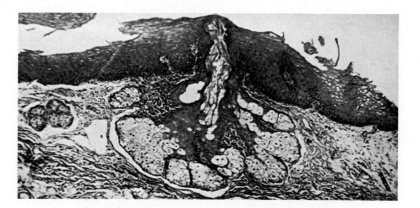

Fig. 9-34. Sebaceous gland in cheek (Fordyce spot).

the buccinator muscle in the cheeks and orbicularis oris muscle in the lips. In the fornix the mucosa is loosely connected to the underlying structures, and so the necessary movements of the lips and cheeks are permitted. The mucous membrane covering the outer surface of the alveolar process (alveolar mucosa) is attached loosely to the periosteum. It is continuous with, but different from, the gingiva, which is firmly attached to the periosteum of the alveolar crest and to the teeth.

The median and lateral labial frenula are folds of the mucous membrane containing loose connective tissue. No muscle fibers are found in these folds.

Gingiva and alveolar mucosa are separated by the mucogingival junction. The gingiva is stippled, firm, and thick, lacks a separate submucous layer, is immovably attached to bone and teeth by coarse collagen fibers, and has no glands. The gingival epithelium is thick and mostly parakeratinized or keratinized. The epithelial ridges and the papillae of the lamina propria are high.

The alveolar mucosa is thin and loosely attached to the periosteum by a well-defined submucous layer of loose connective tissue (Fig. 9-29, *B*), and it may contain small mixed glands. The epithelium is thin and nonkeratinized, and the epithelial ridges and papillae are low and often entirely missing. These differences cause the variation in color between the pale pink gingiva and the red lining mucosa.

Inferior surface of tongue; floor of oral cavity. The mucous membrane on the floor of the oral cavity is thin and loosely attached to the underlying structures to allow for the free mobility of the tongue. The epithelium is nonkeratinized, and the papillae of the lamina propria are short (Fig. 9-35). The submucosa contains adipose tissue. The sublingual glands lie close to the covering mucosa in the sublingual fold. The sublingual mucosa and the lingual gingiva have a junction corresponding to the mucogingival junction on the vestibular surface. The sublingual mucosa reflects onto the lower surface of the tongue and continues as the ventrolingual mucosa.

The mucosa membrane of the inferior surface of the tongue is smooth and relatively thin (Fig. 9-36). The epithelium is nonkeratinized. The papillae of the connective tissue are numerous but short. Here the submucosa cannot be identified

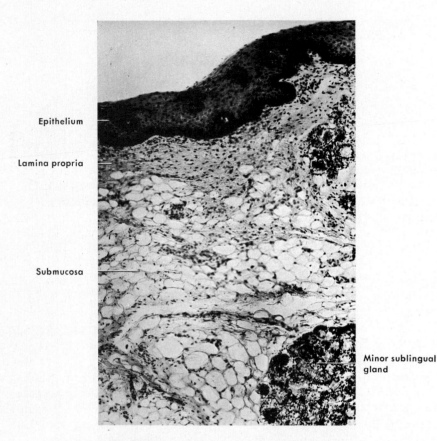

Epithelium

Lamina propria

Submucosa

Minor sublingual gland

Fig. 9-35. Mucous membrane from floor of mouth.

as a separate layer. It binds the mucous membrane tightly to the connective tissue surrounding the bundles of the muscles of the tongue.

Soft palate. The mucous membrane on the oral surface of the soft palate is highly vascularized and reddish in color, noticeably differing from the pale color of the hard palate. The papillae of the connective tissue are few and short. The stratified squamous epithelium is nonkeratinized (Fig. 9-37). The lamina propria shows a distinct layer of elastic fibers separating it from the submucosa. The latter is relatively loose and contains an almost continuous

layer of mucous glands. It also contains taste buds. Typical oral mucosa continues around the free border of the soft palate for a variable distance and is then replaced by nasal mucosa with its pseudostratified, ciliated columnar epithelium.

Specialized mucosa

Dorsal lingual mucosa. The superior surface of the tongue is rough and irregular (Fig. 9-38). A V-shaped line divides it into an anterior part, or body, and a posterior part, or base. The former comprises about two thirds of the length of the organ, and the latter forms the posterior one third. The

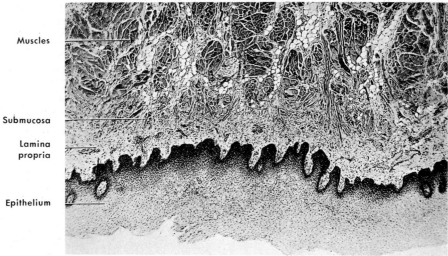

Muscles

Submucosa

Lamina
propria

Epithelium

Fig. 9-36. Mucous membrane on inferior surface of tongue.

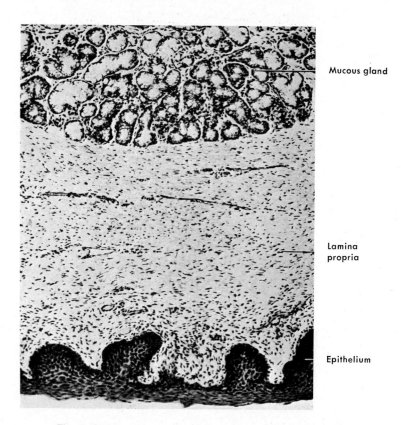

Mucous gland

Lamina
propria

Epithelium

Fig. 9-37. Mucous membrane from oral surface of soft palate.

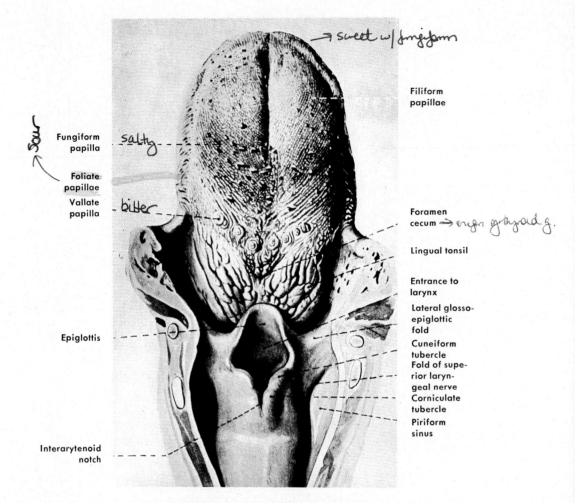

→ sweet w/ fungiform

Filiform
papillae

sour

Fungiform
papilla

salty

Foliate
papillae

Vallate
papilla

bitter

Foramen
cecum → origin of thyroid g.

Lingual tonsil

Entrance to
larynx

Lateral glosso-
epiglottic
fold

Epiglottis

Cuneiform
tubercle

Fold of supe-
rior laryn-
geal nerve

Corniculate
tubercle

Piriform
sinus

Interarytenoid
notch

Fig. 9-38. Surface view of human tongue. (From Sicher H and Tandler J: Anatomie für Zahnärzte, Vienna, 1928, Julius Springer Verlag.)

fact that these two parts develop embryologically from different visceral arches (see Chapter 1) accounts for the different source of nerves of the general senses: the anterior two thirds are supplied by the trigeminal nerve through its lingual branch and the posterior one third by the glossopharyngeal nerve.

The body and the base of the tongue differ widely in the structure of the mucous membrane. The anterior part can be termed the "papillary" and the posterior part the "lymphatic" portion of the dorsolingual mucosa. On the anterior part are found numerous fine-pointed, cone-shaped papillae that give it a velvetlike appearance. These projections, the filiform (thread-shaped) papillae, are epithelial structures containing a core of connective tissue from which secondary papillae protude toward the epithelium (Fig. 9-39, A). The covering epithelium is keratinized and

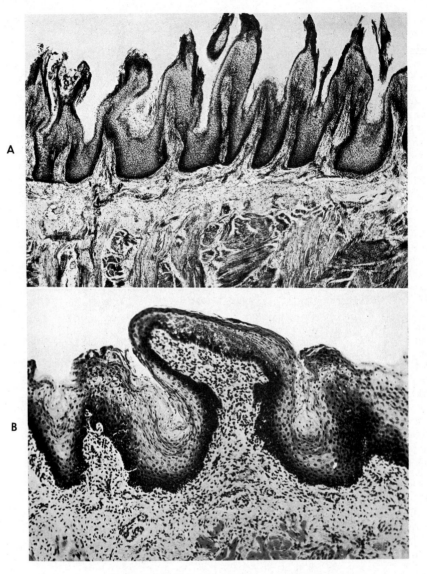

Fig. 9-39. A, Filiform, and **B,** fungiform papillae.

forms tufts at the apex of the dermal papilla. The filiform papillae do not contain taste buds.

Interspersed between the filiform papillae are the isolated fungiform (mushroom-shaped) papillae (Fig. 9-39, *B*), which are round, reddish prominences. Their color is derived from a rich capillary network visible through the relatively thin epithelium. Fungiform papillae contain a few (one to three) taste buds found only on their dorsal surface.

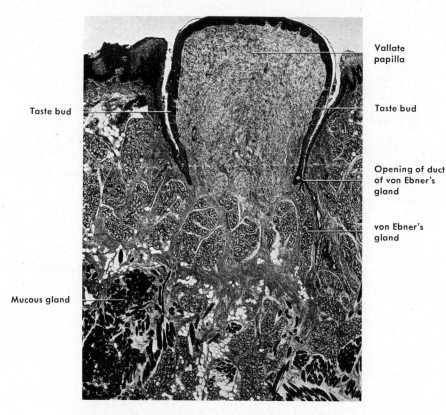

Taste bud

Vallate
papilla

Taste bud

Opening of duct
of von Ebner's
gland

von Ebner's
gland

Mucous gland

Fig. 9-40. Vallate (or circumvallate) papilla.

In front of the dividing V-shaped terminal sulcus, between the body and the base of the tongue, are eight to ten vallate (walled) papillae (Fig. 9-40). They do not protrude above the surface of the tongue but are bounded by a deep circular furrow so that their only connection to the substance of the tongue is at their narrow base. Their free surface shows numerous secondary papillae that are covered by a thin, smooth epithelium. On the lateral surface of the vallate papillae, the epithelium contains numerous taste buds. The ducts of small serous glands called von Ebner's glands open into the trough. They may serve to wash out the soluble elements of

food and are the main source of salivary lipase.

On the lateral border of the posterior parts of the tongue, sharp parallel clefts of varying length can often be observed. They bound narrow folds of the mucous membrane and are the vestige of the large foliate papillae found in many mammals. They contain taste buds.

Taste buds. Taste buds are small ovoid or barrel-shaped intraepithelial organs about 80 μm high and 40 μm thick (Fig. 9-41). They extend from the basal lamina to the surface of the epithelium. Their outer surface is almost covered by a few flat epithelial cells, which surround a small opening,

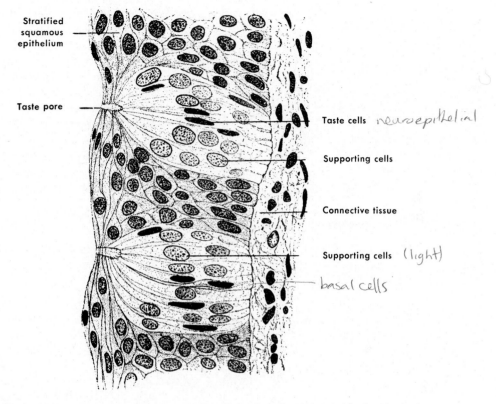

Stratified squamous epithelium

Taste pore

Taste cells neuroepithelial

Supporting cells

Connective tissue

Supporting cells (light)

basal cells

Fig. 9-41. Taste buds from slope of vallate papilla. (From Schaffer J: Lehrbuch der histologie und histogenese, ed 2, Leipzig, 1922, Wilhelm Engelmann.)

the *taste pore* (a taste bud may have more than one taste pore). It leads into a narrow space lined by the supporting cells of the taste bud. The outer supporting cells are arranged like the staves of a barrel. The inner and shorter ones are spindle shaped. Between the latter are arranged 10 to 12 neuroepithelial cells, the receptors of taste stimuli. They are slender, dark-staining cells that carry fingerlike processes at their superficial end. The fingerlike processes are visible at the ultrastructural level and resemble hairs at the light microscope level. The hairs reach into the space beneath the taste pore.

A rich plexus of nerves is found below the taste buds. Some fibers enter the epithelium and end in contact with the sensory cells of the taste bud.

Taste buds are numerous on the inner wall of the trough surrounding the vallate papillae, in the folds of the foliate papillae, on the posterior surface of the epiglottis, and on some of the fungiform papillae at the tip and the lateral borders of the tongue (Fig. 9-42).

The classic view maintains that the primary taste sensations, that is, sweet, salty, bitter, and sour, are perceived in different regions of the tongue and palate (sweet at the tip, salty at the lateral border of the tongue, bitter and sour on the palate and

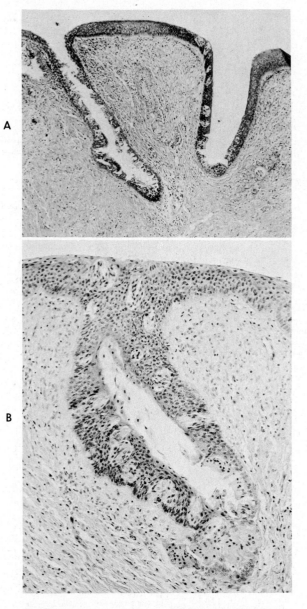

A

B

Fig. 9-42. A, Circumvallate papilla showing trough and numerous taste buds *(light areas)* **B,** Higher magnification of trough and taste buds.

also in the posterior part of the tongue—bitter in the middle and sour in the lateral areas of the tongue). The classic view also diagrammatically and arbitrarily correlates the distribution of the receptors for primary taste qualities with the different types of papillae (vallate papillae with bitter, foliate papillae with sour, taste buds of the fungiform papillae at the tip of the tongue with sweet and at the borders with salty taste). Bitter and sour taste sensations are mediated by the glossopharyngeal nerve, and sweet and salty taste are mediated by the intermediofacial nerve by the chorda tympani.

On the other hand, many authorities believe that taste cannot be broken down into these four primaries, sweet, sour, salty, and bitter, but that it consists of a range of stimuli that form a spectrum of sensations making up all taste senses. Taste occurs when a chemical substance contacts a receptor cell in the taste bud. Each taste bud is innervated by many fibers. The reception of a chemical substance fires the nerve fiber. Thus taste may be a continuum or a composite of the firing of many fibers.

At the angle of the V-shaped terminal groove on the tongue is located the foramen cecum, which represents the remnant of the thyroglossal duct (see Chapter 1). Posterior to the terminal sulcus, the surface of the tongue is irregularly studded with round or oval prominences, the lingual follicles. Each of these shows one or more lymph nodules, sometimes containing a germinal center (Fig. 9-43). Most of these prominences have a small pit at the center, the lingual crypt, which is lined with stratified squamous epithelium. Innumerable lymphocytes migrate into the crypts through the epithelium. Ducts of the small posterior lingual mucous glands open into the crypts. Together the lingual follicles form the lingual tonsil.

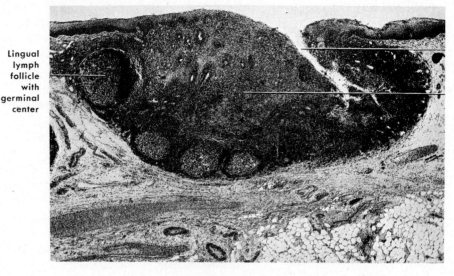

Lingual
lymph
follicle
with
germinal
center

Follicular
crypt

Lingual
follicle

Fig. 9-43. Lingual lymph follicle.

GINGIVAL SULCUS AND DENTOGINGIVAL JUNCTION
Gingival sulcus

The gingival sulcus or crevice is the name given to the invagination made by the gingiva as it joins with the tooth surface. The gingiva does not join the tooth at the gingival margin. It forms a small infolding known as the *sulcus*. The sulcus extends from the free gingival margin to the dentogingival junction. In health its depth is at the approximate level of the free gingival groove on the outer surface of the gingiva. The sulcus may be responsible for the formation of the groove since it leaves the gingival margin without firm support. The groove is believed to be formed by the functional folding of the free gingival margin during mastication. The sulcular (crevicular) epithelium is nonkeratinized in humans. It lacks epithelial ridges and so forms a smooth interface with the lamina propria. It is thinner than the epithelium of the gingiva. The sulcular epithelium is

continuous with the gingival epithelium and the attachment epithelium. These three epithelia have a continuous and coextensive basal lamina.

One view holds that the gingival sulcus is universally and normally present and as it deepens, a pathologic entity, the pocket, is formed. Another view holds that initially the gingiva attaches to the tooth completely and its gradual detachment to form the sulcus is the result of pathologic phenomena.

Dentogingival junction

The junction of the gingiva and the tooth is of great physiologic and clinical importance. This union is unique in many ways and may be a point of lessened resistance to mechanical forces and bacterial attack. The gingiva consists of two tissues maintaining the junction intact. Their biology differs. The dense, resilient lamina propria takes up impacts produced during mastication. In a similar sense so does the keratinized or parakeratinized surface of the gingiva. When the epithelium is injured, the injury is repaired by the turnover of cells and their ability to migrate. When the connective tissue is injured, ribosomes within the fibroblasts form molecules of the precursor protein of collagen (procollagen) and ground substances as well, contributing to repair.

Defense against bacterial injury is a function of the defense mechanism of the body. Macrophages, lymphocytes, plasma cells, polymorphonuclear leukocytes, and Langerhans cells protect against invasion and form antibodies against bacterial antigens in cooperation with keratinocytes through the keratinocyte's ability to form interferon. The lysosomes of the junctional epithelium may have a phagocytic function.

Both epithelium and connective tissue are attached to the tooth, and in health each contributes to the integrity of the dentogingival junction. Again the firmness of this junction is maintained by the gingival portion of the periodontal ligament. It is weakened by any situation that causes the collagen to break down (collagenolysis). The adherence of epithelium to the tooth is a function of the attachment (junctional) epithelium. It is weakened by any cause that injures the epithelium.

Development of junctional (attachment) epithelium. When the ameloblasts finish formation of the enamel matrix, they leave a thin membrane on the surface of the enamel, the *primary enamel cuticle*. This cuticle may be connected with the interprismatic enamel substance and the ameloblasts. The ameloblasts shorten after the primary enamel cuticle has been formed, and the epithelial enamel organ is reduced to a few layers of flat cuboid cells, which are then called *reduced enamel epithelium*. Under normal conditions it covers the entire enamel surface, extending to the cementoenamel junction (Fig. 9-44), and remains attached to the primary enamel cuticle. During eruption, the tip of the tooth approaches the oral mucosa, and the reduced enamel epithelium and the oral epithelium meet and fuse (Fig. 9-45). The remnant of the primary enamel cuticle after eruption is referred to as Nasmyth's membrane.

The epithelium that covers the tip of the crown degenerates in its center, and the crown emerges through this perforation into the oral cavity (Fig. 9-46). The reduced enamel epithelium remains organically attached to the part of the enamel that has not yet erupted. Once the tip of the crown has emerged, the reduced enamel epithelium is termed the *primary attachment epithelium.** Changes in keratin expression, as demonstrated by monoclonal antibody reactions to intermediate filaments, suggest that during the transition from ameloblast to junctional epithelium the changes in keratin expression occur as a form of all differentiations.

At the margin of the gingiva the attachment epithelium is continuous with the oral epithelium (Fig. 9-47). As the tooth erupts, the reduced enamel epithelium grows gradually shorter. A shallow groove, the *gingival sulcus* (Fig. 9-47), may develop between the gingiva and the surface of the tooth and extend around its circum-

---

*Some confusion may result if the student refers to the older literature in which the attachment epithelium is referred to as the epithelial attachment. It was first named the epithelial attachment *(Epithelansatz)* by Gottlieb, but after it was examined electron microscopically, it was renamed the junctional, or attachment, epithelium by Stern. This epithelium synthesizes the material that attaches it to the tooth. This material, its morphology, mode, and mechanism of function, is what is now called the epithelial attachment. Thus the cellular structure is referred to as junctional or attachment epithelium, and its extracellular tooth-attaching substance is referred to as the epithelial attachment.

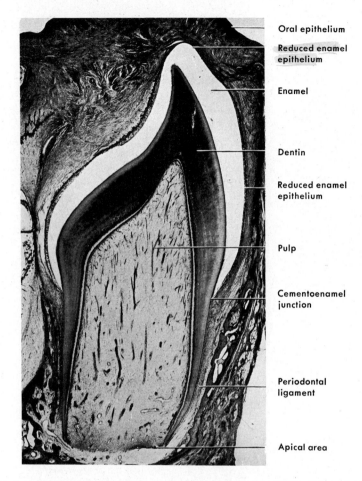

Oral epithelium

Reduced enamel epithelium

Enamel

Dentin

Reduced enamel epithelium

Pulp

Cementoenamel junction

Periodontal ligament

Apical area

Fig. 9-44. Human permanent incisor. Entire surface of enamel is covered by reduced enamel epithelium. Mature enamel is lost by decalcification. (From Gottlieb B and Orban B: Biology of the investing structures of the teeth. In Gordon SM, editor: Dental science and dental art, Philadelphia, 1938, Lea & Febiger.)

ference. It is bounded by the attachment epithelium at its base and by the gingival margin laterally. The gingiva encompassing the sulcus is the free, or marginal, gingiva.

Although the firmness and mechanical strength of the dentogingival junction is mainly attributable to the connective tissue attachment, the attachment of the epithelium to the enamel is by no means loose or weak. This can be demonstrated with ground histologic sections of frozen specimens where enamel and soft tissues are retained in their normal relation. When an attempt is made to detach the gingiva from the tooth in these preparations, the epithelium tears but does not peel off from the enamel surface (Fig. 9-48).

Shift of dentogingival junction. The position of the gingiva on the surface of the

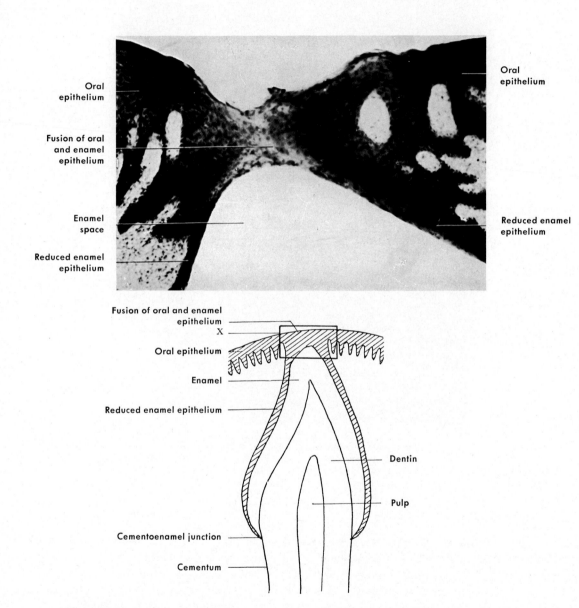

Oral
epithelium

Fusion of oral
and enamel
epithelium

Enamel
space

Reduced enamel
epithelium

Oral
epithelium

Reduced enamel
epithelium

Fusion of oral and enamel
epithelium

X

Oral epithelium

Enamel

Reduced enamel epithelium

Dentin

Pulp

Cementoenamel junction

Cementum

Fig. 9-45. Reduced enamel epithelium fuses with oral epithelium. X in diagram indicates area from which photomicrograph was taken.

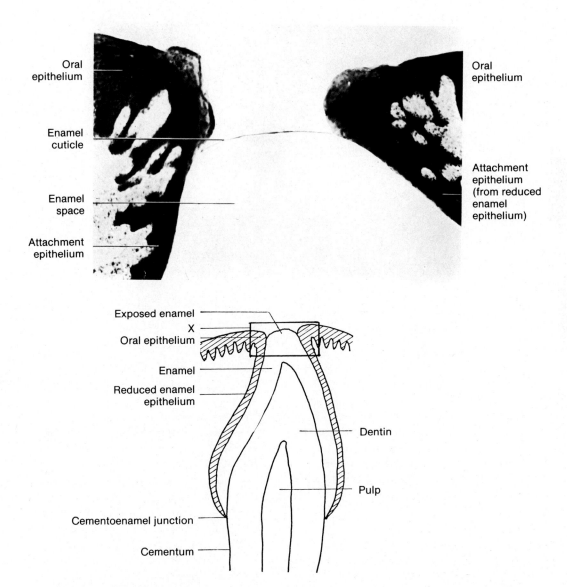

Fig. 9-46. Tooth emerges through perforation in fused epithelia. X in diagram indicates area from which photomicrograph was taken.

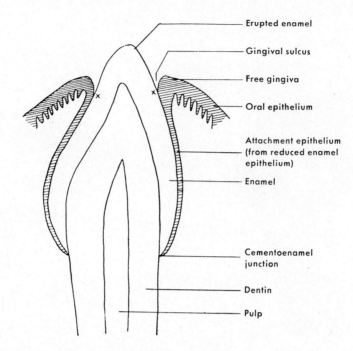

— Erupted enamel

— Gingival sulcus

— Free gingiva

— Oral epithelium

— Attachment epithelium (from reduced enamel epithelium)

— Enamel

— Cementoenamel junction

— Dentin

— Pulp

Fig. 9-47. Diagram of attached epithelial cuff and gingival sulcus at an early stage of tooth eruption. Bottom of sulcus at X.

tooth changes with time. When the tip of the enamel first emerges through the mucous membrane of the oral cavity, the epithelium covers almost the entire enamel (Fig. 9-49). The tooth erupts until it reaches the plane of occlusion (see Chapter 11). The attachment epithelium separates from the enamel surface gradually while the crown emerges into the oral cavity. When the tooth first reaches the plane of occlusion, one third to one fourth of the enamel still remains covered by the gingiva (Fig. 9-50). A gradual exposure of the crown follows. The actual movement of the teeth toward the occlusal plane is termed active eruption. This applies to the preclinical phase of eruption also. The separation of the primary attachment epithelium from the enamel is termed passive eruption. Further recession exposing the cementum

may ultimately occur. When the reduced enamel epithelium has disappeared, the primary attachment epithelium is replaced by a *secondary attachment epithelium* derived from the gingival epithelium.

There is a conceptual construct, called passive eruption, that may be useful in describing the various levels of attachment that may occur as the gingiva recedes onto the cementum. Some persons believe passive eruption to be a normal occurrence with aging. The belief that this is a "normal" occurrence is probably incorrect. Crown exposure involving passive eruption and further recession has been described in four stages. The first two may be physiologic. Many conceive of the last two as normal also, but they are probably pathologic.

First stage. The bottom of the gingival sulcus remains in the region of the enamel-

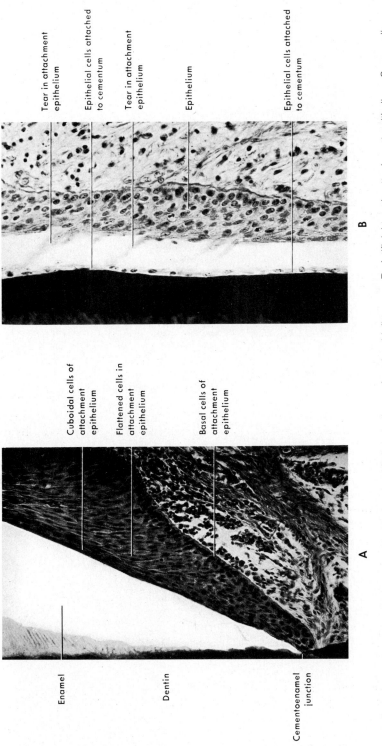

Tear in attachment epithelium

Epithelial cells attached to cementum

Tear in attachment epithelium

Epithelium

Epithelial cells attached to cementum

B

Cuboidal cells of attachment epithelium

Flattened cells in attachment epithelium

Basal cells of attachment epithelium

Enamel

Dentin

Cementoenamel junction

A

Fig. 9-48. A, Arrangement of cells in attachment epithelium indicates functional influences. **B,** Artificial tear in attachment epithelium. Some cells remain attached to cementum, while others bridge tear. (**A** from Orban B: Z Stomatol 22:353, 1924; **B** from Orban B and Mueller E: J Am Dent Assoc 16:1206, 1929.)

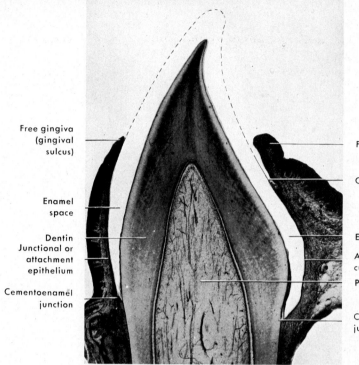

Free gingiva
(gingival
sulcus)

Enamel
space

Dentin
Junctional or
attachment
epithelium

Cementoenamel
junction

Free gingiva

Gingival sulcus

Enamel space

Attachment epithelium
cuff

Pulp

Cementoenamel
junction

Fig. 9-49. Attachment epithelium and gingival sulcus in erupting tooth. *Dotted line,* Erupted part of enamel. Enamel is lost in decalcification. (From Kronfeld R: J Am Dent Assoc 18:382, 1936.)

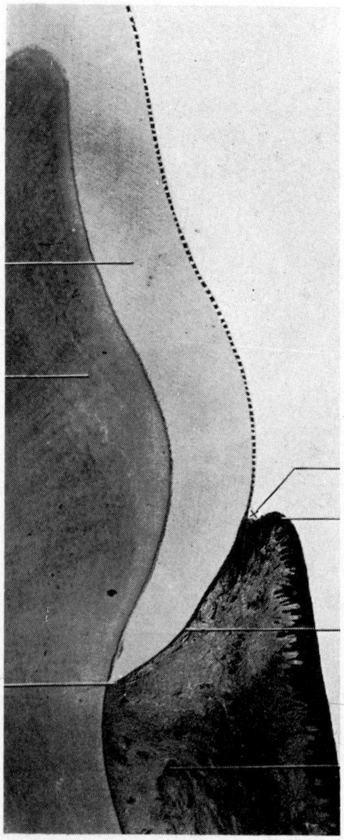

Fig. 9-50. Tooth in occlusion. One fourth of enamel is still covered by attachment epithelium. (From Kronfeld R: J Am Dent Assoc 18:382, 1936.)

Enamel
space

Dentin

Gingival sulcus

Free gingiva

Attachment
epithelium

Cementoenamel
junction

Alveolar crest

covered crown for some time, and the apical end of the attachment epithelium (reduced enamel epithelium) stays at the cementoenamel junction (Fig. 9-51). This relation persists in primary teeth almost up to 1 year of age before shedding and in permanent teeth, usually to the age of 20 or 30 years. However, this relation is subject to a wide range of variation (Fig. 9-52).

Second stage. The bottom of the gingival sulcus is still on the enamel, and the apical end of the attachment epithelium has shifted to the surface of the cementum (Fig. 9-53).

The downgrowth of the attachment epithelium along the cementum is but one facet of the shift of the dentogingival junction. This entails dissolution of fiber bundles that were anchored in the cervical parts of the cementum, now covered by the epithelium, and an apical shift of the gingival and transseptal fibers. The destruction of the fibers may be caused by enzymes formed by the epithelial cells, by plaque

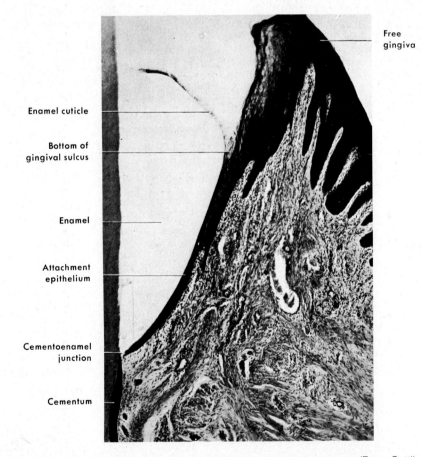

Fig. 9-51. Attachment epithelium on enamel. First stage of crown exposure. (From Gottlieb B and Orban B: Biology and pathology of the tooth [translated by M Diamond], New York, 1938, The Macmillan Co.)

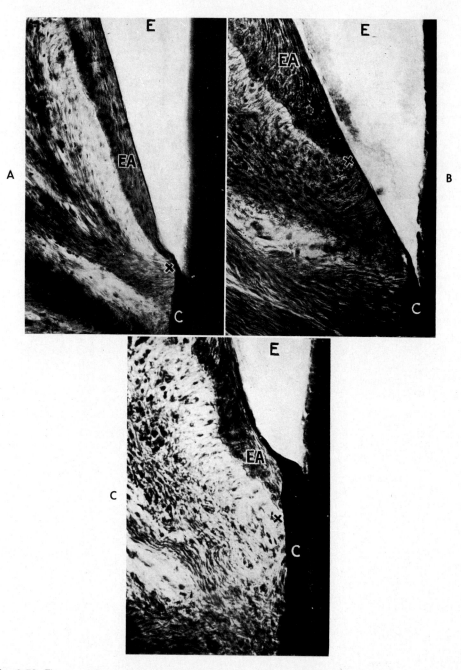

Fig. 9-52. Three sections of same tooth showing different relations of tissues at cementoenamel junction. **A,** Attachment epithelium reaching to cementoenamel junction. **B,** Attachment epithelium ends coronally to cementoenamel junction. **C,** Attachment epithelium covers part of cementum. Cementum overlaps edge of enamel. *C,* Cementum; *E,* enamel (lost in decalcification); *EA,* attachment epithelium; *X,* end of attachment epithelium. (From Orban B: J Am Dent Assoc 17:1977, 1930.)

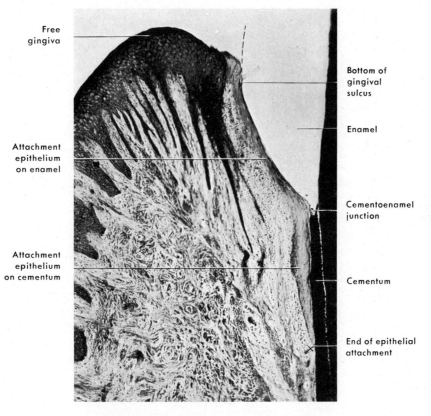

Fig. 9-53. Attachment epithelium partly on enamel and partly on cementum. Second stage of passive tooth exposure. (From Gottlieb B and Orban B: Biology and pathology of the tooth [translated by M Diamond], New York, 1938, The Macmillan Co.)

metabolites or enzymes, or by immunologic reactions as manifestations of periodontal disease. This stage of tooth exposure may persist to the age of 40 years or later.

Third stage. When the bottom of the gingival sulcus is at the cementoenamel junction, the epithelium attachment is entirely on the cementum, and the enamel-covered crown is fully exposed (Fig. 9-54). This stage in the exposure of a tooth no longer is a passive manifestation. The epithelium shifts along the surface of the tooth and does not remain at the cementoenamel junction. This discontinuous and slow process is regarded as the body's attempt to maintain an intact dentogingival junction in the face of factors that cause its deterioration.

Fourth stage. The fourth stage represents recession of the gingiva. When the entire attachment is on cementum, the gingiva may appear normal but is believed to have receded as a result of pathology (Figs. 9-55 and 9-56). It may occur without other clinical evidence of inflammatory periodontal disease.

The rates of crown exposure and reces-

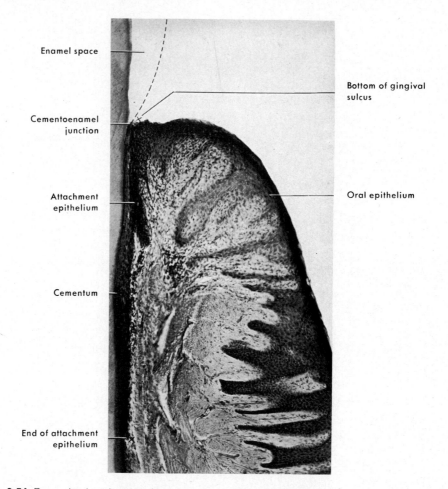

Enamel space

Cementoenamel junction

Attachment epithelium

Cementum

End of attachment epithelium

Bottom of gingival sulcus

Oral epithelium

Fig. 9-54. Recession is at bottom of gingival sulcus at cementoenamel junction, and attachment epithelium is on cementum. (From Gottlieb B: J Am Dent Assoc 14:2178, 1927.)

sion vary in different persons. In some cases the fourth stage is observed in persons during their twenties. In others, even at 50 years of age or older the teeth are still in the first or second stage. The rate varies also in different teeth of the same jaw and on different surfaces of the same tooth. One side may be in the first stage and the other in the second or even the fourth stage (Fig. 9-56).

Gradual exposure of the tooth makes it necessary to distinguish between the anatomic and the clinical crowns of the tooth (Fig. 9-57). That part of the tooth covered by enamel is the anatomic crown. The clinical crown is the part of the tooth exposed in the oral cavity. In the first and second stages the clinical crown is smaller than the anatomic crown. With recession (third stage) the entire enamel-covered part of the tooth is exposed, and the clinical crown is equal to the anatomic crown. Later the

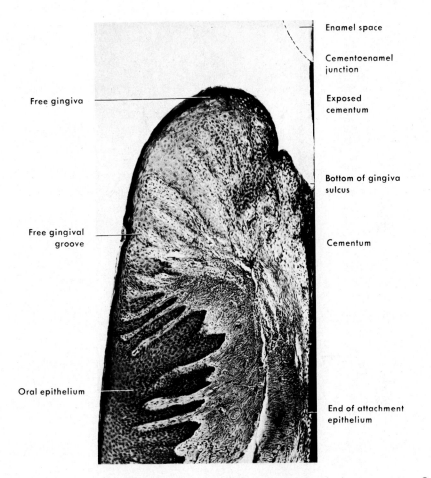

Enamel space

Cementoenamel
junction

Free gingiva

Exposed
cementum

Bottom of gingiva
sulcus

Free gingival
groove

Cementum

Oral epithelium

End of attachment
epithelium

Fig. 9-55. Recession. Bottom of gingival sulcus and attachment epithelium both on cementum. Continued recession may reduce the width of gingiva. (From Gottlieb B: J Am Dent Assoc 14:2178, 1927.)

clinical crown is larger than the anatomic crown because parts of the root have been exposed (fourth stage). This type of crown exposure is to be differentiated from crown exposure that is produced by periodontal disease, loss of attachment (bone), and pocket formation.

Sulcus and cuticles. For a long time the epithelium was believed only to contact but not attach to the enamel. The contact was supposed to be maintained by the turgor of the connective tissue elements of the gingiva. Thus a capillary space was supposed to exist between the gingiva and enamel to the cementoenamel junction. Gottlieb and Orban demonstrated the presence of an organic attachment, which they termed the epithelial attachment. The mode or mechanism of the epithelial attachment is very important. The classic

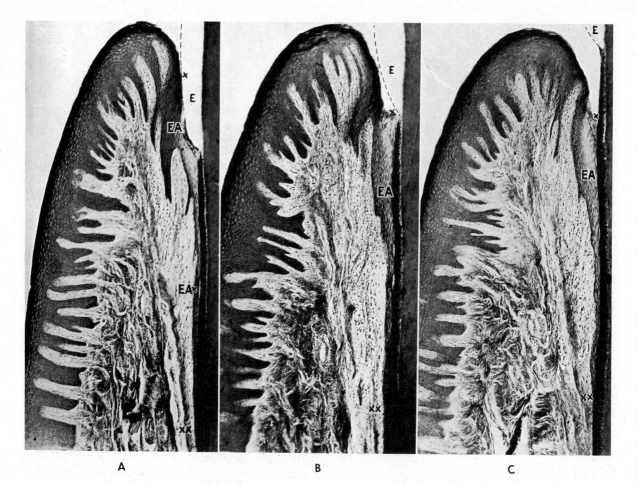

Fig. 9-56. Three sections of same tooth showing different relation of soft to hard tissues. **A,** Bottom of sulcus on enamel (second stage). **B,** Bottom of sulcus at cementoenamel junction (third stage). **C,** Bottom of sulcus on cementum (fourth stage). *E,* Enamel lost in decalcification *(dotted line); EA,* attachment epithelium; X, bottom of gingival sulcus; XX, end of attachment epithelium.

view proposed by Gottlieb and Orban involves the primary cuticle mediating an organic union between ameloblasts and the enamel. When the ameloblasts are replaced by the oral epithelium, a secondary cuticle is formed. When the epithelium proliferates beyond the cementoenamel junction, the cuticle extends along the cementum (Figs. 9-58 and 9-59). Secondary enamel cuticle and the cemental cuticle are re-

ferred to as dental cuticle. These cuticles are microscopically evident as an amorphous material between the attachment epithelium and the tooth.

Deepening of sulcus (pocket formation). The gingival sulcus forms when the tip of the crown emerges through the oral mucosa. It deepens as a result of separation of the reduced dental epithelium from the actively erupting tooth. At first after the tip of the

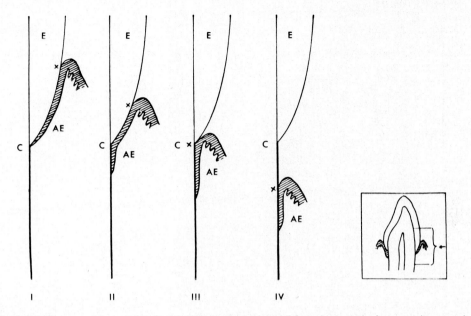

Fig. 9-57. Diagram of four stages in eruption. In stages I and II (passive eruption), anatomic crown is larger than clinical crown. III and IV represent recession. In stage III, anatomic and clinical crowns are equal. In stage IV, clinical crown is larger than anatomic crown. Arrow in small diagram indicates area from which drawings were made. *C*, Cementoenamel junction; *E*, enamel; *AE*, attachment epithelium; *X*, bottom of gingival sulcus.

crown has appeared in the oral cavity, the epithelium separates rapidly from the surface of the tooth. Later, when the tooth comes to occlude with its antagonist, the separation of the attachment from the surface of the tooth slows down.

The formation and relative depth of the gingival sulcus at different ages is a subject of considerable interest. At one time it was believed that from the time the tip of the crown had pierced the oral mucosa, the gingival sulcus extended to the cementoenamel junction (Fig. 9-60, I). It was assumed that the attachment of the gingival epithelium to the tooth occurred only at the cementoenamel junction. The concept of the epithelial attachment introduced by Gottlieb and Orban showed that no cleft existed between epithelium and enamel

and that these tissues were organically connected. The gingival sulcus was shown to be a shallow groove, the bottom of which is at the point of separation of attached epithelium from the tooth (Fig. 9-60, II).

Some investigators contended that the deepening of the gingival sulcus was caused by a tear in the attached epithelium (Fig. 9-60, III). Others believed, however, that deepening occurred as a result of the downgrowth of the oral epithelium alongside the reduced enamel epithelium (primary attachment epithelium), as shown in Fig. 9-60, IV.

What the depth of a normal gingival sulcus should be has been a frequent source of argument. Under normal conditions the depth of the sulcus is variable; 45% of all measured sulci are below 0.5 mm. The av-

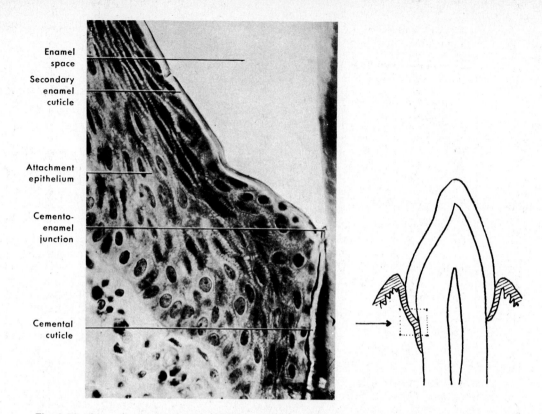

Enamel
space

Secondary
enamel
cuticle

Attachment
epithelium

Cemento-
enamel
junction

Cemental
cuticle

Fig. 9-58. "Secondary enamel cuticle" follows attachment epithelium to cementum forming the dental cuticle. Arrow in diagram indicates area from which photomicrograph was taken.

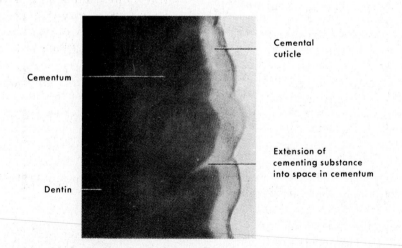

Cementum

Dentin

Cemental
cuticle

Extension of
cementing substance
into space in cementum

Fig. 9-59. Cemental cuticle extending into cementum. (From Gottlieb B and Orban B: Biology and pathology of the tooth [translated by M Diamond], New York, 1938, The Macmillan Co.)

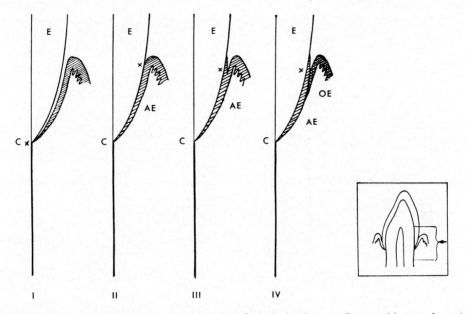

Fig. 9-60. Diagram of different views on formation of gingival sulcus as discussed in text. Arrow in small diagram indicates area from which drawings were made.

erage sulcus is 1.8 mm. The more shallow a sulcus, the more likely that the gingival margin is not inflamed.

Lymphocytes and plasma cells are routinely seen in the connective tissue at the bottom of the gingival sulcus and below the attachment epithelium. Langerhans cells migrate to the sulcular and oral epithelium when infection or inflammation is present. These defense reactions to the bacteria in the gingival sulcus constitute barriers against the invasion of bacteria and the penetration of toxins. The bacterial products may act directly or indirectly via the immune responses.

Epithelial attachment. The ultrastructural attachment of the ameloblasts (primary attachment epithelium) to the tooth was first shown by Stern and confirmed by Listgarten and Schroeder, among others, to be basal lamina to which hemidesmosomes are attached (Fig. 9-6, *A*). This mode of attachment is referred to as the *epithelial attachment*. The secondary attachment epithelium composed of cells derived from the oral epithelium forms an epithelial attachment identical with that of the primary attachment epithelium, that is, a basal lamina and hemidesmosomes. Both reduced ameloblasts and gingival epithelial cells have been shown to form an electron microscopic basal lamina on enamel and cementum. Hemidesmosomes of these cells attach to the basal lamina in the same manner as all basal cells. Thus there is an epithelial attachment. It is submicroscopic, approximately 40 nm (400 Å) wide, and formed by the attachment epithelium. Its exact biochemical nature is unknown, but some of its constituents have been grossly identified. Apparently these constituents are produced by the epithelium. The adhe-

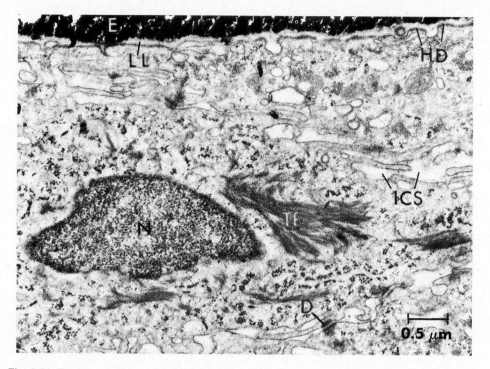

Fig. 9-61. Electron micrograph of cells of attachment epithelium of rat incisor adjacent to enamel, *E.* Hemidesmosomes, *HD,* abut on and attach to lamina lucida, *LL.* Lamina densa is fully calcified and cannot be demonstrated in this calcified specimen. Lamina lucida is approximately 40 nm (400 Å) wide. Note that intercellular space, *ICS,* is wider than lamina lucida. Cells are attached to each other by desmosomes, *D. N,* Nucleus; *Tf,* a bundle of tonofilaments. (From Grant DA, Stern IB, and List-garten MA: Periodontics in the tradition of Orban and Gottlieb, ed 6, St Louis, 1988, The CV Mosby Co.)

sive forces in this zone are molecular in nature and act across a distance smaller than 40 nm (400 Å).

The epithelial attachment resembles an electron microscopic basal lamina. The cells of the attachment epithelium are held to this structure by hemidesmosomes (Fig. 9-61).

Migration of attachment epithelium. Mitotic figures have been observed in cells adjacent to the tooth. When tritiated thymidine is administered to experimental animals, cells about to undergo DNA synthesis pick up radioactive thymidine. The radioactivity can be detected in histologic sections by the use of photographic emulsion. After the administration of the tritiated thymidine, labeled cells are found in the attachment epithelium. Can it be that the cells of the attachment epithelium adjacent to the tooth are basal cells?

When cells leave the stratum germinativum, they become specialized. For instance, in oral epithelium cells specialize and undergo keratinization. In attachment epithelium the cells may remain relatively unspecialized and synthesize a basal lamina (the epithelial attachment). They then migrate over it, with their attachment being maintained by the hemidesmosomes. In general, a cell once specialized neither synthesizes DNA nor divides.

The time it takes for labeled attachment epithelial cells to migrate and desquamate is called transit time. It is less than 144 hours for the continuously growing incisor of rodents (Fig. 9-62), about 72 to 120 hours for primates, and presumably much the same for humans.

How can the cells be attached to the tooth if they are actively migrating? The same mechanism is present at the epidermis—connective tissue junction. The epithelial cells are affixed to the connective tissue through the basal lamina, yet they can detach from it and migrate toward the surface. Similarly, in healing wounds the epithelial cells form a basal lamina on the connective tissue and migrate over it to epithelialize the wound. At no time is the epithelium loose from the connective tissue. The two tissues are in intimate connection. Picture the epithelial attachment as the basal lamina of the attachment (junctional) epithelium. It turns about the most apical cell and extends up along the tooth surface. The cells can then migrate along this basal lamina (Fig. 9-61). The hemidesmosomes hold the cells to this structure so that the strength of the attachment is not diminished despite the migration. The physical integrity of the attachment is maintained during the four stages of tooth exposure by this same biologic mechanism.

The reduced ameloblasts do not divide; however, on the other hand, basal cells adjacent to the tooth do divide and then migrate up and along the tooth, desquamating in 4 to 6 days. They seem to migrate from a mitotically DNA-synthetic active area, a locus of proliferation, in the basal layer at the junction of the oral and the attachment epithelia. There are differences in the blood group carbohydrates of the junctional epithelium, indicating that it is

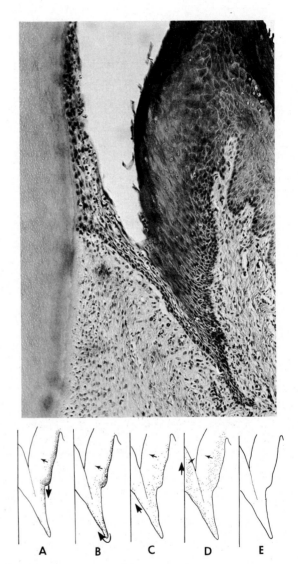

Fig. 9-62. Composite of labeled cells and their positions: **A,** ½ hour; **B,** 6 hours; **C,** 24 hours; **D,** 72 hours; and **E,** 144 hours after administration of tritiated thymidine to rats. Diagram of morphology of attachment epithelium and adjacent tissues is representative of gingiva on cemental (oral) surface of continuously growing rat incisor. *Large arrows,* Migration of attachment (junctional) epithelium toward and along tooth surface. *Small arrows,* Migration of cells toward sulcus. (From Anderson GC and Stern IB: Periodontics 4:115, 1966.)

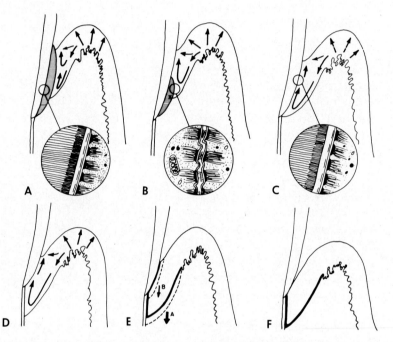

Fig. 9-63. Dynamics of migration of tissues of dentoepithelial junction. **A,** Dentoepithelial junction first consists of reduced ameloblasts attached by hemidesmosomes to lamina lucida. Oral epithelial cells migrate to gingival surface and keratinize *(arrows)*. Some cells join reduced enamel epithelium, to which they attach. **B,** Reduced ameloblasts are gradually displaced by junctional epithelium, cells of which are joined by desmosomes and by tight and gap junctions. When reduced enamel epithelium gives rise to junctional epithelium *(x)*, mitotic activity is increased. Here cells of outer enamel epithelium, and possibly stratum intermedium, form a locus of proliferation. **C,** With complete replacement of reduced enamel epithelium by junctional epithelium, attachment occurs by same mechanism as shown in **A, D,** In time junctional epithelium may be found attaching to both enamel and cementum. How does this apical migration occur? **E,** Junctional epithelium renews itself in a matter of days, as does gingival epithelium. Cells migrate in pathways denoted by arrows in **D.** Cells of junctional epithelium travel from basal lamina to epithelial attachment. In inflammation, basal cells at *a* migrate apically and laterally into areas of collagenolysis. They form new basal lamina. Arrow at *b* represents deepening of sulcus. **F,** Even when junctional epithelium has completely migrated onto cementum, attachment is still mediated by basal lamina and by hemidesmosomes.

a still-dividing, relatively undifferentiated tissue.

While the reduced ameloblasts are still present, the cells of the oral epithelium join them by forming desmosomes. Gradually the reduced enamel epithelium is lost, and the cells of the oral epithelium contact the tooth surface, there forming hemidesmosomes and a lamina lucida, by means of which the cells attach themselves to the tooth. The apical migration of the sulcus is the result of a detachment of basal cells and a reestablishment of their epithelial attachment at a more apical level. It is not the result of degeneration and peeling off of the most coronal cells of the attachment epithelium. The mechanism of sulcus deepening by the deepening of splits and so forth (Fig. 9-62) is not accurate since the attachment is formed by the more deeply located basal cells (Fig. 9-63). The intercellular spaces of the junctional epithelium are large. There are relatively few tight junctions. The spaces are easily penetrated by cells and proteins in transit. Perhaps toxic or inflammatory influences diminish the ability of the basal cells to synthesize DNA or otherwise interfere with the physiology of these cells. Perhaps collagenolysis destroys the subjacent collagen fibers, permitting the epithelium to migrate apically. Perhaps immunologically competent cells or antibody complexes produce tissue damage and permit the epithelium to migrate apically. In any event the junctional epithelium moves apically, replicates a new basal lamina, and reestablishes the epithelial attachment. If this results in a deepening of the sulcus, as gauged by a difference in the position of the top of the epithelial attachment relative to the marginal gingiva, a pocket will have formed.

The junctional epithelium is best regarded as a nondifferentiating, nonkeratinizing tissue lacking a gradient of change in cell types such as is present in the gingival epithelium. The intermediate filaments found in the junctional epithelium differ from those found in the keratinizing oral epithelia.

CLINICAL CONSIDERATIONS

It is essential to be thoroughly familiar with the structure and biologic interrelations of the various periodontal tissues in order to understand the pathogenesis of periodontal disease. Periodontal disturbances produce a deepened gingival sulcus as a response to plaque toxins and the subsequent immunologic response. Reduction in pocket depth is the primary objective of treatment. Treatment methods should be judged by their ability to reduce the depth of pockets and to prevent their recurrence.

The level of the gingival attachment to the tooth plays an important role in restorative dentistry. In young persons the clinical crown is smaller than the anatomic crown. It is therefore very difficult to prepare a tooth properly for an abutment or crown in young individuals. Moreover, when recession occurs at a later time, the restoration may require replacement.

When the root is exposed by recession and a restoration is to be placed, the preparation need not extend to the gingiva. The first requirement is that the restoration be adapted to mechanical needs. In extension of the gingival margin of any restoration the following rules should be observed. If the gingiva is still on the enamel and the gingival papilla fills the entire interdental space, the gingival margin of a cavity should be placed at the sulcus. Special care should be taken to avoid injury to the gingiva and the dentogingival junction and to prevent premature recession of the gingiva. When periodontal disease is present, treatment should precede the placing of a restoration. If the gingiva has receded to the cementum and the gingival papilla does not fill the interdental space, the margin of a cavity need not necessarily be carried to the gingiva.

With gingival recession and exposure of the cervical part of the anatomic root, cemental caries or abrasion may occur. Improperly constructed clasps, overzealous scaling, and strongly abrasive dentrifices may result in pronounced abrasion. After loss of the cementum, the dentin may be extremely sensitive to thermal or chemical stimuli. Desensitizing drugs, judiciously applied, may be used to accelerate sclerosis of the tubules and reparative dentin formation.

The difference in the structure of the submucosa in various regions of the oral cavity is of great clinical importance. Whenever the submucosa consists of a layer of loose connective tissue, edema or hemorrhage can cause much swelling, and infection can spread speedily and extensively.

Injections should be made into loose submucous connective tissue (i.e., the fornix and the alveolar mucosa). The only place in the palate where larger amounts of fluid can be injected without damaging the tissues is the loose connective tissue in the furrow between the palatal and the alveolar processes (Fig. 9-21).

The gingiva is exposed to heavy mechanical stresses during mastication. Moreover, the epithelial attachment to the tooth is relatively weak, and injuries or infections can cause permanent damage. Keratinization of the gingiva may afford relative protection. Therefore steps taken to increase keratinization can be considered preventive measures. One of the methods of including keratinization is by massage or brushing, which acts directly by stimulation and by minimizing plaque accumulation.

Unfavorable mechanical irritation of the gingiva may ensue from sharp edges of carious cavities, overhanging fillings or crowns, and accumulation of plaque. These may cause chronic inflammation of the gingival tissue.

Many systemic diseases cause characteristic changes in the oral mucosa. For instance, metal poisoning (lead, bismuth) causes characteristic discoloration of the gingival margin. Leukemia, pernicious anemia, and other blood dyscrasias can be diagnosed by characteristic infiltrations of the oral mucosa. In the first stages of measles, small red spots with bluish white centers can be seen in the mucous membrane of the cheeks, even before the skin rash appears. They are known as Koplik's spots. Endocrine disturbances, including those of the sex hormones and of the pancreas, may be reflected in the oral mucosa.

Changes of the tongue are sometimes diagnostically significant. In scarlet fever the atrophy of the lingual mucosa causes the peculiar redness of the strawberry tongue. Systemic diseases such as pernicious anemia and vitamin deficiencies, especially vitamin B—complex deficiency, lead to characteristic changes such as magenta tongue and beefy red tongue.

In denture construction it is important to observe the firmness or looseness of the mucous membrane. In denture-bearing areas the mucosa should be firm.

In old age the mucous membrane of the mouth may atrophy. It is then thin and parchmentlike. The atrophy of the lingual papillae leaves the upper surface of the tongue smooth, shiny and varnished in appearance. Atrophy of the major and minor salivary glands may lead to xerostomia (dry mouth) and sometimes to a secondary atrophy of the mucous membrane. In a large percentage of individuals the sebaceous glands of the cheek are visible as fairly large, yellowish patches called Fordyce spots. They do not represent a pathologic change (Fig. 9-33).

REFERENCES

Adams D: Surface coatings of cells in the oral epithelium of the human fetus, J Anat 118:61, 1974.

Ainamo J and Löe H: Anatomical characteristics of gingiva. A clinical and microscopic study of the free and attached gingiva, J Periodontol 37:5, 1966.

Altman LC et al.: Culture and characterization of rat junctional epithelium, J Periodont Res 23:91, 1988.

Anderson GS and Stern IB: The proliferation and migration of the attachment epithelium on the cemental surface of the rat incisor, Periodontics 4:115, 1966.

Andersson A, Klinge B, and Warfvinge K: New views on the construction of the human gingival epithelium, J Clin Periodontal 14:63, 1987.

Arvidson D and Friberg U: Human taste: response and tastebud number in fungiform papillae, Science 209:807, 1980.

Barker DS: The dendritic cell system in human gingival epithelium, Arch Oral Biol 12:203, 1967.

Barnett ML: Mast cells in the epithelial layer of human gingiva, J Ultrastruct Res 43:247, 1973.

Barnett ML and Szabó G: Gap junctions in human gingival keratinized epithelium, J Periodont Res 8:117, 1973.

Baume LJ: The structure of the epithelial attachment revealed by phase contrast microscopy, J Periodontol 24:99, 1953.

Beagrie GS and Skougaard MR: Observations in the life cycle of the gingival epithelial cells of mice as revealed by autoradiography, Acta Odontol Scand 20:15, 1962.

Beidler LN and Smallman RLS: Renewal of cells within taste buds, J Cell Biol 27:263, 1965.

Bergstrasser PR, Tigelaar RE, and Streilein JW: Thy-1 antigen-bearing dendritic cells in murine epidermis are derived from bone marrow precursors, J Invest Dermatol 83:83, 1984.

Bergstrasser PR et al.: Origin and function of Thy-1[+] dendritic epidermal cells in mice, J Invest Dermatol (suppl 1)85:85, 1985.

Bickenbach JR and Mackenzie IC: Identification and localization of label-retaining cells in hamster epithelia, J Invest Dermatol 82:618, 1984.

Bjercke S, Elgo J, Braathen L, and Thorsby E: Enriched epidermal cells are potent antigen-presenting cells for T cells, J Invest Dermatol 83:286, 1984.

Bolden TE: Histology of oral pigmentation, J Periodontol 31:361, 1960.

Bradley RM and Mistretta CM: The morphological and functional development of fetal gustatory recep-tors. In Emmelin N and Zotterman Y, editors: Oral physiology, Oxford, England, 1972, Pergamon Press, Ltd.

Bradley RM and Stern IB: The development of the human taste bud during the foetal period, J Anat 101:743, 1967.

Breathnach SM, Fox PA, Neises GR, Stanley JR, et al.: A unique epithelial basement membrane antigen defined by a monoclonal antibody (KF-1), J Invest Dermatol 80:392, 1983.

Buck D: The uptake of H[3] proline in the guinea pig gingiva and palate, J Periodontol 4:94, 1969.

Carlos JP, Brunelle JA, and Wolfe MD: Attachment loss vs. pocket depth as indicators of periodontal disease: a methologic note, J Periodont Res 22:524, 1987.

Chen S-Y, Gerson S, and Meyer J: The fusion of Merkel cell granules with a synapse-like structure, J Invest Dermatol 61:290, 1973.

Clark RAF: Fibronectin in the skin, J Invest Dermatol 81:475, 1983.

Clausen H et al.: Differentiation-dependent expression of keratins in human oral epithelia, J Invest Dermatol 86:249, 1986.

Cleaton-Jones P and Fleisch L: A comparative study of the surface of keratinized and non-keratinized oral epithelia, J Periodont Res 8:366, 1973.

Cohen RL, Crawford JM, and Chambers DA: Thy-1[+] epidermal cells are not demonstrable in rat and human skin, J Invest Dermatol 87:30, 1986.

Dale BA: Purification and characterization of a basic protein from the stratum corneum of mammalian epidermis, Biochem Biophys Acta 491:193, 1977.

Dale BA, Holbrook KA, and Steinert PM: Assembly of stratum corneum basic protein and keratin filaments in macrofibrils, Nature 276:729, 1978.

Dale BA and Ling S-Y: Evidence of a precursor form of stratum corneum basic protein in rat epidermis, Biochemistry 18:35, 1979.

Dale BA and Ling S-Y: Immunologic cross-reaction of stratum corneum basic protein and a keratohyalin granule protein, J Invest Dermatol 72:257, 1979.

Dale BA, Lonsdale-Eccles JD, and Lynley AM: Two dimensional analysis of rat oral epithelium and epidermis, Arch Oral Biol 27:529, 1982.

Dale BA, Resing KA, and Lonsdale-Eccles JD: Filaggrin: a keratin filament associated protein, Ann NY Acad Sci 455:330, 1985.

Dale BA, Smith S, Clausen H, et al.: Use of antibodies to epithelial keratins and keratohyalin, IADR Abst 63:167, (special issue), 1984 (abstract).

Dale BA and Stern IB: Keratohyalin granule proteins, J Dent Res 53:143, 1975.

Dale BA and Stern IB: SDS polyacrylamide electrophoresis of proteins of newborn rat skin. I. Cell strata and nuclear proteins. J Invest Dermatol 65:220, 1975.

Dale BA and Stern IB: SDS polyacrylamide electrophoresis of proteins of newborn rat skin. II. Keratohyalin and stratum corneum proteins, J Invest Dermatol 65:223, 1975.

Dale BA, Stern IB, and Clagett J: Initial characterization of the proteins of keratinized epithelium of rat oral mucosa. Arch Oral Biol 22:75, 1977.

Dale BA, Stern IB, Rabin M, et al.: The identification of fibrous proteins in fetal rat epidermis by electrophoretic and immunologic techniques, J Invest Dermatol 66:230, 1976.

Dale BA and Thompson WL: Stratum corneum basic protein of keratinized rat oral epithelia, J Dent Res 57:222, 1978.

Dale BA, Thompson WB, and Stern IB: Distribution of histidine-rich basic protein, a possible keratin matrix protein, in the oral epithelium, Arch Oral Biol 27:535, 1982.

Daniels TE: Human mucosal Langerhans cells: postmortem identification of regional variations in oral mucosa, J Invest Dermatol 82:21, 1984.

DeHan R and Graziadei PPC: Functional anatomy of frog's taste organs, Experientia 27:823, 1971.

Desjardins RP, Winkelmann RK, and Gonzalez JB: Comparison of nerve endings in normal gingiva with those in mucosa covering edentulous alveolar ridges, J Dent Res 50:867, 1971.

DeWaal RMW, Semeijn JT, Cornelissen IMH, et al.: Epidermal Langerhans cells contain intermediate sized filaments of the Vimentin type: an immunocytologic study, J Invest Dermatol 82:602, 1984.

Dezutter-Dambuyant C: Immunogold technique applied to simultaneous identification of T6 and HLA-DR antigens on Langerhans cells by electron microscopy, J Invest Dermatol 84:465, 1985.

Dixon AD: The position, incidence and origin of sensory nerve terminations in oral mucous membrane, Arch Oral Biol 7:39, 1962.

Edelson RL and Fink JM: The immunologic function of skin, Sci Am 252:46, 1985.

Egelberg J: The blood vessels of the dentogingival junction, J Periodont Res 1:163, 1966.

El-Labban NG and Kramer IRH: On the so-called microgranules in the non-keratinized buccal epithelium, J Ultrastruct Res 48:377, 1974.

Emslie RD and Weinmann JP: The architectural pattern of the boundary between epithelium and connective tissue of the gingiva in the rhesus monkey, Anat Rec 105:35, 1949.

Farbman AI: Electron microscope study of a small cytoplasmic structure in rat oral epithelium, J Cell Biol 21:491, 1964.

Farbman AI: Electron microscope study of the developing taste bud in rat fungiform papillae, Dev Biol 11:110, 1965.

Farbman AI: Plasma membrane changes during keratinization, Anat Rec 156:269, 1966.

Farbman AI: Structure of chemoreceptors. In Symposium on foods. Chemistry and physiology of flavors, Westport, Conn, 1967, Avi Publishing Co.

Flotte TJ, Murphy GF, and Bhan AK: Demonstration of T-200 on human Langerhans cell surface membranes, J Invest Dermatol 82:535, 1984.

Fortman GJ and Winkelmann RK: The Merkel cell in oral human mucosa, J Dent Res 56:1303, 1977.

Frank RM and Cimasoni G: Electron microscopic study of the human epithelial attachment, J Dent Res 49:691, 1970.

Frank RM and Cimasoni G: Ultrastructure de l'épithélium cliniquement normal du sillon et de la jonction gingivo-dentaires, Z Zellforsch Mikrosk Anat 109:356, 1970.

Franke WW, Moll R, Mueller H, et al.: Immunocytochemical identification of epithelium-derived human tumors with antibodies to desmosomal plaque proteins, Proc Natl Acad Sci USA 80:543, 1983.

Frithiof L: Ultrastructural changes in the plasma membrane in human oral epithelium, J Ultrastruct Res 32:1, 1970.

Frithiof L and Wersall J: A highly ordered structure in keratinizing human oral epithelium, J Ultrastruct Res 12:371, 1965.

Gavin JB: The ultrastructure of the crevicular epithelium of cat gingiva, Am J Anat 123:283, 1968.

Geisenheimer J and Han SS: A quantitative electron microscopic study of desmosomes and hemidesmosomes in human crevicular epithelium, J Peridontol 42:396, 1971.

Gorbsky G and Steinberg MS: Isolation of intercellular glycoproteins of desmosomes, J Cell Biol 90:243, 1981.

Gottlieb B: Der Epithelansatz am Zähne, Dtsch Monatsschr Zahnheilkd 39:142, 1921.

Gottlieb B: Zur Biologie des Epithelansatzes und des Alveolarrandes, Dtsch Zahnaerztl Wochenschr 25:434, 1922.

Gottlieb B and Orban B: Biology and pathology of the tooth (translated by M Diamond), New York, 1938, The MacMillan Co.

Grant DA and Orban B: Leukocytes in the epithelial attachment, J Periodontol 31:87, 1960.

Grant DA, Stern IB, and Listgarten MA: Periodontics in the tradition of Orban and Gottlieb, ed 6, St. Louis, 1988, The CV Mosby Co.

Grossman ES and Austin JC: The ultrastructural response to loading of the oral mucosa of the vervet monkey, J Periodont Res 18:474, 1983.

Grossman ES and Austin JC: A quantitative electron microscopic study of desmosomes and hemidesmosomes in vervet monkey oral mucosa, J Periodont Res 18:580, 1983.

Hamilton AI and Blackwood HJJ: Cell renewal of oral mucosal epithelium of the rat, J Anat 117:313, 1974.

Hansen ER: Mitotic activity of the gingival epithelium in colchicinized rats, Odont Tidskr 74:229, 1966.

Hashimoto K: The fine structure of the Merkel cell in human oral mucosa, J Invest Dermatol 58:381, 1972.

Hashimoto K, Dibella RJ, and Shklar G: Electron microscopic studies of the normal human buccal mucosa, J Invest Dermatol 47:512, 1966.

Hashimoto S, Yamamura T, and Shimono M: Morphometric analysis of the intercellular space and desmosomes of rat junctional epithelium, J Periodont Res 21:510, 1986.

Hayward AF and Hackemann MM: Electron microscopy of membrane-coating granules and a cell surface coat in keratinized and nonkeratinized human oral epithelium, J Ultrastruct Res 43:205, 1973.

Hayward AF, Hamilton AI, and Hackemann MM: Histological and ultrastructural observations on the keratinizing epithelia of the palate of the rat, Arch Oral Biol 18:1041, 1973.

Hedin CA and Larsson A: Large melanosome complexes in the human gingival epithelium, J Periodont Res 22:108, 1987.

Huang LY, Stern IB, Clagett JA, et al.: Two polypeptide chain constituents of the major protein of the cornified layer of newborn rat epidermis, Biochemistry 14:3573, 1975.

Hutchens LM, Sagebiel RW, and Clark MA: Oral epithelial cells of the Rhesus monkey—histologic demonstration, fine structure and quantitative distribution. J Invest Dermatol 56:325, 1971.

Ito H, Enomoto S, and Kobayashi K: Electron microscopic study of the human epithelial attachment, Bull Tokyo Med Dent Univ 14:267, 1967.

Karring T and Löe H: The three dimensional concept of the epithelium-connective tissue boundary of gingiva, Acta Odontol Scand 28:917, 1970.

Katz SI, Tamaki K, and Sachs DI.: Epidermal Langerhans cells are derived from cells originating in bone marrow, Nature 282:324, 1979.

Klavan B, Genco R, Löe H, et al.: Proceedings of the International Conference on Research in the Biology of Periodontal Disease, Chicago, 1977, University of Illinois College of Dentistry.

Kobayashi K, Rose GG, and Mahan CJ: Ultrastructure of the dento-epithelial junction, J Periodont Res 11:313, 1976.

Kobayashi K, Rose GG, and Mahan CJ: Ultrastructural histochemistry of the dento-epithelial junction, I.J Periodont Res 12:351, 1977.

Korman M, Rubinstein A, and Gargiulo A: Preservation of palatal mucosa. I. Ultrastructural changes and freezing technique, J Periodontol 44:464, 1973.

Kubo M, Norris DA, Howell SE, et al.: Human keratinocytes synthesize, secrete, and deposit fibronectin in the pericellular matrix, J Invest Dermatol 82:580, 1984.

Kurahashi Y and Takuma S: Electron microscopy of human gingival epithelium, Bull Tokyo Dent Col 3:29, 1962.

Landay MA and Schroeder HE: Quantitative electron microscopic analysis of the stratified epithelium of normal human buccal mucosa, Cell Tissue Res 177:383, 1977.

Lange D and Schroeder HE: Cytochemistry and ultrastructure of gingival sulcus cells, Helv Odontol Acta 15:65, 1971.

Lavker RM: Membrane coating granules: the fate of the discharged lamellae, J Ultrastruc Res 55:79, 1976.

Lavker RM and Sun TT: Heterogeneity in epidermal basal keratinocytes: morphological and functional correlations, Science 215:1239, 1982.

Lavker RH and Sun TT: Epidermal stem cells, J Invest Dermatol 81(suppl):121s, 1983.

Listgarten MA: The ultrastructure of human gingival epithelium, Am J Anat 114:49, 1964.

Listgarten MA: Electron microscopic study of the gingivo-dental junction of man, Am J Anat 119:147, 1966.

Listgarten MA: Phase contrast and electron microscopic study of the junction between reduced enamel epithelium and enamel in unerupted human teeth, Arch Oral Biol 11:999, 1966.

Listgarten MA: Changing concepts about the dentoepithelial junction, J Can Dent Assoc 36:70, 1970.

Löe H, Karring T, and Hara K: The site of mitotic activity in rat and human oral epithelium, Scand J Dent Res 80:111, 1972.

Loening T, Caselitz J, Seifert G, et al.: Identification of Langerhans cells: simultaneous use of sera to intermediate filaments, T6 and HLA-DR antigens on oral mucosa, human epidermis and their tumors. Virchows Arch (Pathol Anat) 398:119, 1982.

Luzardo-Baptista M: Intraepithelial nerve fibers in the human oral mucosa, Oral Surg 35:372, 1973.

Mackenzie IC: Nature and mechanisms of regeneration of the junctional epithelia phenotype, J Periodont Res 22:243, 1987.

Mahrle G and Orfanos CE: Merkel cells as human cutaneous neuroceptor cells. Their presence in dermal neural corpuscles and in the external hair root sheath of human adult skin, Arch Dermatol Forsch 251:19, 1974.

Marikova Z: Ultrastructure of normal and newly formed dento-epithelial junction in rats, J Periodont Res 18:459, 1983.

Massoth DL and Dale BA: Immunohistochemical study of structural proteins in developing functional epithelium, J Periodont 57:756, 1986.

Mattern CFT, Daniel WA, and Henkin RI: The ultrastructure of the human circumvallate papilla. I. Cilia of the papillary crypt, Anat Rec 167:175, 1970.

Matusim DF, Takahashi Y, Labib RS, et al.: A pool of bullous pemphigoid antigen(s) is intracellular and associated with the basal cell cytoskeleton–hemidesmosome complex, J Invest Dermatol 84:47, 1985.

McDougall WA: pathways of penetration and effects of horseradish peroxidase in rat molar gingiva, Arch Oral Biol 15:621, 1970.

McHugh WD: Keratinization of gingival epithelium in laboratory animals, J Periodontol 35:338, 1964.

McMillan MD: A scanning electron study of keratinized epithelium of the hard palate of the rat, Arch Oral Biol 19:225, 1974.

McMillan MD: The complementary structure of the superficial and deep surfaces of the cells of the stratum corneum of the hard palate of the rat. A scanning and transmission electron microscope study, J Periodont Res 14:492, 1979.

Melcher AH and Bowen WH: Biology of the periodontium, London, 1969, Academic Press, Inc.

Meyer J and Gerson SJ: A comparison of human palatal and buccal mucosa, Periodontics 2:284, 1964.

Meyer M and Schroeder HE: A quantitative electron microscopic analysis of the keratinizing epithelium of normal human hard palate, Cell Tissue Res 158:177, 1975.

Mignon ML: Ultrastructure of the gingival epithelium in the newborn cat—some characteristics of the intercellular junctions, J Dent Res 53:1484, 1974.

Mihara M, Hashimoto K, Ueda K, et al.: The specialized junctions between Merkel cell and neurite: an electron microscopic study, J Invest Dermatol 73:325, 1979.

Mueller H and Franke W: Biochemical and immunological characterization of desmoplakin I and II, the major polypeptides of the desmosomal plaque, J Mol Biol 163:647, 1983.

Munger B: Neural-epithelial interactions in sensory receptors, J Invest Dermatol 69:27, 1977.

Murphy GF: Cytokeratin typing of cutaneous tumors: Q new immunocytochemical probe for cellular differentiation and malignant transformation, J Invest Dermatol 84:1, 1985.

Murray RG, Murray A, and Fujimoto S: Fine structure of gustatory cells in rabbit taste buds, J Ultrastruct Res 27:444, 1969.

Necomb GH and Powell RN: Human gingival Langerhans cells in health and disease, J Periodont Res 21:640, 1986.

Negus VE: The comparative anatomy of the nose and paranasal sinuses, London, 1958, E and S Livingstone.

Ness KH, Morton TH, and Dale BA: Identification of Merkel cells in oral epithelium using antikeratin and antineuroendocrine monoclonal antibodies, J Dent Res 66:1154, 1987.

Newcomb GM, Seymour GJ, and Powell RN: Association between plaque accumulation and Langerhans cell numbers in the oral epithelium of attached gingiva, J Clin Periodontol 9:197, 1982.

Nuki K and Hock J: The organization of the gingival vasculature, J Periodont Res 9:305, 1974.

Orban B: Zahnfleischtasche und Epithelansatz, Z Stomatol 22:353, 1924.

Orban B: Hornification of the gums, J Am Dent Assoc 17:1977, 1930.

Orban B: Clinical and histologic study of the surface characteristics of the gingiva, Oral Surg 1:827, 1948.

Orban B, Bhatia H, et al.: Epithelial attachment (the attached gingival cuff), J Periodontol 27:167, 1956.

Orban B and Mueller E: The gingival crevice, J Am Dent Assoc 16:1206, 1929.

Orban B and Sicher H: The oral mucosa, J Dent Educ 10:94, 1946.

Osborn M: Components of the cellular cytoskeleton: a new generation of markers of histogenetic origin? J Invest Dermatol 82:443, 1984.

Palade GE and Farquhar MG: A special fibril of the dermis, J Cell Biol 27:215, 1965.

Peterson LI, Zettergren JG, and Wuepper KD: Biochemistry of transglutaminases and cross-linking in the skin, J Invest Dermatol 81(suppl):95s, 1983.

Petitet NF and Stern IB: Ultrastructure de l'épithélium gingival humain. In Favard P, editor: Microscopie électronique, vol 3, Paris, 1970, Société Française de Microscopie Électronique.

Pfaff DA, editor: Taste, olefaction and the central nervous system, New York, 1987, Rockefeller University Press.

Pruniéras M, Régnier M, Fougère S, et al.: Keratinocytes synthesize basal-lamina proteins in culture, J Invest Dermatol 81(suppl):28s, 1983.

Romani W et al.: Morphological and phenotypical characterization of bone marrow—derived dendritic Thy-1-positive epidermal cells of the mouse, J Invest Dermatol 85(suppl 1):91, 1985.

Romanowski AW, Squier CA, and Lesch CA: Permeability of rodent junctional epithelium to exogenous protein, J Periodont Res 23:81, 1988.

Rowat JS and Squier CA: Rates of epithelial cells proliferation in the oral mucosa and skin of the Tamarin monkey *(Saguinus fuscicollis)*, J Dent Res 65:1326, 1986.

Sage H: Collagens of basement membranes, J Invest Dermatol 79:515, 1982.

Saglie FR, Pertuiset JH, Smith CT, et al.: The presence of bacteria in the oral epithelium in periodontal disease. III. Correlation with Langerhans cells, J Periodontol 58:417, 1987.

Saito I, Watanabe O, Kawahara H, et al.: Intercellular junctions and the permeability barrier in the junctional epithelium. A study with freeze-fracture and thin sectioning, J Periodont Res 16:467, 1981.

Salonen J: Sampling and preliminary analysis of the extra- and intra-cellular material involved in the attachment of human oral epithelium in vitro, J Periodont Res 21:279, 1986.

Salonen J and Santti R: Ultrastructural and immunohistochemical similarities in the attachment of human oral epithelium to the tooth in vivo and to an inert substrate in an explant culture, J Periodont Res 20:176, 1985.

Sauder DN: Biologic properties of epidermal cell thymocyte-activating factor, J Invest Dermatol 85(suppl 1):176, 1985.

Sauder DN, Carter CS, Katz SJ, et al.: Epidermal cell production of thymocyte activating factor (ETAF), J Invest Dermatol 79:34, 1982.

Sauder DN, Dinerello CA, and Morhenn VB: Langerhans cell production of interleukin-1, J Invest Dermatol 82:605, 1984.

Sauder DN, Monick MM, and Hunninghake GW: Epidermal cell-derived thymocyte activating factor (ETAF) is a potent T-cell chemoattractant, J Invest Deramtol 85:431, 1985.

Sauder DN et al.: Epidermal cell production of thymocyte activating factor (ETAF), J Invest Dermatol 79:35, 1982.

Saurat J-H, Merot Y, Didierjean L, et al.: Normal rabbit Merkel cells do not express neurofilament proteins, J Invest Dermatol 82:641, 1984.

Saurat J-H, Didierjean L, Skalli O, et al.: The intermediate filaments of rabbit normal epidermal Merkel cells and cytokeratins, J Invest Dermatol 83:431, 1984.

Schroeder HE: Differentiation of human oral stratified epithelia, Basel, Switzerland, 1981, Karger.

Schroeder HE: Melanin-containing organelles in cells of the human gingiva. I. Epithelial melanocytes, J Periodont Res 4:1, 1969.

Schroeder HE and Listgarten MA: Fine structure of the developing epithelial attachment of human teeth (Monographs in developmental biology, vol 2), ed 2, Basel, Switzerland, 1977, Karger.

Schroeder HE and Munzel-Pedrazzoli S: Correlated morphometric and biochemical analysis of gingival tissue, J Microscopy 99:301, 1973.

Schroeder HE and Theilade J: Electron microscopy of normal human gingival epithelium, J Periodont Res 1:95, 1966.

Schuler G: The dendritic Thy-1-positive cell of murine epidermis: a new epidermal cell type of bone marrow origin, J Invest Dermatol 83:81, 1984.

Schweizer J and Marks F: A developmental study of the distribution and frequency of Langerhans cells in relation to formation and patterning in mouse tail epidermis, J Invest Dermatol 69:198, 1977.

Silberberg-Sinakin I, Thorbecke GJ, Baer RL, et al.: Antigen-bearing Langerhans cells in the skin, dermis and in lymph developments. Cell Immunol 25:137, 1976.

Skillen WG: The morphology of the gingiva of the rat molar, J Am Dent Assoc 17:645, 1930.

Skougaard MR: Cell renewal, with special reference to the gingival epithelium, Adv Oral Biol 4:261, 1970.

Smith CJ: Gingival epithelium. In Melcher AH, and Bowen WH, editors: Biology of the periodontium, New York, 1969, Academic Press, Inc.

Smith SA and Dale BA: Immunologic localization of filaggrin in human oral epithelia and correlation with keratinization, J Invest Dermatol 86(2):168, 1986.

Squier CA: The permeability of keratinized and nonkeratinized oral epithelium to horseradish peroxidase, J Ultrastruct Res 43:160, 1973.

Squier CA and Meyer J: Current concepts of the histology of oral mucosa, Springfield, Ill, 1971, Charles C Thomas, Publisher.

Squier CA and Waterhouse LP: The ultrastructure of the melanocyte in human gingival epithelium, J Dent Res 46:112, 1967.

Stanley JR, Hawley-Nelson P, Yaar M, et al.: Laminin and bullous pemphigoid antigen are distinct basement membrane proteins synthesized by epidermal cells, J Invest Dermatol 78:457, 1982.

Steffenson B et al.: Blood group substances as differentiation markers in human dento-gingival epithelium, J Periodont Res 22:451, 1987.

Stern IB: Electron microscopic observations of oral epithelium. I. Basal cells and the basement membrane, Periodontics 3:224, 1965.

Stern IB: The fine structure of the ameloblast-enamel junction in rat incisors, epithelial attachment and cuticular membrane, vol B, Fifth International congress for Electron Microscopy, New York, 1966, Academic Press, Inc.

Stern IB: Further electron microscopic observations of the epithelial attachment, Int Assoc Dent Res Abstr no 325, 45th general meeting, 1967, p 118.

Stern IB: Current concepts of the dentogingival junction: the epithelial and connective tissue attachments to the tooth, J Periodontol 52:465, 1981.

Stern IB, Dayton L, and Duecy J: The uptake of tritiated thymidine by the dorsal epidermis of the fetal and newborn rat, Anat Rec 170:225, 1971.

Stern IB and Sekeri-Pataryas KH: The uptake of ^{14}C-leucine and ^{14}C-histidine by cell suspension of isolated strata of neonatal rat epidermis, J Invest Dermatol 59:251, 1972.

Streilein JW: Circuits and signals of the skin-associated lymphoid tissues (SALT), J Invest Dermatol 85(suppl 1):10s-13s, 1985.

Streilein JW: Skin-associated lymphoid tissue (SALT): origins and functions, J Invest Dermatol 80(suppl): 12s, 1983.

Susi FR: Histochemical, autoradiographic and electron microscopic studies of keratinization in oral mucosa, PhD thesis, Tufts University, October 1967.

Susi FR: Studies of cellular renewal and protein synthesis in mouse oral mucosa utilizing H^3-thymidine and H^3-cystine, J Invest Dermatol 51:403, 1968.

Susi FR: Anchoring fibrils in the attachment of epithelium to connective tissue in oral mucous membranes, J Dent Res 48:144, 1969.

Susi FR, Belt WD, and Kelly JW: Fine structure of fibrillar complexes associated with the basement membrane in human oral mucosa, J Cell Biol 34:686, 1967.

Svejda J and Janota M: Scanning electron microscopy of the papillae foliatae of the human tongue, Oral Surg 37:208, 1974.

Takata T et al.: Ultrastructure of regenerated junctional epithelium after surgery of the rat molar gingiva, J Periodontol 57:776, 1986.

Takehana S et al.: Ultrastructural observation on Langerhans cells in the rat gingival epithelium, J Periodont Res 20:276, 1985.

Terranova VP and Lyall RM: Chemotaxis of human gingival epithelial cells to laminin. A mechanism for epithelial cell apical migration, J Periodontol 57:311, 1986.

Thilander H and Bloom GD: Cell contacts in oral epithelia, J Periodont Res 3:96, 1968.

Toto PD and Grundel ER: Acid mucopolysaccharides in the oral epithelium, J Dent Res 45:211, 1966.

Toto PD and Sicher H: The epithelial attachment, Periodontics 2:154, 1964.

Vidic B et al.: The structure and prenatal morphology of the nasal septum in the rat, J Morphol 137:131, 1972.

Volc-Platzer B et al.: Human epidermal cells synthesize HLA-DR allo-antigens in vitro upon stimulation with J interferon, J Invest Dermatol 85:16, 1985.

Walsh LJ and Seymour GJ: Interleukin-1 induces CD1 antigen expression on human gingival epithelial cells, J Invest Dermatol 90:13, 1988.

Walsh LJ, Seymour GJ, and Powell RN: Interleukin-1 modulates T6 expression on a putative intra-epithelial Langerhans cell precursor population, J Dent Res 65:1425, 1986.

Walsh LJ et al.: In vitro modulation of T6 expression on gingival Langerhans cells by interleukin-1 inhibition and ETAF, J Dent Res 66:766, 1987.

Weinmann JP: The keratinization of the human oral mucosa, J Dent Res 19:57, 1940.

Weinmann JP and Meyer J: Types of keratinization in the human gingiva, J Invest Dermatol 32:9, 1959.

Weinstock M and Wilgram GF: Fine structural observations on the formation and enzymatic activity of keratinosomes in mouse tongue filiform papilla, J Ultrastruct Res 30:262, 1970.

Wentz FM, Maier AW, and Orban B: Age changes and sex differences in the clinically "normal" gingiva, J Periodontol 23:13, 1952.

Wertz PW, and Downing DT: Glycolipids in mammalian epidermis: structure and function in the water barrier, Science 217:1261, 1982.

Wiebkin OW and Thonard JC: Mucopolysaccharide localization in gingival epithelium. I. An autoradiographic demonstration, J Periodont Res 16:600, 1981.

Winkelmann RK: The Merkel cell system and a comparison between it and the neurosecretory or APUD cell system, J Invest Dermatol 69:41, 1977.

Wolff K and Stingl G: The Langerhans cell, J Invest Dermatol 80:(suppl):17s, 1983.

Yamasaki A et al.: Cytochemical identification of lysosomal system of rat junctional epithelium, J Periodont Res 20:591, 1985.

10
SALIVARY GLANDS

The salivary glands are exocrine glands whose secretions flow into the oral cavity. There are three pairs of large glands located extraorally known as the major salivary glands and numerous small glands widely distributed in the mucosa and submucosa of the oral cavity, known as the minor salivary glands. Both the major and minor glands are composed of parenchymal elements invested in and supported by connective tissue. The parenchymal elements are derived from the oral epithelium and consist of terminal secretory units leading into ducts that eventually open into the oral cavity. The connective tissue forms a capsule around the gland and extends into it, dividing groups of secretory units and ducts into lobes and lobules. The blood and lymph vessels and nerves that supply the gland are contained within the connective tissue. The production of saliva is the most important function of the salivary glands. Saliva contains various organic and inorganic substances, provides the primary natural protection for the teeth and soft tissues of the oral cavity, and assists in the mastication, deglutition, and digestion of food.

STRUCTURE AND FUNCTION OF SALIVARY GLAND CELLS

The terminal secretory units are composed of serous, mucous, and myoepithelial cells arranged into acini or secretory tubules (Fig. 10-1). The secretions of these units are collected by the intercalated ducts, which empty into the striated ducts. The structure and function of each of these

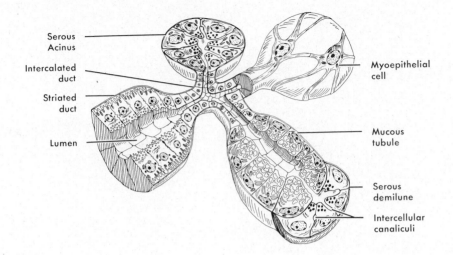

Fig. 10-1. Main features of parenchymal cells of salivary glands and their arrangement to form ducts and terminal secretory units.

components will be considered in detail, followed by a description of the connective tissue elements and nerves.

Serous cells

Serous cells are specialized for the synthesis, storage, and secretion of proteins.

The typical serous cell is pyramidal in shape, with its broad base resting on a thin basal lamina and its narrow apex bordering on the lumen (Figs. 10-1 and 10-2). The spherical nucleus is located in the basal region of the cell; occasionally binucleated cells are observed.

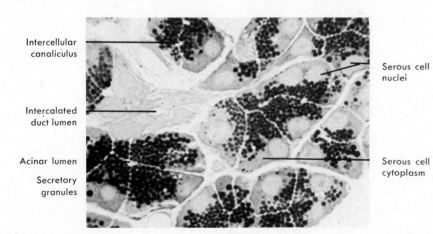

Fig. 10-2. Light micrograph of rat parotid gland illustrating general arrangement and cytologic features of serous cells. Gland was incubated in cytochemical medium to demonstrate the secretory enzyme peroxidase, resulting in unstained nuclei, lightly stained cytoplasm, and heavily stained secretory granules. Cells of intercalated duct are unreactive. (1 μm; × 990.)

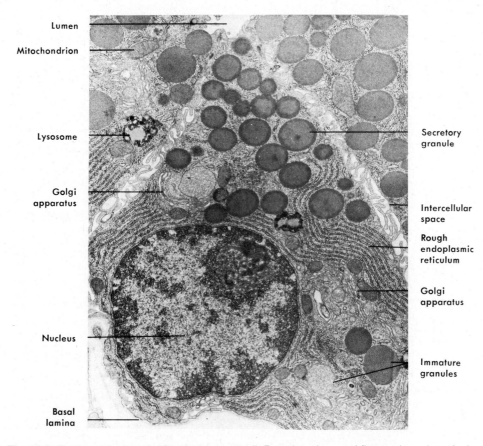

Lumen

Mitochondrion

Lysosome

Golgi apparatus

Nucleus

Basal lamina

Secretory granule

Intercellular space

Rough endoplasmic reticulum

Golgi apparatus

Immature granules

Fig. 10-3. Electron micrograph of typical serous cell. Round nucleus and flattened rough endoplasmic reticulum cisternae are located in basal half of cell. Golgi apparatus and immature granules are located apical and lateral to nucleus, and dense secretory granules are located in cell apex. Folds of cell membranes interdigitate in intercellular spaces. Note faint basal lamina. (Rat parotid gland; ×10,500.) (From Hand AR: Am J Anat 135:71, 1972; reprinted by permission of the Wistar Institute Press.)

The most prominent feature of the serous cell is the accumulation of secretory granules in the apical cytoplasm (Fig. 10-2). These granules are about 1 μm in diameter and by electron microscopy are observed to have a distinct limiting membrane and a dense content (Fig. 10-3). In some salivary glands, including those of humans, the serous granules may contain a dense core or a twisted skeinlike structure within a lighter matrix. The granules may be very closely apposed to one another, the plasma membrane, or other organelles, but in unstimulated cells they retain their individual nature and do not fuse with other structures. In routine histologic preparations, the serous granules are usually not well resolved because of section thickness and the conditions of fixation, and the apical portion of the cell may appear as an acidophilic mass.

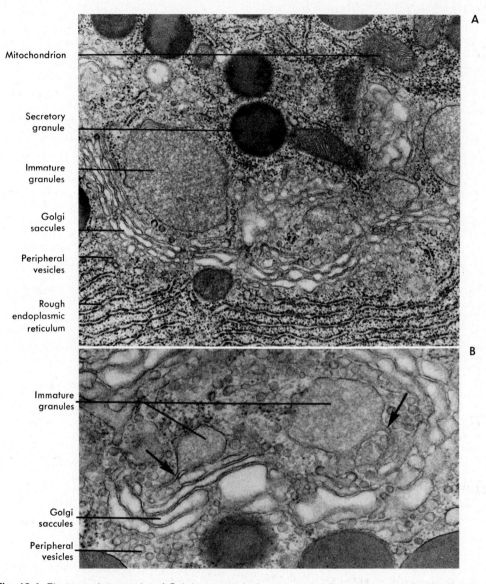

Mitochondrion

Secretory
granule

Immature
granules

Golgi
saccules

Peripheral
vesicles

Rough
endoplasmic
reticulum

A

Immature
granules

Golgi
saccules

Peripheral
vesicles

B

Fig. 10-4. Electron mictrographs of Golgi apparatus of serous cells. Saccules at *cis* face of Golgi apparatus are wider than saccules at *trans* face. Immature granules, located at *trans* face, are frequently larger than the mature granules and are often connected to membranes in Golgi region *(arrows).* Numerous vesicles are present between rough endoplasmic reticulum and *cis* saccules and at the *trans* face. (Rat parotid gland; **A,** ×25,400; **B,** ×46,400.)

However, in semithin (1 μm) sections of plastic-embedded tissue, stained with toluidine blue or by specific cytochemical techniques (Fig. 10-2), the secretory granules are clearly seen.

The basal portion of the cytoplasm is filled with ribosome-studded (rough) endoplasmic reticulum (RER), a closed system of membranous sacs or cisternae (Figs. 10-3 and 10-4, A). The ribosomes, consisting of ribonucleic acid (RNA) and proteins, are the basic units of protein synthesis. Acting under the direction of messenger RNA from the nucleus, the ribosomes translate the encoded message, adding the appropriate amino acids in their proper sequence in the protein being synthesized. Proteins destined for secretion are synthesized as *pre*proteins, with an NH_2-terminal extension of about 16 to 30 amino acids, called a signal sequence. As the signal sequence emerges from the ribosome, it is recognized by specific proteins in the RER membrane, which direct attachment of the ribosome to the membrane. The signal sequence also assists in transfer of the growing polypeptide chain across the RER membrane. When the newly synthesized protein reaches the cisternal space of the RER, the signal sequence is removed by a proteolytic enzyme called signal peptidase, and the protein assumes its characteristic three-dimensional structure. In cells that produce large amounts of protein for secretion, the RER is well developed and arranged in parallel stacks, usually basal and lateral to the nucleus.

A second system of membranous cisternae, the Golgi apparatus, is located apical or lateral to the nucleus (Figs. 10-3 and 10-4). The Golgi apparatus consists of several stacks of four to six smooth-surfaced saccules that are slightly curved or cup shaped, with the concave or *trans* face usually oriented toward the secretory surface of the cell. The Golgi apparatus is functionally interconnected with the RER through vesicles budding from the ends of the RER cisternae that approach the periphery (convex or *cis* face) of the Golgi apparatus (Fig. 10-4, A). The newly synthesized secretory proteins within the RER are transported to the Golgi apparatus via these small vesicles. Although the exact route followed by the secretory proteins has not been firmly established, it is believed that in most cells the RERderived vesicles fuse with the *cis* Golgi saccule, contributing their content to it. The proteins apparently then move through the Golgi saccules toward the *trans* face of the Golgi apparatus, where they are packaged into vacuoles of variable size and density (Figs. 10-3 and 10-4). These vacuoles are the forming secretory granules and are called *immature granules, prosecretory granules,* or *condensing vacuoles.* The immature granules have direct connections with smooth membranes at the *trans* face of the Golgi apparatus (Fig. 10-4, B); additionally, their limiting membrane is frequently irregular, suggesting that some secretory material may reach the immature granules through fusion with small vesicles. The smaller immature granules have a light flocculent content; as they increase in size, their content increases in density until it is near that of the mature granules. The increase in density of the secretory material suggests that it is being concentrated as it is being transported and packaged for storage in granules.

Following their synthesis, many secretory proteins undergo one or more covalent structural modifications prior to their secretion. The most common modification of salivary proteins is glycosylation (i.e., the addition of carbohydrate side chains to the amino acids asparagine, serine, and threonine in the protein). The carbohydrates of secretory glycoproteins include galactose, mannose, fucose, glucosamine, galactosamine, and sialic acid. Glycosylation is a multistep process that begins in the RER and is completed in the Golgi apparatus. Other modifications of the secretory proteins may include the addition of phosphate or sulfate groups and specific proteolytic cleavage to produce the final secretory product.

The completed secretory proteins are stored in the secretory granules in the cell apex. Secretion or discharge of the granule content occurs by a process called exocytosis. This involves fusion of the granule membrane with the plasma membrane at the lumen or intercellular canaliculus, followed by the opening of the fused portion (Fig. 10-5). In this manner, the granule membrane becomes continuous with the plasma membrane, and the granule content is exteriorized without loss of cytoplasm. During rapid secretion, such as that occurring after stimulation by various pharmacologic agents, a second granule may fuse with the membrane of a previously dis-

charged granule; continuation of this process, termed compound exocytosis, can lead to a long string of interconnected granule profiles extending into the cytoplasm. The addition of granule membranes results in a great enlargement of the plasma membrane at the secretory surface; during recovery, this excess membrane is retrieved by the cell as small vesicles. A portion of these vesicles fuses with lysosomes (see below) where the membrane may be degraded, while some may return to the Golgi apparatus where the membrane may be reutilized during the formation of new secretory granules. The proportion of the membrane undergoing degradation or reutilization has not been established.

In summary, secretory proteins are synthesized by membrane-bound ribosomes, are transferred to the cisternal space of the RER, and migrate to the Golgi apparatus where carbohydrate addition and other posttranslational modifications are completed and they are packaged into secretory granules. After a variable period of storage

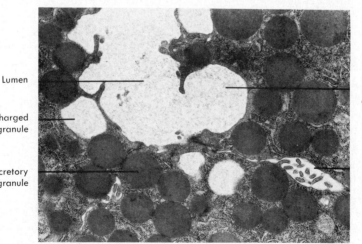

Lumen

Discharged granule

Secretory granule

Discharged granules

Intercellular space

Fig. 10-5. Electron micrograph of three serous cells illustrating exocytosis of secretory granules induced by isoproterenol. Flask-shaped invaginations of lumen into cell apices mark sites of granule discharge. (Rat lingual serous gland; ×12,800.)

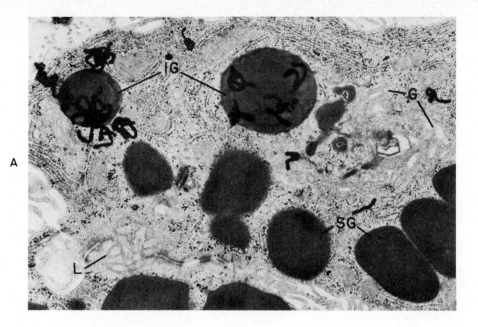

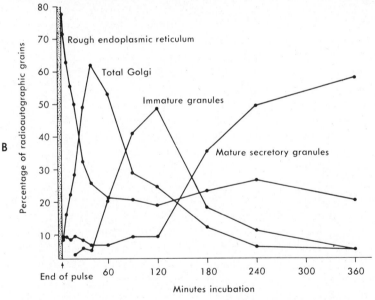

Fig. 10-6. A, Electron microscope radioautograph of serous cell of rabbit parotid gland, pulse labeled with ^{3}H-leucine for 4 minutes and incubated in vitro for 116 minutes. Radioautographic grains, indicating presence of radioactive leucine incorporated into newly synthesized proteins, are concentrated over immature granules, *IG*. A few grains are present over rough endoplasmic reticulum (RER) and Golgi apparatus, *G*, but none are localized over mature secretory granules, *SG*. Lumen, *L*.**B,** Radioautographic grain counts of rabbit parotid serous cells after pulse-labeling with ^{3}H-leucine and in vitro incubation. Newly synthesized proteins move in wavelike fashion from RER, through Golgi apparatus, and into immature and finally mature secretory granules. About 20% of label remains with RER as nonsecretory proteins. (**A,** ×17,100.) (**A** and **B** from Castle JD, Jamieson JD, and Palade GE: J Cell Biol 53:290, 1972; reprinted by permission of the Rockefeller University Press.)

in the cell apex, they are discharged by exocytosis at the secretory surface of the cell. The incorporation of amino acids into the secretory proteins and the movement of the proteins through the various compartments of the cell has been studied by electron microscope radioautography (Fig. 10-6, *A*). Counts of the radioautographic grains at various times after administration of radioactive amino acids reveal the sequential flow of proteins from the RER to the Golgi apparatus, their accumulation in immature granules, and finally storage in the mature secretory granules (Fig. 10-6, *B*). Enzyme and immunocytochemical studies have confirmed the presence of specific secretory proteins in these various intracellular compartments.

The serous cell contains several other cytoplasmic organelles, which are also found in most other salivary gland cells. Free or unattached ribosomes are located in the cytoplasm throughout the cell; they are concerned with the synthesis of nonsecretory cellular proteins. Mitochondria are also found throughout the cell, most frequently between the RER cisternae, around the Golgi apparatus, and along the lateral and basal plasma membranes. The mitochondria contain the enzymes of the citric acid cycle, electron transport, and oxidative phosphorylation; hence they are the major source of high-energy compounds necessary for the numerous synthetic and transport processes that occur in the cell. Lysosomes, organelles that contain potent hydrolytic enzymes, are also occasionally seen. They function to destroy foreign materials taken up by the cells, as well as portions of the cells themselves such as worn-out mitochondria or other membranous organelles. Their typical heterogeneous content of granular and membranous debris and lipidlike droplets probably reflects the role of lysosomes in this latter process. A few peroxisomes (microbodies), small organelles containing the enzyme catalase and other oxidative enzymes, can be demonstrated in the serous cells by cytochemical techniques; their exact functions are unknown, but they probably participate in certain aspects of lipid metabolism. Bundles of tonofilaments, associated with desmosomes, and microfilaments may be seen in the cytoplasm, as well as an occasional microtubule.

Mucous cells

The mucous cell, like the serous cell, is specialized for the synthesis, storage, and secretion of a secretory product. However, its structure differs from that of the serous cell. In routine histologic preparations the apex of the cell appears empty except for thin strands of cytoplasm forming a trabecular network (Fig. 10-7, *A*). The nucleus and a thin rim of cytoplasm are compressed against the base of the cell.

In the electron microscope the mucous cell is seen to be filled with pale, electron-lucent secretory droplets containing scattered flocculent material (Fig. 10-8). These droplets are usually larger than serous granules and may be irregular or compressed in shape. Adjacent mucous droplets are separated by thin strands of cytoplasm, or they may be so closely apposed that their membranes fuse. During fixation and processing of the tissue for microscopy, these tenuous partitions are often disrupted; several droplets may thus form a larger mass. The secretory products of most mucous cells differ from those of serous cells in two important respects: (1) they have little or no enzymatic activity and probably serve mainly for lubrication and protection of the oral tissues, and (2) the ratio of carbohydrate to protein is greater, and larger amounts of sialic acid and occasionally sulfated sugar residues are

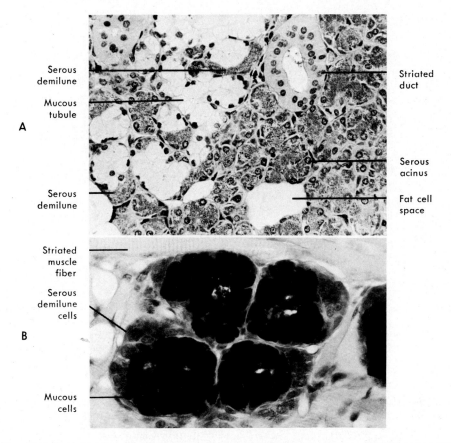

Serous
demilune

Mucous
tubule

A

Serous
demilune

Striated
muscle
fiber

Serous
demilune
cells

B

Mucous
cells

Striated
duct

Serous
acinus

Fat cell
space

Fig. 10-7. A, Light micrograph of human submandibular gland illustrating different appearance of mucous and serous cells. Mucous tubules are capped by serous demilunes. Two striated ducts are cut in cross section. **B,** Light micrograph of posterior lingual mucous gland of rat, stained with alcian blue and periodic acid–Schiff (PAS). Mucous secretory glycoprotein stains with both alcian blue and PAS, indicating acidic carbohydrate residues. Granules of serous demilune cells stain only with PAS, indicating neutral glycoproteins. (**A,** ×265; **B,** ×420.)

present. The differences in the carbohydrate content of the secretory material of mucous and serous cells can be demonstrated by histochemical staining techniques (Fig. 10-7, *B*).

The nucleus of the mucous cell is oval or flattened in shape and located just above the basal plasma membrane (Fig. 10-8). The RER is limited to a narrow band of cytoplasm along the base and lateral borders

of the cell and to an occasional patch of cytoplasm between the mucous droplets. The mitochondria and other organelles are also primarily limited to this band of basal and lateral cytoplasm. The Golgi apparatus is large, consisting of several stacks of 10 to 12 saccules sandwiched between the basal RER and mucous droplets forming from the *trans* face. The Golgi apparatus plays an important role in these cells because of the

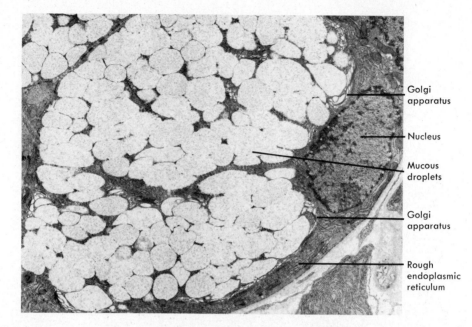

Golgi apparatus

Nucleus

Mucous droplets

Golgi apparatus

Rough endoplasmic reticulum

Fig. 10-8. Electron micrograph of mucous cell. Pale mucous droplets have flocculent content and tend to coalesce into larger masses. Golgi apparatus is well developed; rough endoplasmic reticulum and nucleus are compressed against base of cell. (×7000.)

large amount of carbohydrate that it adds to the secretory products.

The secretion of mucous droplets occurs by a somewhat different mechanism than the exocytotic process seen in the serous cells. When a single droplet is discharged, its limiting membrane fuses with the apical plasma membrane, resulting in a single membrane separating the droplet from the lumen. This separating membrane may then fragment, being lost with the discharge of mucus, or the droplet may be discharged with the membrane intact, surrounding it. During rapid droplet discharge, the apical cytoplasm may not seal itself off, and the entire mass of mucus may be spilled into the lumen.

Myoepithelial cells

Myoepithelial cells are closely related to

the secretory and intercalated duct cells, lying between the basal lamina and the basal membranes of the parenchymal cells (Figs. 10-1 and 10-9). The body of the cell is small, filled mostly with a flattened nucleus, and numerous branching cytoplasmic processes radiate out to embrance the parenchymal cells. Myoepithelial cells are difficult to identify in routine histologic preparations, but their typical stellate shape can be observed in sections stained by special histochemical or immunofluorescent techniques (Fig. 10-9, *A*). Their appearance is reminiscent of a basket cradling the secretory unit; hence the name "basket cell" in the older literature.

The usual appearance of myoepithelial cells in electron micrographs is a section through one of their processes lying in a groove on the surface of a secretory or duct cell (Fig. 10-11, *B*). The processes are filled

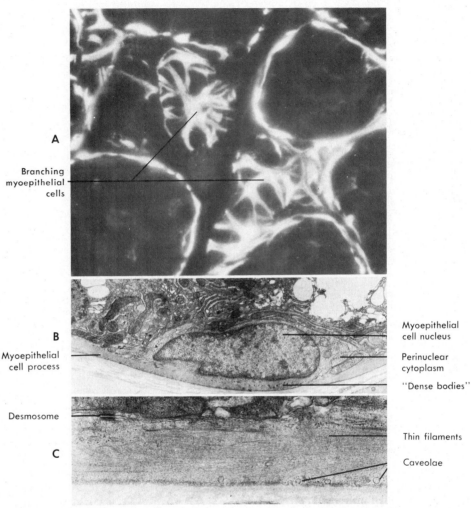

A

Branching
myoepithelial
cells

B

Myoepithelial
cell process

Desmosome

C

Myoepithelial
cell nucleus

Perinuclear
cytoplasm

"Dense bodies"

Thin filaments

Caveolae

Fig. 10-9. A, Fluorescent micrograph of rat sublingual gland treated with antibody to smooth muscle myosin, to localize myosin present in myoepithelial cells. Tangential sections of acini reveal branching nature of myoepithelial cells; myoepithelial cell processes cut in cross and longitudinal section surround adjacent acini. **B,** Electron micrograph of myoepithelial cell body showing concentration of organelles in perinuclear cytoplasm and processes filled with fine filaments. The "dense bodies" are characteristic of myoepithelium and smooth muscle. Rat sublingual gland. **C,** Higher magnification of myoepithelial cell process filled with longitudinally arranged thin filaments. Several caveolae are located along basal surface of cell, and a desmosome attaches the process to mucous cell. (Rat sublingual gland; **A,** ×700; **B,** ×6000; **C,** ×19,100.) (**A** courtesy D. Drenckhahn, Kiel, Federal Republic of Germany.)

with longitudinally oriented fine filaments about 6 nm (60 Å) thick (Fig. 10-9, *C*). Small dense bodies are frequently present between the thin filaments; these are also present in smooth muscle cells, where they appear to form a cytoskeletal network in association with 10 nm (100 Å) diameter filaments. The usual cytoplasmic organelles are largely restricted to the perinuclear cytoplasm. The body of the cell, containing the nucleus, often lies in the space where the basal regions of two or three parenchymal cells come together (Fig. 10-9, *B*). The plasma membrane of the myoepithelial cell closely parallels the basal membrane of the parenchymal cell, and the two are joined by occasional desmosomes. Numerous micropinocytotic vesicles, or caveolae, are located on the plasma membranes of the myoepithelial cells.

Myoepithelial cells are considered to have a contractile function, helping to expel secretions from the lumina of the secretory units and ducts. Although direct evidence is lacking for the salivary glands, the following observations suggest that this may be the case: (1) the structure of myoepithelium is similar to that of smooth muscle; (2) immunofluorescent studies indicate the presence of actin, myosin, and related proteins in myoepithelial cells (Fig. 10-9, *A*); (3) measurements of ductal pressure after appropriate stimulation suggest a contractile process; and (4) cinemicrography of individual secretory units stimulated to secrete in vitro reveals a regular pulsatile movement of the entire unit. Studies of sweat and mammary glands, where myoepithelial cells are abundant, also support a contractile function.

Arrangement of cells in the terminal secretory units

The structure of the terminal secretory units is different for different glands. When the gland consists entirely of serous secretory units such as the human parotid, the serous cells are clustered in a roughly spherical fashion around a central lumen, forming an acinus (Fig. 10-1). At the apical ends of adjoining cells, the lumen is sealed off from the lateral intercellular spaces by junctional complexes, consisting of a tight junction (zonula occludens), an intermediate junction (zonula adherens), and one or more desmosomes (maculae adherens). These junctions serve to hold the cells together as well as prevent leakage of the luminal contents into the intercellular spaces. Experimental studies have demonstrated, however, that following secretory stimulation the tight junctions may become more permeable to macromolecules and other organic substances. Fingerlike branches of the lumen, called intercellular canaliculi, extend between adjacent cells almost to their base (Fig. 10-10); they increase the area of the secretory surface and are sealed by junctional complexes along their length. A fine microfilament network, containing actin and myosin (Fig. 10-10), is located in the apical cytoplasm adjacent to the secretory surface. The remainder of the apposed lateral surfaces are joined by frequent desmosomes and an occasional gap junction.

In glands composed entirely of mucous secretory units the arrangement of the secretory cells is similar. Rather than a spherical acinus, however, a tubular secretory end piece may be formed (Fig. 10-1). The central lumen is usually larger than in serous acini, and intercellular canaliculi are not usually present, although they have been observed between the mucous cells of the human labial glands.

In mixed glands the proportion of serous and mucous cells may vary from predominantly serous, as in the human submandibular gland, to predominantly mucous, as in

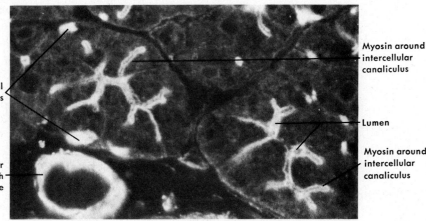

Fig. 10-10. Fluorescent micrograph of rat parotid gland treated with antibody to smooth muscle myosin. Myosin is located in myoepithelial cell processes, cut in cross section, and in apical cytoplasm of acinar cells, outlining lumen and intercellular canaliculi. (×900.) (From Drenckhahn D, Gröschel-Stewart U, and Unsicker K: Cell Tissue Res 183:273, 1977; reprinted by permission of Springer-Verlag.)

the human sublingual gland. Separate serous and mucous units may exist, in addition to secretory units composed of both cell types. In the latter arrangement, the mucous cells form a typical tubular portion that is capped at the blind end by crescents of several serous cells, known as demilunes (Figs. 10-1 and 10-7). The secretion of the serous demilune cells reaches the lumen through the intercellular canaliculi.

The disposition of the myoepithelium in relation to the parenchymal cells has already been described. In some glands the cell bodies may be restricted to the intercalated ducts with only the branching processes reaching the acini. Myoepithelial cells are not usually present along the striated ducts.

Ducts

The duct system of the salivary glands is formed by the confluence of small ducts into ones of progressively larger caliber. Within a lobule, the smallest ducts are the intercalated ducts (Fig. 10-1); they are thin branching tubes of variable length that connect the terminal secretory units to the next larger ducts, the striated ducts. In the interlobular connective tissue the ducts continue to join one another, increasing in size until the main excretory duct is formed.

Intercalated ducts. The intercalated ducts (Figs. 10-1, 10-2, and 10-11, *A*) are lined by a single layer of low cuboid cells with relatively empty-appearing cytoplasm. They are often difficult to identify in the light microscope because they are compressed between secretory units. In electron micrographs the intercalated duct cells share several characteristics of serous cells (Fig. 10-11, *B*). A small amount of RER is located in the basal cytoplasm, and a Golgi apparatus of moderate size is found apically. In proximally located cells (near the secretory units) a few small secretory granules may be found. The lateral membranes of adjacent cells are joined apically by junctional complexes and several desmosomes. One or two areas of prominent in-

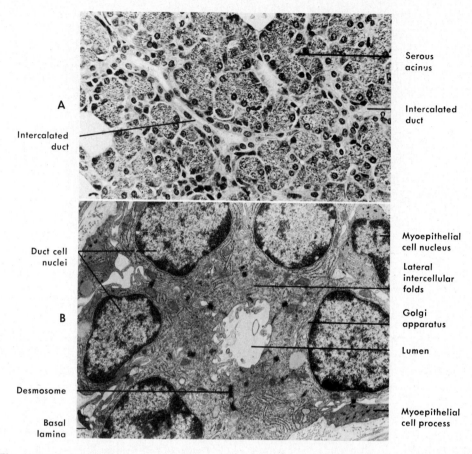

A

Intercalated
duct

B

Duct cell
nuclei

Desmosome

Basal
lamina

Serous
acinus

Intercalated
duct

Myoepithelial
cell nucleus

Lateral
intercellular
folds

Golgi
apparatus

Lumen

Myoepithelial
cell process

Fig. 10-11. A, Light micrograph of human parotid gland showing long branching intercalated ducts between serous acini. **B,** Electron micrograph of intercalated duct cut in cross section. Duct cells contain a moderate amount of rough endoplasmic reticulum and a prominent Golgi apparatus but few or no secretory granules. Prominent desmosomes and interlocking folds are present between adjacent cells. Myoepithelial cell processes extend longitudinally along duct, inside basal lamina. (Rat parotid gland. **A,** ×265; **B,** ×9600.)

terlocking folds of the lateral surface are located further basally. At the periphery of the duct, processes and cell bodies of myoepithelial cells may be found, attached by desmosomes to the duct cells.

Striated ducts. The striated ducts are lined by a layer of tall columnar epithelial cells with large, spherical, centrally placed nuclei (Figs. 10-1, 10-7, A, and 10-12). The cytoplasm is abundant and eosinophilic

and shows prominent striations at the basal ends of the cells, perpendicular to the basal surface. An occasional basally located cell can be identified by the position of its nucleus, below the level of those of the other cells (Fig. 10-7, A).

In electron micrographs the basal cytoplasm of the striated duct cells is partitioned by deep infoldings of the plasma membrane, producing numerous sheetlike

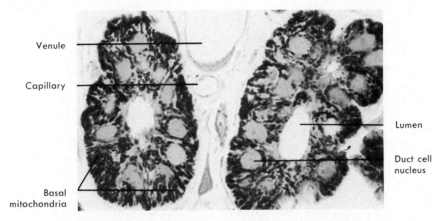

Fig. 10-12. Light micrograph of two striated ducts cut in cross section. Large, primarily radially oriented mitochondria, stained for cytochrome oxidase activity, fill basal regions of duct cells. Unstained nuclei are centrally located, and small mitochondria are found in apical cytoplasm. (Rat parotid gland; ×990.)

folds that extend beyond the lateral boundaries of the cell and interdigitate with similar folds of adjacent cells (Figs. 10-13 and 10-14, *B*). Abundant large mitochondria, usually radially oriented, are located in portions of the cytoplasm between the membrane infoldings (Figs. 10-12 to 10-14). The combination of infoldings and mitochondria accounts for the striations seen in the light microscope. A few short RER cisternae and a small Golgi apparatus are found in the perinuclear cytoplasm. Apically the cytoplasm may contain a variable amount of branching, tubular, smooth endoplasmic reticulum, small secretory granules of moderate density (Fig. 10-14, *A*) or small, empty-appearing vesicles. Several lysosomes, numerous small peroxisomes, bundles of cytoplasmic filaments, free ribosomes, and a moderate amount of glycogen are also usually present. Numerous short microvilli on the apical surfaces project into the lumen, and adjacent cells are joined by apical junctional complexes and several desmosomes along their lateral surfaces.

In the interlobular (excretory) ducts the epithelium becomes pseudostratified, with increasing numbers of smaller basal cells between the tall columnar cells. The characteristics of the striated cells are maintained to a variable degree, becoming less pronounced as the duct increases in size. In the largest ducts occasional mucous goblet cells and ciliated cells may be found, and the epithelium of the main duct gradually becomes stratified as it merges with the epithelium of the oral cavity.

Functions of salivary ducts. The main function of the salivary gland ducts is to convey the primary saliva secreted by the terminal secretory units to the oral cavity. The ducts are not just passive conduits, however; they actively modify the primary saliva by secretion and reabsorption of electrolytes and secretion of proteins. The intercalated duct cells often contain secretory granules in their apical cytoplasm, and two of the antibacterial proteins present in saliva, lysozyme and lactoferrin, have been localized to these ducts by immunofluorescent procedures. The striated duct cells contain

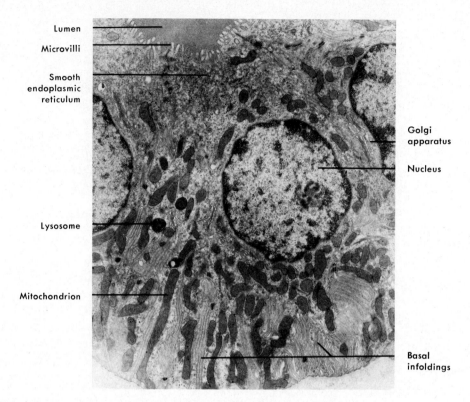

Lumen
Microvilli
Smooth endoplasmic reticulum
Golgi apparatus
Nucleus
Lysosome
Mitochondrion
Basal infoldings

Fig. 10-13. Electron micrograph of striated duct cells of rat parotid gland. Numerous mitochondria are located between infoldings of basal plasma membrane. A few lysosomes and the Golgi apparatus are located in perinuclear region, and smooth endoplasmic reticulum is found in cell apices. Short microvilli project into lumen. (×7400.)

kallikrein, an enzyme found in saliva, and synthesize secretory glycoproteins, which are stored in the apical granules. Studies have shown that both intercalated and striated duct cells are also capable of reabsorbing proteins from the lumen by endocytic mechanisms.

The structure of the striated duct cells (i.e., basal infoldings and numerous mitochondria) is typical of tissues involved in water and electrolyte transport such as the kidney tubules and the choroid plexus. The role of the salivary ducts in electrolyte secretion and reabsorption has been extensively studied in experimental animals un-

der various conditions of secretion. Analysis of the primary secretion, obtained by micropuncture techniques from the lumen of an intercalated duct draining several secretory units, reveals that it is isotonic or slightly hypertonic to plasma, with Na^+ and Cl^- concentrations approximately equal to those in plasma. K^+ concentration is low compared to that of Na^+, but it is significantly higher than the K^+ concentration of plasma. HCO_3^- concentration is variable, depending on the specific gland. Analysis of fluid collected from the excretory ducts reveals that it is hypotonic, with low Na^+ and Cl^- and high K^+ concentrations. Fur-

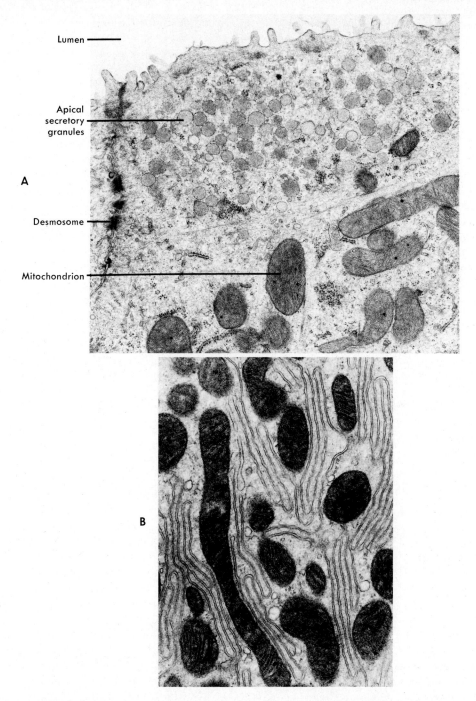

Lumen ——————

Apical
secretory
granules ————

A

Desmosome ——————

Mitochondrion ——————

B

Fig. 10-14. A, Electron micrograph of apical cytoplasm of striated duct cell. Small secretory granules are located near lumen. Mitochondria and smooth and rough endoplasmic reticulum are also present. **B,** Basal region of striated duct cell, showing mitochondria and infolded plasma membranes. (Rat sublingual gland; **A,** ×22,200; **B,** ×23,900.)

thermore, the concentration of these electrolytes varies with the flow rate of the saliva: with increasing flow, Na^+ and Cl^- increase, as does HCO_3^-, whereas K^+ decreases. It is believed that the striated ducts actively reabsorb Na^+ from the primary secretion and secrete K^+ and HCO_3^-; Cl^- tends to follow the electrochemical gradient established by Na^+ reabsorption. At increased flow rates Na^+ reabsorption becomes less efficient and the secretion is in contact with the ductal epithelium for a shorter time; hence Na^+ concentrations of the saliva tend to increase. Supporting this postulated role in Na^+ and Cl^- reabsorption, the basal regions of the striated duct cells contain high concentrations of the transport enzyme $(Na^+ + K^+)$–activated adenosine triphosphatase, as shown by binding of the specific inhibitor ^3H-ouabain. Microperfusion studies of the main excretory duct have shown that it too is able to reabsorb Na^+ and secrete K^+ and HCO_3^-.

Essentially all of the water enters saliva at the level of the terminal secretory units; the striated and excretory ducts appear to be relatively impermeable to water. The ductal reabsorption of Na^+ and Cl^- exceeds the secretion of K^+ and HCO_3^-, leaving a hypotonic luminal fluid. Since active transport of water does not occur, the ducts cannot secrete water against the osmotic gradient to produce the final hypotonic saliva.

Connective tissue elements

The cells found in the connective tissue of the salivary glands are the same as those in other connective tissues of the body and include fibroblasts, macrophages, mast cells, occasional leukocytes, fat cells, and plasma cells. The cells, along with collagen and reticular fibers, are embedded in a ground substance composed of proteogly-cans and glycoproteins. The vascular supply to the glands is also embedded within the connective tissue, entering the glands along the excretory ducts and branching to follow them into the individual lobules. The ducts, to the level of the intralobular striated ducts, are supplied with a dense capillary network; the capillary loops to the intercalated ducts and terminal secretory units are less extensive. A system of arteriovenous anastomoses around the larger interlobular ducts has also been described.

Nerves. The main branches of the nerves supplying the glands follow the course of the vessels, breaking up into terminal plexuses in the connective tissue adjacent to the terminal portions of the parenchyma. Nerve bundles, consisting of unmyelinated axons surrounded by cytoplasmic processes of Schwann cells, are distributed to the smooth muscle of the arterioles, the secretory cells and myoepithelium, and possibly the intercalated and striated ducts.

The secretory cells receive their innervation by one of two patterns. In the intraepithelial type, the axons split off from the nerve bundle and penetrate the basal lamina, lying adjacent to or between the secretory cells (Fig. 10-15, *A*). As the axons pass through the basal lamina, the Schwann cell covering is usually lost; occasionally it may be continued into the parenchyma and lie between the axons and the secretory cell. The site of innervation (neuroeffector site) is considered to be at varicosities of the axon, which contain small vesicles and mitochondria. The vesicles are believed to contain the chemical neurotransmitters norepinephrine and acetylcholine and presumably release them by an exocytosis-like process. The membranes of the axon and secretory cell are separated by a space of only 10 to 20 nm (100 to 200 Å), but no specializations of the plasma membranes have been detected at these sites. A single axon

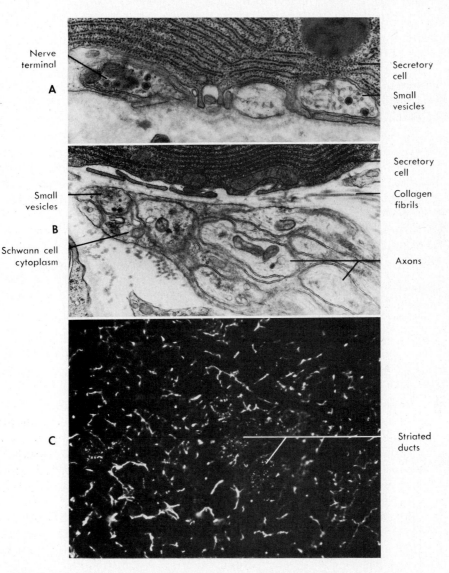

Fig. 10-15. A, Electron micrograph of three nerves of intraepithelial type at base of secretory cell. Axons are on epithelial side of basal lamina, in close contact with secretory cell. Nerve terminals contain mitochondria, small vesicles, a few larger dense-cored vesicles, and microtubules. Rat parotid gland. **B,** Electron micrograph of nerve bundle of subepithelial type in rat submandibular gland. Several axons are enclosed by a Schwann cell; innervation of secretory cell presumably occurs where axonal varicosities are bared of covering Schwann cell cytoplasm. **C,** Light micrograph of human parotid gland treated with formaldehyde vapor, which causes fluorescence of adrenergic nerves. Fluorescent structures seen here are nerve bundles, such as that in Fig. 10-15, *B,* located in connective tissue around parenchymal cells. The extensive nature of the sympathetic innervation of human parotid is evident. Fluorescence of striated ducts is caused by lysosomes. (**A,** ×20,800; **B,** ×15,200; **C,** courtesy J.R. Garrett, London.)

may have several varicosities along its length, making contact with the same cell or with two or more cells.

The second type of innervation is subepithelial. Instead of penetrating the basal lamina, the axons remain associated with the nerve bundle in the connective tissue (Fig. 10-15, *B*). Where the nerve bundles approach the secretory cells, some of the axonal varicosities, which contain the small neurotransmitter vesicles, lose their covering of Schwann cell cytoplasm. Presumably, these bared axonal varicosities are the sites of transmitter release. The axons remain separated from the secretory cells by 100 to 200 nm (1000 to 2000 Å), and the transmitters must diffuse across this space, which includes the basal laminae of the secretory cells and the nerve bundle.

The pattern of innervation varies between glands in the same animal and between the same gland in different species. The parotid serous cells and the sublingual mucous cells of the rat receive an intraepithelial type of innervation, as do the mucous cells of human labial glands. In contrast, the innervation of the secretory cells of the rat submandibular and the serous cells of the human parotid and submandibular glands is of the subepithelial type.

Both divisions of the autonomic nervous system may participate in the innervation of the secretory cells. In some glands both sympathetic (adrenergic) (Fig. 10-15, *C*) and parasympathetic (cholinergic) terminals (distinguished by special fixation and cytochemical techniques) have been observed in proximity to the secretory cells. Similarly, physiologic studies indicate that the cells of some glands respond to both sympathetic and parasympathetic stimulation by changes in their membrane potential. However, the extent of participation by each division varies between glands and animals, and the composition of the saliva

secreted in response to stimulation of each division is distinctly different. In general, a copious flow of watery saliva is secreted in response to parasympathetic stimulation, whereas that produced by sympathetic stimulation is thicker, higher in organic content, and comparatively less in quantity.

The innervation of duct cells is not clear. Intraepithelial terminals in ducts have been observed only rarely, but histochemical studies suggest that cholinergic and adrenergic nerves are found in the connective tissue around the ducts. Physiologic studies indicate that the ductal system is responsive to autonomic stimulation or administration of autonomic drugs: membrane potential changes in duct cells have been recorded, as well as changes in the transductal ion flux.

CLASSIFICATION AND STRUCTURE OF HUMAN SALIVARY GLANDS

The salivary glands have been classified in a variety of ways by different histologists; the two most commonly used groupings are based on (1) the size and location and (2) the histochemical nature of the secretory products. In this chapter the former classification will be used, although the latter is not without considerable merit. To a large extent, the nature of the secretion produced by a gland depends on its cellular makeup in terms of serous and mucous cells. However, all serous cells are not alike; they may differ considerably in the type and amount of enzymes and other proteins they produce and in the amount and nature of the carbohydrates attached to the secretory proteins. Mucous cells show a similar variability in the nature of their carbohydrate component. Furthermore, in salivary glands of some animals, the secretory cells may have a structure that cannot be readily classified as serous or mucous; histochemical characterization of their secretory products is useful for comparisons with other glands.

Major salivary glands

The largest of the glands are the three bilaterally paired major salivary glands. They are all located extraorally, and their secretions reach the mouth by variably long ducts.

Parotid gland. The parotid gland is enclosed within a well-formed connective tissue capsule, with its superficial portion lying in front of the external ear and its deeper part filling the retromandibular fossa. The main excretory duct (Stensen's duct) opens into the oral cavity on the buccal mucosa opposite the maxillary second molar. The opening is usually marked by a small papilla.

The parotid gland is a pure serous gland (Fig. 10-16, *A*); all the acinar cells are similar in structure to the serous cells described earlier. In the infant, however, a few mucous secretory units may be found. Electron microscopic studies indicate that the serous granules may have a dense central core. The intercalated ducts of the parotid are long and branching (Fig. 10-11, *A*), and the pale-staining striated ducts are numerous and stand out conspicuously against the more densely stained acini. The connective tissue septa in the parotid contain numerous fat cells, which increase in number with age and leave an empty space in histologic sections.

Submandibular gland. The submandibular gland is also enveloped by a well-defined capsule; it is located in the submandibular triangle behind and below the free border of the mylohyoid muscle, with a small extension lying above the mylohyoid. The main excretory duct (Wharton's duct) opens at the *caruncula sublingualis*, a small papilla at the side of the lingual frenum on the floor of the mouth. Some isolated smooth muscle cells have been reported around the duct.

The submandibular gland is a mixed gland, with both serous and mucous secretory units (Figs. 10-7, *A*, and 10-16, *B*). The serous units predominate, but the proportions may vary from one lobule to the next. The mucous terminal portions are capped by demilunes of serous cells. Although they appear similar by light microscopy, notable differences between submandibular and parotid serous cells are observed in the electron microscope (Fig. 10-17). The basal and lateral plasma membranes are thrown into numerous folds, interdigitating with similar processes from adjacent cells. The serous granules exhibit a variable substructure, from a granular matrix with a dense core or crescent, to an irregular skein of dense material dispersed in the matrix. The intercalated ducts tend to be somewhat shorter than those of the parotid, whereas the striated ducts are usually longer.

Sublingual gland. The sublingual gland lies between the floor of the mouth and the mylohyoid muscle; it is composed of one main gland and several smaller glands. The main duct (Bartholin's duct) opens with or near the submandibular duct, and several smaller ducts open independently along the sublingual fold. The capsule is poorly developed, but the connective tissue septa are particularly prominent within the gland.

The sublingual is also a mixed gland, but the mucous secretory units greatly outnumber the serous units (Fig. 10-16, *C*). The mucous cells are usually arranged in a tubular pattern; serous demilunes may be present at the blind ends of the tubules. Pure serous acini are rare or absent. The intercalated and striated ducts are poorly developed; mucous tubules may open directly into ducts lined with cuboid or co-

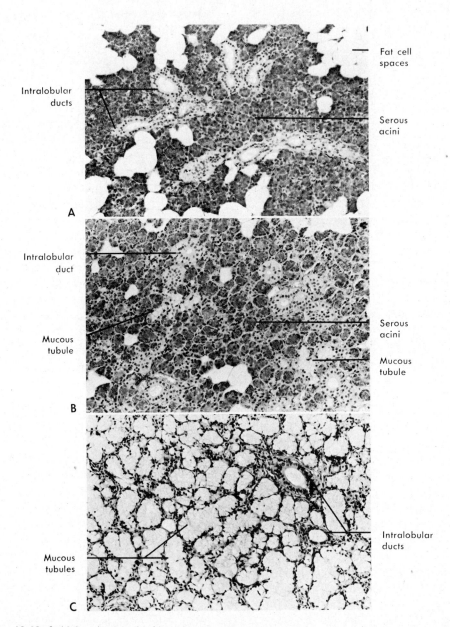

Fat cell spaces

Intralobular ducts

Serous acini

A

Intralobular duct

Mucous tubule

Serous acini

Mucous tubule

B

Intralobular ducts

Mucous tubules

C

Fig. 10-16. A, Light micrograph of human parotid gland, showing serous acini, several intralobular striated ducts, and numerous fat cell spaces. **B,** Light micrograph of human submandibular gland. Serous acini predominate, but a few mucous secretory units are present. Several intralobular striated ducts are cut in cross section. **C,** Light micrograph of human sublingual gland showing large mucous secretory units with typical tubular structure. Serous demilunes are difficult to distinguish at low magnification. Intralobular ducts are poorly developed. (**A** to **C**, ×90.)

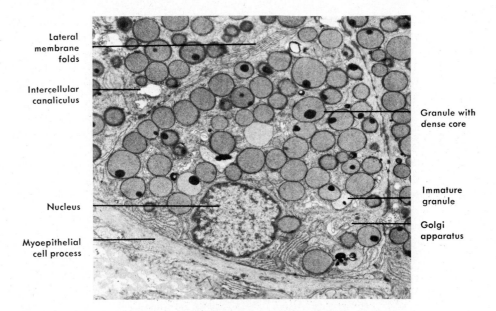

Lateral membrane folds

Intercellular canaliculus

Granule with dense core

Immature granule

Golgi apparatus

Nucleus

Myoepithelial cell process

Fig. 10-17. Electron micrograph of serous cell of human submandibular gland, showing secretory granules with dense core. Immature granules with similar cores are seen in Golgi regions. Several intercellular canaliculi are cut in cross section, and extensive folding of lateral cell membranes occurs between adjacent cells. Myoepithelial cell process is present at base of cell. (×6600.) (From Tandler B and Erlandson RA: Am J Anat 135:419, 1972; reprinted by permission of the Wistar Institute Press.)

lumnar cells without typical basal striations.

Minor salivary glands

The minor salivary glands are located beneath the epithelium in almost all parts of the oral cavity. These glands usually consist of several small groups of secretory units opening via short ducts directly into the mouth. They lack a distinct capsule, instead mixing with the connective tissue of the submucosa or muscle fibers of the tongue or cheek.

Labial and buccal glands. The glands of the lips and cheeks classically have been described as mixed, consisting of mucous tubules with serous demilunes. However, ultrastructural studies of the labial glands have revealed the presence of mucous cells only. Intercellular canaliculi have also

been observed between the mucous cells. The intercalated ducts are variable in length, and the intralobular ducts possess only a few cells with basal striations. Although the buccal glands have not been examined by electron microscopy, they are usually described as a continuation of the labial glands with a similar structure.

Glossopalatine glands. The glossopalatine glands are pure mucous glands. They are principally localized to the region of the isthmus in the glossopalatine fold but may extend from the posterior extension of the sublingual gland to the glands of the soft palate.

Palatine glands. The palatine glands are also of the pure mucous variety. They consist of several hundred glandular aggregates in the lamina propria of the posterolateral region of the hard palate and in the submucosa of the soft palate and uvula. The excretory ducts may have an irregular contour with large distensions as they course through the lamina propria. The openings of the ducts on the palatal mucosa are often large and easily recognizable.

Lingual glands. The glands of the tongue can be divided into several groups. The anterior lingual glands (glands of Blandin and Nuhn) are located near the apex of the tongue. The anterior regions of the glands are chiefly mucous in character, whereas the posterior portions are mixed. The ducts open on the ventral surface of the tongue near the lingual frenum. The posterior lingual mucous glands (Fig. 10-18) are located lateral and posterior to the vallate papillae and in association with the lingual tonsil. They are purely mucous in character, and

their ducts open onto the dorsal surface of the tongue. The posterior lingual serous glands (von Ebner's glands) are an extensive group of purely serous glands located between the muscle fibers of the tongue below the vallate papillae (Fig. 10-18). Their ducts open into the trough of the vallate papillae and at the rudimentary foliate papillae on the sides of the tongue.

Of all of the minor salivary glands, the posterior lingual serous glands are among the most interesting. Classically, their secretions have been described as serving to wash out the trough of the papillae and ready the taste receptors (located in the epithelium of the trough) for a new stimulus. Although this may be a part of their function, studies suggest that these glands have significant protective and digestive functions. Histochemical studies have localized

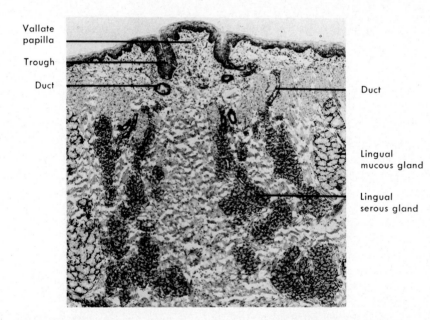

Fig. 10-18. Light micrograph of minor salivary glands of rat tongue. Lingual serous (von Ebner's) gland is located between muscle fibers of tongue below vallate papilla. Its ducts empty into trough around papilla. Posterior lingual mucous glands are located lateral to serous glands; their ducts open onto surface of tongue. (×36.) (From Hand AR: J Cell Biol 44:340, 1970; reprinted by permission of the Rockefeller University Press.)

the antibacterial enzymes peroxidase and lysozyme to these glands in humans. Biochemical studies of the lingual serous glands have demonstrated the presence of a secretory enzyme with lipolytic activity; similar lipolytic activity has been detected in aspirates from the esophagus and stomach. This lingual lipase has an acid pH optimum so that it is capable of hydrolyzing triglycerides in the stomach. The fatty acids, monoglycerides and diglycerides produced by lingual lipase, help to emulsify the remaining fat and increase the efficiency of pancreatic lipase in the intestine. In the newborn, when fat intake is high and levels of pancreatic lipase are low, lingual lipase probably plays a significant role in lipid digestion. Amylase activity has also been detected in the lingual serous glands of some species.

SPECIES VARIATION

From the preceding sections it is obvious that a number of differences exist between the individual salivary glands of humans. Numerous differences in the structure and biochemical makeup of the salivary glands also exist between various mammalian species. Although many of them are relatively minor, such as variations in the proportion of serous to mucous cells or the extent of innervation by each division of the autonomic nervous system, others are important because they represent variations in the structure and biochemistry of the parenchymal cells, they may be a reflection of the particular diet of the animal, or they occur in animals that are widely used for research purposes.

The parotid gland of ruminants is specialized for the production of large amounts of fluid, up to 60 L per day. The structure of the secretory cells reflects this function; they have little RER and few secretory granules, but extensive lateral membrane folds and numerous apical microvilli are present. The submandibular gland of rodents is one of the most interesting and widely studied of the salivary glands. In the rat and mouse the acinar cells are intermediate in structure and carbohydrate content between serous and mucous cells; they are usually termed "seromucous." The rodent submandibular gland, at the time of sexual maturity, also undergoes a specialization of the proximal portion of the intralobular striated ducts (adjacent to the intercalated ducts) to form a granular tubule segment. The cells of the granular tubule are large, with basally situated nuclei and remnants of basal infoldings and a large number of electron-dense granules of various size in the apical cytoplasm. The granular tubules are very sensitive to hormonal influences. They are generally smaller in the female than in the male, but administration of testosterone to females results in development of a malelike structure; conversely, castration of males results in femalelike glands. Interrelationships between the pituitary, thyroid, and submandibular glands have also been shown. The male mouse shows the greatest development of the granular tubules, and several proteins with unique biologic activities are found in the cells of the granular tubules. Many of these proteins exhibit trypsinlike esteroprotease activity or occur as complexes with protein components that have protease activity; however, their effects on tissues and animals are quite different. Nerve growth factor (NGF) stimulates the growth of neurites from embryonic dorsal root ganglia and sympathetic ganglia in culture; injection of antibodies to NGF into mice destroys their sympathetic neurons. Epidermal growth factor (EGF) is a potent mitogen for a variety of cell types and, when injected into newborn mice, causes increased keratinization and premature opening of the eyelids and eruption of the incisors.

Other growth-stimulating properties attributed to extracts of the mouse submandibular gland include mesenchyme stimulating factor, muscle differentiating factor, endothelial growth–stimulating factor, and thymotropic factor. Significant quantities of a glucagon-like substance, capable of producing hyperglycemia after intravenous injection, have been demonstrated in the rodent submandibular gland. Synthesis of an insulin-like substance has also been shown to occur in rodent salivary glands. Renin and kallikrein, proteolytic enzymes that act on plasma proteins to liberate vasoactive peptides, have been localized to the granular tubule cells by immunocytochemical techniques; kallikrein has also been found in the striated duct cells of other salivary glands and in other species. Most of these substances are found in high concentration in mouse submandibular saliva, indicating that they are exocrine secretory products of the granular tubule cells. The presence of many of these biologically active substances in blood plasma suggests that these cells may also have an endocrine function. However, several other tissues also produce these substances, and studies of the effects of gland extirpation on plasma concentrations have been contradictory. Therefore the significance of these substances in the salivary glands still remains obscure.

DEVELOPMENT AND GROWTH

During fetal life each salivary gland is formed at a specific location in the oral cavity through the growth of a bud of oral epithelium into the underlying mesenchyme. The primordia of the parotid and submandibular glands of humans appear during the sixth week, whereas the primordium of the sublingual gland appears after 7 to 8 weeks of fetal life. The minor salivary glands begin their development during the third month. The epithelial bud grows into an extensively branched system of cords of cells that are first solid but gradually develop a lumen and become ducts. The secretory portions develop later than the duct system and form by repeated branching and budding of the finer cell cords and ducts.

Studies of embryonic salivary glands in vitro have provided considerable information on the mechanism of glandular morphogenesis. The mesenchyme into which the glandular rudiment grows produces a factor or factors that stimulate the growth of the gland. If the mesenchyme and epithelium are separated and cultured on opposite sides of a filter, the growth of the epithelium proceeds normally; in the absence of the mesenchyme, the epithelium fails to grow. In the mouse the submandibular gland exhibits a specific requirement for submandibular mesenchyme; however, in the rat, parotid mesenchyme and, to a lesser extent, lung mesenchyme can support morphogenesis of the submandibular epithelium. The rat parotid and sublingual rudiments appear to be somewhat less specific in their mesenchymal requirements. The process of branching morphogenesis, that is, the formation of hollow, tubular glands from an initially flat epithelial surface, appears to be related to the presence of microfilaments in the epithelial cells. Microfilaments about 5 to 7 nm (50 to 70 Å) thick form a network beneath the cell membrane of almost all cells; they consist of the contractile protein actin. In developing salivary epithelium they are particularly prominent at the apical and basal ends of the cells; differential contraction could cause a group of cells to pucker outward or clefts to form in a solid cord or sheet of cells, similar to the effect of pulling a purse string. Addition of the drug cytochalasin B, which disrupts the structure and function of microfilaments, to salivary gland rudiments growing in vitro prevents branching and cleft formation and causes newly formed clefts to disappear. Older clefts are unaffected, probably because they have been stabilized by the presence of mesenchymal cells and extracellular materials.

The presence of a functional innervation is also essential to proper growth and maintenance of salivary gland structure. Parasympathetic denervation of adult animals results in a 30% loss in glandular weight within 2 to 3 weeks. Sympathetic denervation causes variable responses, from atrophy of some glands to hypertrophy of others. Parasympathectomy of the developing rat parotid prevents attainment of adult gland size, cell number and size, and DNA and RNA content; sympathectomy has a moderate effect on cell and gland size only. Normal physiologic activity is also important for the proper growth of developing glands, as well as maintenance of adult structure and enzyme content. Feeding of a liquid diet to rats greatly diminishes the reflexly mediated secretory activity; the parotid rapidly decreases in weight and amylase content, and the normal diurnal pattern of synthesis and secretion is eliminated.

Conversely, chronically increased stimulation can cause an increase in glandular size. For example, increasing the bulk content of the food, which necessitates increased masticatory activity, results in hypertrophy of the rat parotid. Repeated amputation of the incisors, apparently acting reflexly through the superior cervical ganglion, also causes enlargement of the salivary glands. Treatment of mice and rats with isoproterenol, a β-adrenergic drug,

causes several interesting changes in the salivary glands. A single injection results in the rapid and complete discharge of the stored secretory products and stimulation of protein synthesis; 20 to 30 hours after injection an increase in DNA synthesis and a wave of mitoses occur. Daily injections of isoproterenol cause cellular hypertrophy and hyperplasia, resulting in glandular enlargement up to five times that of untreated animals. The synthesis of certain proteins is enhanced, whereas that of others is reduced; additionally, several new proteins are synthesized by the enlarged glands. The effects on the salivary glands of isoproterenol and related adrenergic drugs have found wide application in experimental studies of cellular secretion, protein and nucleic acid synthesis, and regulation of gene expression.

CONTROL OF SECRETION

The physiologic control of salivary gland secretion is mediated through the activity of the autonomic nervous system. The release of neurotransmitters from the vesicles in the nerve terminals adjacent to the parenchymal cells stimulates them to discharge their secretory granules and secrete water and electrolytes. The molecular events that occur during this process, called stimulus-secretion coupling, have been extensively studied in the parotid gland of the rat. The neurotransmitters interact with specific receptors located on the plasma membrane of the acinar cell. Norepinephrine, the sympathetic transmitter, interacts with both α- and β-adrenergic receptors, and acetylcholine interacts with the cholinergic receptor. Protein secretion is mediated primarily through the β-adrenergic receptor; stimulation of the α-adrenergic and cholinergic receptors also causes low levels of protein secretion, but these two receptors appear to be mainly involved in the secretion of water and electrolytes. Receptors for the peptide transmitter substance P are also present on salivary gland cells; substance P stimulates secretion similar to that caused by α-adrenergic and cholinergic agonists. Vasoactive intestinal polypeptide (VIP) is present in nerve endings in the salivary glands and has been shown to induce secretion by some glands.

Receptor stimulation results in increases in the intracellular concentration of "second messengers," which trigger additional events leading to the cellular response. In the case of α-adrenergic, cholinergic, and substance P receptors, the membrane permeability to Ca^{++} is increased and a marked influx of Ca^{++} into the cell occurs. Recent experiments have linked the activation of these receptors to rapid changes in membrane phospholipid metabolism and release of Ca^{++} from intracellular stores such as the endoplasmic reticulum or the plasma membrane. The increased cytoplasmic Ca^{++} concentration causes K^+ efflux, water and electrolyte secretion, and a low level of exocytosis. Stimulation of the β-adrenergic receptor activates the plasma membrane enzyme adenylate cyclase, which catalyzes the formation of 3′,5′-cyclic adenosine monophosphate (cyclic AMP) from adenosine triphosphate. The increased intracellular concentration of cyclic AMP activates cyclic AMP–dependent protein kinase, an enzyme that phosphorylates other proteins, which in turn may be involved in the process of exocytosis. Cyclic AMP may also stimulate release of Ca^{++} from intracellular stores, thereby increasing its cytoplasmic concentration. Thus Ca^{++} may be the common intracellular mediator for all of the receptors; the different cellular responses may reflect the different sources of Ca^{++} or differing local concentration or both. Ca^{++} may have ad-

ditional effects, including stimulation of guanylate cyclase activity and an increase in the concentration of 3′,5′-cyclic guanosine monophosphate (cyclic GMP). However, the role of cyclic GMP in the secretory process has not yet been determined.

Adjacent secretory cells are joined to one another by specialized intercellular junctions called *gap junctions*. These junctions are permeable to ions and small molecules; thus changes in the intracellular concentration of these substances in one cell are reflected by parallel changes in the adjacent cells. Therefore physiologic stimulation probably results in a response by secretory units (acini) rather than individual cells.

The discharge of secretory granules involves translocation to the luminal cell surface and fusion of the granule membrane with the plasma membrane. Considerable evidence suggests that microtubules and microfilaments may act as a cytoskeletal framework or contractile mechanism for granule movement. Colchicine and vinblastine, drugs that disrupt microtubules, and cytochalasin B inhibit amylase release from rat parotid gland in vitro; similar effects are observed in several other tissues. However, contradictory results have been reported for some secretory cells, and definite associations of microtubules and microfilaments with secretory granules have been observed only rarely. Conclusions regarding the involvement of these organelles in salivary secretion cannot be made at present. The molecular mechanisms responsible for granule–plasma membrane fusion are poorly understood. Evidence for the presence of a Ca^{++}-dependent protein called synexin, which is involved in the initial fusion of granules with the plasma membrane, has been obtained for certain secretory cells. Other studies have indicated structural and compositional differences between the luminal membrane and the remainder of the plasma membrane, which may account for the specificity of the exocytotic process, as well as structural modifications of the membrane that may precede or occur concomitantly with exocytosis. These and other processes involved in exocrine secretion are currently under active investigation in a number of laboratories.

SALIVA: COMPOSITION AND FUNCTIONS

The most important function of the salivary glands is the production and secretion of saliva. It is important to make a distinction between pure glandular secretions, collected by special devices from the ducts, and whole saliva obtained from the mouth, usually by expectoration. In addition to the components contributed by the glands, whole saliva contains desquamated oral epithelial cells, leukocytes, microorganisms and their products, fluid from the gingival sulcus, and food remnants. The total volume of saliva secreted daily by humans is approximately 750 ml, of which about 60% is produced by the submandibular glands, 30% by the parotids, 5% or less from the sublinguals, and about 7% from the minor salivary glands. These proportions may change considerably with stimulation of various intensities, however. Water accounts for 99% or more of the saliva; inorganic ions, secretory proteins and glycoproteins, certain serum constituents, and other substances make up the remaining 1% or less. The major inorganic ions of saliva are Na^+, K^+, Cl^-, and HCO_3^-; the levels of these ions are variable, depending on the type of stimulation and rate of salivary flow. Other ions found in smaller amounts include Ca^{++}, Mg^{++}, HPO_4^{--}, I^-, SCN^-, and F^-. The pH of whole saliva varies from 6.7 to about 7.4, whereas parotid saliva may vary over a greater range, from pH 6.0 to 7.8. The primary buffering system of saliva

is formed by HCO_3^-, but certain salivary proteins may also provide some buffer capacity.

Secretory proteins represent the main category of organic substances in the saliva. These include various enzymes, large carbohydrate-rich glycoproteins or mucins, antibacterial substances, and a group of proteins involved principally in enamel pellicle formation and calcium phosphate homeostasis in the saliva. Certain serum constituents such as albumin, blood clotting factors, β_2-microglobulin, and immunoglobulins are also found in saliva. Other organic molecules present in saliva include cyclic AMP and cyclic AMP−binding proteins, amino acids, urea, uric acid, various lipids, and corticosteroids.

Saliva participates in digestion by providing a fluid environment for solubilization of food and taste substances and through the action of its digestive enzymes, principally amylase. Several isoenzymes of amylase have been identified in humans; two of these, representing 25% to 30% of the total amylase protein, have small amounts of bound carbohydrate. The action of amylase on ingested carbohydrates to produce glucose and maltose begins in the mouth and may continue for up to 30 minutes in the stomach before the amylase is inactivated by the acid pH and proteolysis. Lingual lipase, produced by the lingual serous glands, initiates the digestion of dietary lipids, hydrolyzing triglycerides to monoglycerides and diglycerides and fatty acids. Other hydrolytic enzymes have been detected in saliva, but their significance in food digestion has not been established.

Saliva has several protective functions. It keeps the oral tissues moist and facilitates swallowing and speaking. The mucous glycoproteins, which may have up to 800 oligosaccharide groups attached to the protein core, provide lubrication for the movement of the oral tissues against each other, as well as protection from chemical and thermal insults. Saliva also helps to protect the teeth from dental caries by means of both the cleansing and buffering action of saliva and the control of calcium and phosphate concentrations in the saliva and around the teeth. A large group of salivary proteins, called proline-rich proteins because of their high content of the amino acid proline, and statherin, a small tyrosine-rich protein, inhibit the precipitation of calcium phosphate from the saliva. Along with other salivary glycoproteins, statherin and certain of the proline-rich proteins bind to the tooth surface, forming the acquired enamel pellicle. The resulting localized supersaturation of calcium and phosphate reduces dissolution and promotes remineralization of the tooth enamel.

Several substances that are capable of inhibiting the growth of microorganisms and possibly preventing infection are found in saliva. Certain of the high-molecular-weight salivary glycoproteins aggregate specific strains of oral microorganisms or prevent their adherence to oral tissues, facilitating clearance from the mouth by swallowing. The secretion of peroxidase by the acinar cells and thiocyanate by the duct system establishes a bactericidal system in saliva. In the presence of hydrogen peroxide, peroxidase catalyzes the formation of hypothiocyanite ($OSCN^-$), which is inhibitory to bacteria. Another antibacterial protein present in saliva is lysozyme, an enzyme that hydrolyzes the polysaccharide of bacterial cell walls, resulting in cell lysis. An important group of defensive substances in saliva are the immunoglobulins. The predominant salivary immunoglobulin is IgA. Salivary or secretory IgA differs from serum IgA in that it is produced locally by plasma cells in the connective tissue stroma of the glands and consists of a

dimer of two IgA molecules and a protein called J chain. There is an additional glycoprotein produced by the parenchymal cells, called secretory component, that is also a part of the secretory IgA molecule. Secretory component, acting as a specific receptor in the parenchymal cell membrane for dimeric IgA, facilitates the transfer of the IgA to the lumen, either by translation in the cell membrane or by endocytosis and secretion along with the secretory products of the parenchymal cells. Secretory component may also increase the resistance of the IgA molecule to denaturation or proteolysis in the oral cavity. Small amounts of IgG and IgM have also been detected in saliva, and occasional plasma cells in the glandular stroma can be stained by fluorescent antibodies specific for these immunoglobulins. Serum immunoglobulins may also enter the saliva through the gingival crevice. Salivary immunoglobulins may act primarily through their ability to inhibit the adherence of microorganisms to oral tissues. Another antibacterial substance found in saliva is lactoferrin, an iron-binding protein. In the presence of specific antibody, lactoferrin that is not saturated with iron enhances the inhibitory effect of the antibody on the microorganisms.

The salivary glands of animals other than humans have additional specialized functions such as thermoregulation in mammals lacking sweat glands. In some reptiles and amphibians the homologous venom glands produce a variety of toxic substances. The salivary glands, as are many other tissues, are affected by secretions of the endocrine glands. The pronounced sexual dimorphism of the rodent submandibular gland has already been discussed. Thyroid and pituitary hormones have also been implicated in structural and functional changes of the salivary glands. The sodium and potassium content of saliva can be influenced by the administration of adrenocorticotropic hormone or mineralocorticoids, and alterations of salivary $Na^+:K^+$ ratios are observed in patients with Addison's disease and Cushing's syndrome. The possibility that the salivary glands may have an endocrine function in addition to their role in saliva production was discussed in relation to the variety of biologically active substances found in the rodent submandibular gland. There is some evidence, although not yet thoroughly accepted, that the human parotid gland produces a hormone called parotin. Parotin is said to promote the growth of mesenchymal tissues; it also lowers serum calcium levels in rabbits, stimulates calcification of rat incisor dentin, and increases bone marrow temperature with an accompaning increase in circulating leukocytes.

CLINICAL CONSIDERATIONS

An understanding of the anatomy, histology, and physiology of the salivary glands is essential for good dental practice. There is hardly any aspect of clinical practice in which salivary glands and saliva do not play an obvious or hidden role.

With the exception of a portion of the anterior part of the hard palate, salivary glands are seen everywhere in the oral cavity. They may, by developmental coincidence, even be included within the jaws. In the mandible this occurs in an area just posterior to the third molar teeth. In the maxilla salivary glands may be present in the nasopalatine canal. Because of these features, lesions of salivary glands, including tumors, can occur almost anywhere within the mouth. In a differential diagnosis of oral lesions therefore a salivary gland origin must always be kept in mind.

The salivary glands are subject to a number of pathologic conditions. These include inflammatory diseases such as viral, bacterial, or allergic sialadenitis, a variety of benign and malignant tumors, autoimmune diseases such as Sjögren's syndrome, and genetic diseases such as cystic fibrosis. One of the most common surface lesions of the oral mucosa is a vesicular elevation called mucocele. This is produced from the severance of the duct of a minor salivary gland and pooling of the saliva in the tissues. A blockage of a salivary gland duct may occur after formation of a mucous or calcified plug within the duct. If this occurs in a minor salivary gland, it usually causes no symptoms, but in major glands such obstruction can be very painful and may require surgical treatment.

The salivary glands may also be affected by a variety of systemic and metabolic diseases. The major glands, especially the parotid, may become enlarged during starvation, protein deficiency, alcoholism, pregnancy, diabetes mellitus, and liver disease. The association of the major salivary glands with the cervical lymph nodes, brought about by a common area of development, necessitates the differentiation of pathologic conditions of these lymph nodes from salivary gland diseases.

Alteration of salivary gland function during disease states may have profound influences on the oral tissues. The quality and quantity of saliva have a relationship to the incidence of dental caries. In conditions associated with the reduction or absence of salivary flow (xerostomia) the incidence of decay increases. Reduction in salivary flow is most often seen in patients with sicca syndrome, or Sjögren's syndrome, after irradiation of the head and neck region, or because of the use of various therapeutic pharmacologic agents. Inflammation and ulceration of the oral mucosa and frequent oral infections may also occur when salivary flow is reduced. Age changes in the salivary glands, particularly prominent in the parotid, consist of a gradual replacement of parenchyma with fatty tissue. Since the parotid is the major source of serous saliva, with advancing age patients often complain of dryness and an increase in the viscosity of saliva. Studies have shown that in the aged the flow of saliva is reduced during resting conditions, but in quantity and composition stimulated saliva in healthy, aged individuals is similar to that of young adults.

Determination of the quantity and composition of the saliva, sialochemistry, is often of value in the diagnosis of glandular or systemic disease. Experimentally, sialochemistry has also been used to determine ovulation time. Saliva is frequently used to monitor plasma concentrations of certain drugs that exhibit consistent saliva: plasma ratios.

REFERENCES

Amsterdam A, Ohad I, and Schramm M: Dynamic changes in the ultrastructure of the acinar cell of the rat parotid gland during the secretory cycle, J Cell Biol 41:753, 1969.

Archer FL and Kao VCY: Immunohistochemical identification of actomyosin in myoepithelium of human tissues, Lab Invest 18:669, 1968.

Aub DL, McKinney JS, and Putney JW Jr: Nature of the receptor-regulated calcium pool in the rat parotid gland, J Physiol 331:557, 1982.

Ball WD: Development of the rat salivary glands. III. Mesenchymal specificity in the morphogenesis of the embryonic submaxillary and sublingual glands of the rat, J Exp Zool 188:277, 1974.

Barka T: Biologically active polypeptides in submandibular glands, J Histochem Cytochem 28:836, 1980.

Batzri S, Selinger Z, Schramm M, et al.: Potassium release mediated by the epinephrine α-receptor in rat parotid slices. Properties and relation to enzyme secretion, J Biol Chem 248:361, 1973.

Bdolah A and Schramm M: The function of 3'5'-cyclic AMP in enzyme secretion, Biochem Biophys Res Commun 18:452, 1965.

Bennick A: Salivary proline-rich proteins, Mol Cell Biochem 45:83, 1982.

Bhaskar SN: Synopsis of oral pathology, ed 5, St. Louis, 1977, The CV Mosby Co.

Bhaskar SN: Radiographic interpretation for the dentist, ed 3, St. Louis, 1979, The CV Mosby Co.

Bienenstock J, Tourville D, and Tomasi TB Jr: The secretion of immunoglobulins by the human salivary glands. In Botelho SY, Brooks FP, and Shelley WB, editors: The exocrine glands, Philadelphia, 1969, University of Pennsylvania Press.

Blobel G: Synthesis and segregation of secretory proteins: the signal hypothesis. In Brinkley BR and Porter KR, editors: International cell biology, 1976-1977, New York, 1977, Rockefeller University Press.

Brandtzaeg P: Mucosal and glandular distribution of immunoglobulin components: differential localization of free and bound SC in secretory epithelial cells, J Immunol 112:1553, 1974.

Bullen JJ, Rogers HJ, and Griffiths E: Iron binding proteins and infection, Br J Haematol 23:389, 1972.

Bundgaard M, Møller M, and Poulsen JH: Localization of sodium pump sites in cat salivary glands, J Physiol 273:339, 1977.

Case RM: Synthesis, intracellular transport and discharge of exportable proteins in the pancreatic acinar cell and other cells, Biol Rev 53:211, 1978.

Castle JD, Jamieson JD, and Palade GE: Radioautographic analysis of the secretory process in the parotid acinar cell of the rabbit, J Cell Biol 53:290, 1972.

Clamp JR, Allen A, Gibbons RA, and Roberts GP: Chemical aspects of mucus, Br Med Bull 34:25, 1978.

Code CF, editor: Handbook of Physiology, section 6, vol 2, Washington, DC, 1967, American Physiological Society.

Creutz CE, Pazoles CJ, and Pollard HB: Identification and purification of an adrenal medullary protein (synexin) that causes calcium-dependent aggregation of isolated chromaffin granules, J Biol Chem 253:2858, 1978.

Dardick I et al.: Immunohistochemistry and ultrastructure of myoepithelium and modified myoepithelium of the ducts of human major salivary glands: histogenetic implications for salivary gland tumors, Oral Surg 64:703, 1987.

De Camilli P, Peluchetti D, and Meldolesi J: Dynamic changes of the luminal plasmalemma in stimulated parotid acinar cells. A freeze-fracture study, J Cell Biol 70:59, 1976.

Drenckhahn D, Gröschel-Stewart U, and Unsicker K: Immunofluorescence-microscopic demonstration of myosin and actin in salivary glands and exocrine pancreas of the rat, Cell Tissue Res 183:273, 1977.

Ekfors TO, and Hopsu-Havu VK: Immunofluorescent localization of trypsin-like esteropeptidases in the mouse submandibular gland, Histochem J 3:415, 1971.

Farquhar MG, and Palade GE: The Golgi apparatus (complex)—(1954-1981)—from artifact to center stage, J Cell Biol 91:77s, 1981.

Garrett JR: The innervation of normal human submandibular and parotid salivary glands. Demonstrated by cholinesterase histochemistry, catecholamine fluorescence and electron microscopy, Arch Oral Biol 12:1417, 1967.

Garrett JR: Neuro-effector sites in salivary glands. In Emmelin N and Zotterman Y, editors: Oral physiology, Oxford, England, 1972, Pergamon Press.

Gill G: Metabolic and endocrine influences on the salivary glands, Otolaryngol Clin North Am 10:363, 1977.

Gresik E, Michelakis A, Barka T, et al.: Immunocytochemical localization of renin in the submandibular gland of the mouse, J Histochem Cytochem 26:855, 1978.

Grobstein C: Epithelio-mesenchymal specificity in the morphogenesis of mouse submandibular rudiments in vitro, J Exp Zool 124:383, 1953.

Hall HD and Schneyer CA: Salivary gland atrophy in rat induced by liquid diet, Proc Soc Exp Biol Med 117:789, 1964.

Hammer MG and Sheridan JD: Electrical coupling and dye transfer between acinar cells in rat salivary glands, J Physiol 275:495, 1978.

Hamosh M: The role of lingual lipase in neonatal fat digestion. In Harries JT, editor: Pre- and post-natal development of mammalian absorptive processes. Ciba Found Symp 70:69, 1979.

Hamosh M and Scow RO: Lingual lipase and its role in the digestion of dietary fat, J Clin Invest 52:88, 1973.

Hand AR: The fine structure of von Ebner's gland of the rat, J Cell Biol 44:340, 1970.

Hand AR: Morphology and cytochemistry of the Golgi apparatus of rat salivary gland acinar cells, Am J Anat 130:141, 1971.

Hand AR: Synthesis of secretory and plasma membrane glycoproteins by striated duct cells of rat salivary glands as visualized by radioautography after ^{3}H-fucose injection, Anat Rec 195:317, 1979.

Hand AR and Ball WD: Ultrastructural immunocytochemical localization of secretory proteins in autophagic vacuoles of parotid acinar cells of starved rats, J Oral Pathol 17:279, 1988.

Hand AR and Jungmann RA: Localization of cellular regulatory proteins using postembedding immunogold labeling, Am J Anat 185:183, 1989.

Hand AR and Oliver C: Cytochemical studies of GERL and its role in secretory granule formation in exocrine cells, Histochem J 9:375, 1977.

Hand AR and Oliver C, editors: Basic mechanisms of cellular secretion: Methods in cell biology, vol 23, New York, 1981, Academic Press, Inc.

Hansson HA and Tunhall S: Epidermal growth factor and insulin-like growth factor I are localized in different compartments of salivary gland duct cells. Immunohistochemical evidence, Acta Physiol Scand 134:383, 1988.

Ichikawa M, Sasaki K, and Ichikawa A: Immunocytochemical localization of amylase in gerbil salivery gland acinar cells processed by rapid freezing and freeze-substitution fixation, J Histochem Cytochem 37:185, 1989.

Ito Y: Parotin: a salivary gland hormone, Ann NY Acad Sci 85:228, 1960.

Jamieson JD and Palade GE: Intracellular transport of secretory proteins in the pancreatic exocrine cell. I. Role of the peripheral elements of the Golgi complex, J Cell Biol 34:577, 1967.

Jamieson JD and Palade GE: Intracellular transport of secretory proteins in the pancreatic exocrine cell. II. Transport to condensing vacuoles and zymogen granules, J Cell Biol 34:597, 1967.

Jamieson JD and Palade GE: Production of secretory proteins in animal cells. In Brinkley BR and Porter KR, editors: International cell biology, 1976-1977, New York, 1977, Rockefeller University Press.

Johnson DA and Sreebny LM: Effect of food consistency and starvation on the diurnal cycle of the rat parotid gland, Arch Oral Biol 16:177, 1971.

Johnson DA and Sreebny LM: Effect of increased mastication on the secretory process of the rat parotid gland, Arch Oral Biol 18:1555, 1973.

Kauffman DL, Zager NI, Cohen E, et al: The isoenzymes of human parotid amylase, Arch Biochem Biophys 137:325, 1970.

Kim SK, Nasjleti CE, and Han SS: The secretion processes in mucous and serous secretory cells of the rat's sublingual gland, J Ultrastruct Res 38:371, 1972.

Klebanoff SJ and Luebke RG: The antilactobacillus system of saliva. Role of salivary peroxidase, Proc Soc Exp Biol Med 118:483, 1965.

Kleinberg I, Ellison SA, and Mandel ID, editors: Saliva and dental caries, (special suppl) Microbiology Abstracts, New York, 1979, Information Retrieval Inc.

Korsrud FR and Brandtzaeg P: Characterization ofepithelial elements in human major salivary glands by functional markers: localization of amylase, lactoferrin, lysozyme, secretory component, and secretory immunoglobulins by paired immunofluorescence staining, J Histochem Cytochem 30:657, 1982.

Kurth BE et al.: Cell culture and characterization of human minor salivary gland duct cells, J Oral Pathol 18:214, 1989.

Lawrence AM, Tan S, Hojvat S, et al.: Salivary gland hyperglycemic factor: an extrapancreatic source of glucagon-like material, Science 195:70, 1977.

Lawson D, Raff MC, Gomperts B, et al.: Molecular events during membrane fusion. A study of exocytosis in rat peritoneal mast cells, J Cell Biol 72:242, 1977.

Lawson KA: The role of mesenchyme in the morphogenesis and functional differentiation of rat salivary epithelium, J Embryol Exp Morphol 27:497, 1972.

Leblond CP and Bennett G: Role of the Golgi apparatus in terminal glycosylation. In Brinkley BR and Porter KR, editors: International cell biology, 1976-1977, New York, 1977, Rockefeller University Press.

Leslie BA, Putney JW Jr, and Sherman JM: α-Adrenergic, β-adrenergic and cholinergic mechanisms for amylase secretion by rat parotid gland *in vitro*, J Physiol 260:351, 1976.

Levi-Montalcini R and Angeletti PU: Nerve growth factor, Physiol Rev 48:534, 1968.

Liang T and Cascieri MA: Substance P receptor on parotid cell membranes, J Neurosci 1:1133, 1981.

Lotti LV and Hand AR: Endocytosis of parotid salivary proteins by striated duct cells in streptozotocin-diabetic rats, Anat Rec 221:802, 1988.

Mandel ID: Human submaxillary, sublingual, and parotid glycoproteins and enamel pellicle. In Horowitz MI and Pigman W, editors: The glycoconjugates. Vol 1. Mammalian glycoproteins and glycolipids, New York, 1977, Academic Press Inc.

Mandel ID: Sialochemistry in diseases and clinical situations affecting salivary glands, CRC Crit Rev Clin Lab Sci 12:321, 1980.

Mason DK and Chisholm DM: Salivary glands in health and disease, London, 1975, WB Saunders Co.

Masson PL, Heremans JL, and Dive C: An iron-binding protein common to many external secretions, Clin Chim Acta 14:735, 1966.

Mayo JW and Carlson DM: Protein composition of human submandibular secretions, Arch Biochem Biophys 161:134, 1974.

Mayo JW and Carlson DM: Isolation and properties of four α-amylase isozymes from human submandibular saliva, Arch Biochem Biophys 163:498, 1974.

Mazariegos MR and Hand AR: Regulation of tight junctional permeability in the rat parotid gland by autonomic agonists, J Dent Res 63:1102, 1984.

Mednieks MI and Hand AR: Cyclic AMP-dependent protein kinase in stimulated rat parotid gland cells: compartmental shifts after in vitro treatment with isoproterenol, Eur J Cell Biol 28:264, 1982.

Mednieks MI and Hand AR: Cyclic AMP binding proteins in saliva, Experientia 40:945, 1984.

Mestecky J and Lawton AR, editors: The immunoglobulin A system, New York, 1974, Plenum Press.

Moreira JE et al.: Light and electron microscopic immunolocalization of rat submandibular gland mucin glycoprotein and glutamine/glutamic acid-rich proteins, J Histochem Cytochem 37:515, 1989.

Murakami K, Tanaguchi H, and Baba S: Presence of insulin-like immunoreactivity and its biosynthesis in rat and human parotid gland, Diabetologia 22:358, 1982.

Murphy RA, Saide JD, Blanchard MH, et al.: Molecular properties of the nerve growth factor secreted in mouse saliva, Proc Natl Acad Sci USA 74:2672, 1977.

Myant NB: Iodine metabolism of salivary glands, Ann NY Acad Sci 85:208, 1960.

Nakamura T, Nagura H, Watanabe K, et al.: Immunocytochemical localization of secretory immunoglobulins in human parotid and submandibular glands, J Electron Microsc 31:151, 1982.

Neutra M and Leblond CP: Synthesis of the carbohydrate of mucus in the Golgi complex shown by electron microscope radioautography of goblet cells from rats injected with glucose-H^3, J Cell Biol 30:119, 1966.

Nustad K, Ørstavik TB, Gautvik KM, et al.: Glandular kallikreins, Gen Pharmacol 9:1, 1978.

Oliver C and Hand AR: Uptake and fate of luminally administered horseradish peroxidase in resting and isoproterenol stimulated rat parotid acinar cells, J Cell Biol 76:207, 1978.

Ørstavik TB, Brandtzaeg P, Nustad K, et al.: Cellular localization of kallikreins in rat submandibular and sublingual salivary glands, Acta Histochem 54:183, 1975.

Palade G: Intracellular aspects of the process of protein secretion, Science 189:347, 1975.

Parks HF: On the fine structure of the parotid gland of mouse and rat, Am J Anat 108:303, 1961.

Petersen OH: The electrophysiology of gland cells. London, 1980, Academic Press, Inc.

Pinkstaff CA: The cytology of salivary glands, Int Rev Cytol 63:141, 1980.

Poggioli J and Putney JW Jr: Net calcium fluxes in rat parotid acinar cells. Evidence for a hormone-sensitive calcium pool in or near the plasma membrane, Pflügers Arch 392:239, 1982.

Putney JW Jr: Inositol lipids and cell stimulation in mammalian salivary gland, Cell Calcium 3:369, 1982.

Putney JW Jr, Weiss SJ, Leslie BA, et al.: Is calcium the final mediator of exocytosis in the rat parotid gland? J Pharmacol Exp Ther 203:144, 1977.

Rasmussen H: Cell communication, calcium ion, and cyclic adenosine monophosphate, Science 170:404, 1970.

Riva A and Riva-Testa F: Fine structure of acinar cells of human parotid gland, Anat Rec 176:149, 1973.

Riva A, Testa-Riva F, Del Fiacco M, et al.: Fine structure and cytochemistry of the intralobular ducts of the human parotid gland, J Anat 122:627, 1976.

Scott BL and Pease DC: Electron microscopy of the salivary and lacrimal glands of the rat, Am J Anat 104:115, 1959.

Scott J and Gradwell E: A quantitative study of the effects of chronic hypoxia on the histological structure of the rat major salivary glands, Arch Oral Biol 34:315, 1989.

Schneyer CA and Hall HD: Autonomic regulation of postnatal changes in cell number and size of rat parotid gland, Am J Physiol 219:1268, 1970.

Schneyer LH, Young JA, and Schneyer CA: Salivary secretion of electrolytes, Physiol Rev 52:720, 1972.

Schramm M and Selinger Z: The functions of cyclic AMP and calcium as alternative second messengers in parotid gland and pancreas, J Cyclic Nucleotide Res 1:181, 1975.

Selye H, Veilleux R, and Cantin M: Excessive stimulation of salivary gland growth by isoproterenol, Science 133:44, 1961.

Shackleford JM and Klapper CE: Structure and carbohydrate histochemistry of mammalian salivary glands, Am J Anat 111:25, 1962.

Simson JAV, Hazen D, Spicer SS, et al.: Secretagogue-mediated discharge of nerve growth factor from granular tubules of male mouse submandibular glands: an immunocytochemical study, Anat Rec 192:375, 1978.

Smith PH and Patel DG: Immunochemical studies of the insulin-like material in the parotid gland of rats, Diabetes 33:661, 1984.

Spooner BS and Wessells NK: An analysis of salivary gland morphogenesis: role of cytoplasmic microfilaments and microtubules, Dev Biol 27:38, 1972.

Sreebny LM, Johnson DA, and Robinovitch MR: Functional regulation of protein synthesis in the rat parotid gland, J Biol Chem 246:3879, 1971.

Suddick RP and Dowd FJ: The microvascular architecture of the rat submaxillary gland: possible relationship to secretory mechanisms, Arch Oral Biol 14:567, 1969.

Sumi LA et al.: Immunoelectron microscopical localization of immunoglobulins, secretory component and J chain in the human minor salivary glands, J Oral Pathol 17:390, 1988.

Tabak LA, Levine MJ, Mandel ID, et al.: Role of salivary mucins in the protection of the oral cavity, J Oral Pathol 11:1, 1982.

Tamarin A and Sreebny LM: The rat submaxillary salivary gland. A correlative study by light and electron microscopy, J Morphol 117:295, 1965.

Tandler B: Ultrastructure of the human submaxillary gland. I. Architecture and histological relationships of the secretory cells, Am J Anat 111:287, 1962.

Tandler B: Ultrastructure of the human submaxillary gland. III. Myoepithelium, Z Zellforsch 68:852, 1965.

Tandler B, Denning CR, Mandel ID, et al.: Ultrastructure of human labial salivary glands. I. Acinar secretory cells, J Morphol 127:383, 1969.

Tandler B and Erlandson RA: Ultrastructure of the human submaxillary gland. IV. Serous granules, Am J Anat 135:419, 1972.

Taubman MA and Smith DJ: Secretory immunoglobulins and dental disease. In Han SS, Sreebny L, and Suddick R, editors: Symposium on the mechanism of exocrine secretion, Ann Arbor, 1973, University of Michigan Press.

Taylor T and Erlandsen SL: Peroxidase localization in von Ebner's gland of man, J Dent Res 52:635, 1973.

Testa-Riva F: Ultrastructure of human submandibular gland, J Submicrosc Cytol 9:251, 1977.

Testa-Riva F, Puxeddu P, Riva A, et al.: The epithelium of the excretory duct of the human submandibular gland: a transmission and scanning electron microscope study, Am J Anat 160:381, 1981.

Tomasi TB Jr, Tan EM, Solomon A, et al.: Characteristics of an immune system common to certain external secretions, J Exp Med 121:101, 1965.

Vigneswaran N, Haneke E, and Hornstein OP: A comparative lectin histochemical study of major and minor salivary glands with special reference to the labial glands, Arch Oral Biol 34:739, 1989.

Wells H: Functional and pharmacological studies on the regulation of salivary gland growth. In Schneyer LH and Schneyer CA, editors: Secretory mechanisms of salivary glands, New York, 1967, Academic Press, Inc.

Young JA and Schneyer CA: Composition of saliva in mammalia, Aust J Exp Biol Med Sci 59:1, 1981.

Young JA and van Lennep EW: The morphology of salivary glands, London, 1978, Academic Press.

Young JA and van Lennep EW: Transport in salivary and salt glands. In Giebisch G, Tosteson DC, and Ussing HH, editors: Membrane transport in biology, vol 4B, Berlin, 1979, Springer-Verlag.

11

TOOTH ERUPTION

Although the word "eruption" properly refers to the cutting of the tooth through the gum (from the Latin *erumpere*, meaning "to break out"), it is generally understood to mean the axial or occlusal movement of the tooth from its developmental position within the jaw to its functional position in the occlusal plane. However, eruption is only part of the total pattern of physiologic tooth movement, because teeth also undergo complex movements related to maintaining their position in the growing jaws and compensating for masticatory wear. Physiologic tooth movement is described as consisting of the following:

1. Preeruptive tooth movement
2. Eruptive tooth movement
3. Posteruptive tooth movement

Superimposed on these movements is the replacement of the entire deciduous dentition by the permanent dentition.

PATTERN OF TOOTH MOVEMENT

Preeruptive tooth movement. When deciduous tooth germs first differentiate, they are very small and a good deal of space is between them. This space is soon used because of the rapid growth of the tooth germs, and crowding results, especially in the incisor and canine region. This crowding is then relieved by growth of the jaws in length, which permits drifting of the tooth germs.

Permanent teeth with deciduous predecessors also move before they reach the position from which they will erupt, but analysis and description of such movements are complicated by the fact that change in position of the tooth germ is the result of a number of factors involving body move-

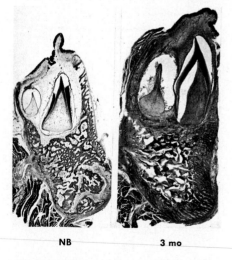

NB   3 mo

Fig. 11-1. For legend see opposite page.

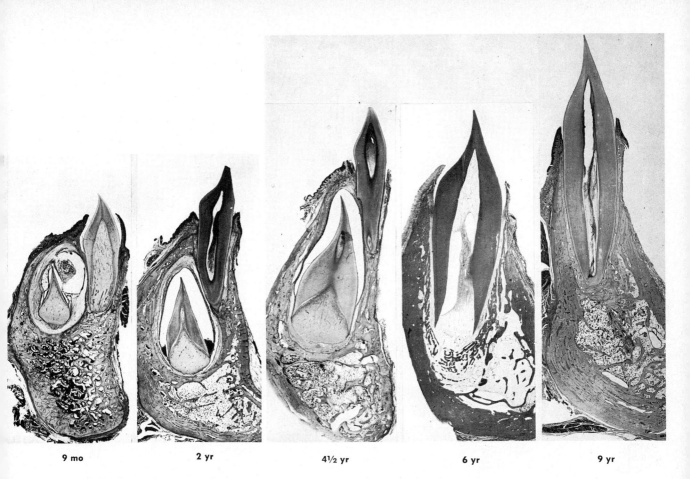

9 mo **2 yr** **4½ yr** **6 yr** **9 yr**

Fig. 11-1. Buccolingual sections through central incisor region of mandible at representative stages of development from birth to 9 years of age. At birth both deciduous and permanent tooth germs occupy same bony crypt. Notice how, by eccentric growth and eruption of deciduous tooth, permanent tooth germ comes to occupy its own bony crypt apical to erupted incisor. At 4½ years, resorption of deciduous incisor has begun. At 6 years, deciduous incisor has been shed and its successor is erupting. Notice active deposition of new bone at base of socket at this time.

ment of the tooth germ, its growth, or a relative change in position of associated deciduous and permanent tooth germs. For example, in Fig. 11-1 there appears to be a considerable change in position between the permanent incisor tooth germ and its deciduous predecessor in the first 2 years of life. But whether there has been much body movement of the tooth germ in its crypt is doubtful because the changes in the relative positions can be ascribed to growth of the permanent tooth and eruptive movement of the deciduous tooth. The

same also holds for the permanent molars (Fig. 11-2).

The permanent molars, which have no deciduous predecessors, also exhibit movement. For example, the upper permanent molars, which develop in the tuberosity of the maxilla, at first have their occlusal surfaces facing distally (Fig. 11-3) and swing around only when the maxilla has grown sufficiently to provide the necessary space. Similarly, mandibular molars develop with their occlusal surfaces inclined mesially and only become upright as room becomes

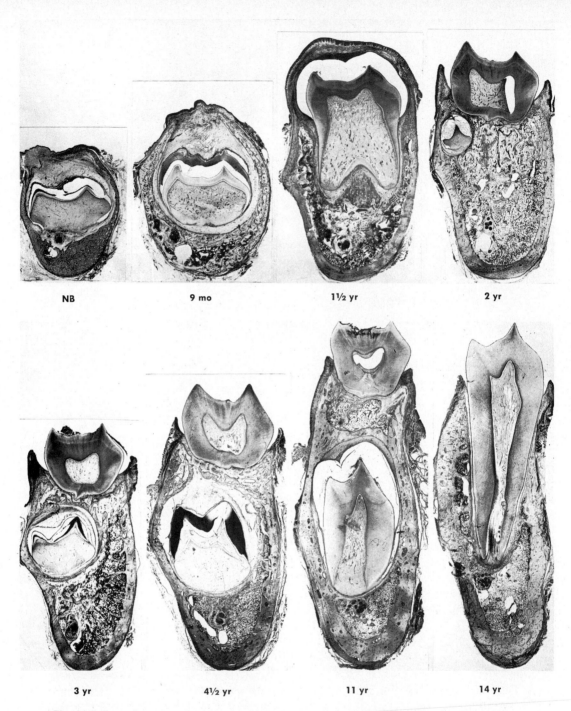

Fig. 11-2. Buccolingual sections through deciduous first molar and first permanent premolar of mandible at representative stages of development from birth to 14 years. Notice how permanent tooth germ shifts its position. In section of 4½-year mandible, gubernacular canal is clearly visible. Lack of roots in the 2-, 3-, 4½-, and 11-year sections is not the result of resorption but of the section's being cut in midline of tooth with widely divergent roots.

NB   9 mo   1½ yr   2 yr

3 yr   4½ yr   11 yr   14 yr

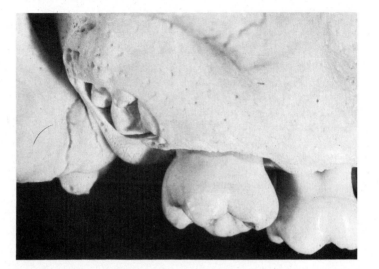

Fig. 11-3. Region of maxillary tuberosity of dried skull of 4-year-old child. At this stage of development, first permanent molar is still within its bony crypt. Notice how occlusal surface faces backward. With further growth of maxilla, molar swings down so that it eventually erupts into occlusal plane.

available.

All these movements occur in association with growth of the jaws, which makes analysis of individual tooth movement even more difficult. For the beginning student preeruptive tooth movement should be considered as movement positioning the tooth and its crypt within the growing jaws preparatory to tooth eruption.

Eruptive tooth movement. During the phase of eruptive tooth movement the tooth moves from its position within the bone of the jaw to its functional position in occlusion, and the principal direction of movement is occlusal or axial. However, as in the case of preeruptive tooth movement, jaw growth is still occurring while most teeth are erupting so that movement in planes other than axial movement is superimposed on eruptive movement.

Posteruptive tooth movement. Posteruptive tooth movements are those that (1) maintain the position of the erupted tooth while the jaw continues to grow and (2) compensate for occlusal and proximal wear. The former movement, like eruptive movement, occurs principally in an axial direction to keep pace with the increase in height of the jaws. It involves both the tooth and its socket and ceases when jaw growth is completed. The movements compensating for occlusal and proximal wear continue throughout life and consist of axial and mesial migration, respectively.

HISTOLOGY OF TOOTH MOVEMENT

Preeruptive phase. Preeruptive tooth movement, whether it involves drifting or growth of the tooth germ, demands remodeling of the bony wall of the crypt. This is achieved by the selective deposition and removal of bone by osteoblastic and osteoclastic activity, but whether such bony remodeling is the cause of preeruptive tooth movements or reflects a response to forces produced by other factors is not known. It is of interest that there are instances that indicate normal skeletal morphogenesis might be involved in determining tooth position. Thus marrow spaces of consistent configuration develop in bones, and, as will be described later, eruptive pathways through bone form even in the absence of associated teeth.

Eruptive phase. During the eruptive phase of physiologic tooth movement, significant developmental events occur that are associated with eruptive tooth movement. They include the formation of the roots, the periodontal ligament, and the dentogingival junction.

Root formation is initiated by growth of Hertwig's epithelial root sheath, which initiates the differentiation of odontoblasts from the dental papilla. The odontoblasts then form root dentin, bringing about an overall increase in length of the tooth that is largely accommodated by eruptive tooth movement, which begins at approximately the same time as root formation is initiated. Shortly after the onset of root formation cementum, periodontal ligament, and the

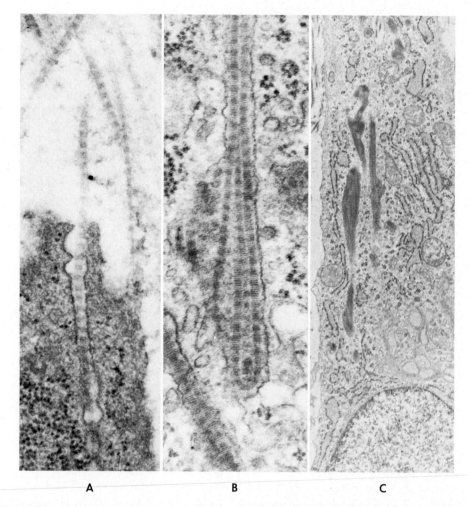

A   B   C

Fig. 11-4. Three electron micrographs illustrating role of fibroblast in periodontal ligament remodeling and turnover. **A,** Phagocytosis (ingestion) of collagen fibril. **B,** Once within fibroblast, lysosomes containing catabolic enzymes fuse with vesicle containing collagen, and **C,** degradation continues in phagolysosomes. (From Ten Cate AR: Anat Rec 182:1, 1975.)

bone lining the crypt wall are formed (see Chapter 7). In addition, a number of structural changes are seen within the periodontal ligament, which could be responsible for tooth movement. Fibroblasts of the periodontal ligament possess as part of their cytoskeleton intermediate filaments that consist of contractile proteins. They also exhibit frequent cell-to-cell contacts of the adherence type and a further specialization involving the cell membrane, the fibronexus. This describes a morphologic relationship between the intracellular filaments of the fibroblast, transmembrane proteins, which produce an increased density of fibroblast cell membrane, extracellular filaments, and fibronectin. Fibronectin is a sticky glycoprotein that can stick to a number of extracellular components, including collagen. Finally, the ligament fibroblast has the ability to ingest and degrade extracellular collagen while forming new collagen fibrils (Fig. 11-4). How these morphologic features might be related to tooth movement is discussed later in the section dealing with mechanisms.

Significant histologic changes also occur in the tissues overlying the erupting tooth. Bone removal is necessary for permanent teeth to erupt. In the case of those teeth with deciduous predecessors there is an additional anatomic feature, the *gubernacular canal* and its contents, the *gubernacular cord,* which may have an influence on eruptive tooth movement. When the successional tooth germ first develops within the came crypt as its deciduous predecessor, bone surrounds both tooth germs but does not completely close over them. As the deciduous tooth erupts, the permanent tooth germ becomes situated apically and is entirely enclosed by bone (Figs. 11-1 and 11-2) except for a small canal that is filled with connective tissue and often contains epithelial remnants of the dental lamina. This connective tissue mass is termed the "gubernacular cord" (Figs. 11-5 and 11-6), and it may have a function in guiding the permanent tooth as it erupts. After removal of any overlying bone there is loss of

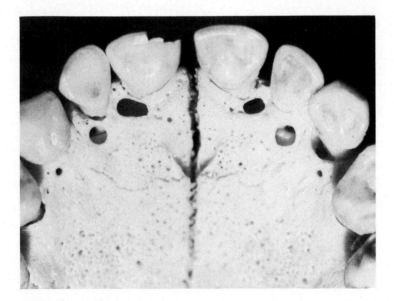

Fig. 11-5. Incisor region of dried maxilla of 4-year-old child. Notice foramina lingual to deciduous teeth. These are gubernacular canals.

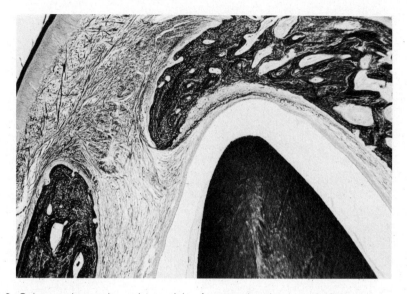

Fig. 11-6. Gubernacular cord consists mainly of connective tissue and often contains a central strand of epithelium surrounded by connective tissue.

the intervening soft connective tissue between the reduced enamel epithelium covering the crown of the tooth and the overlying oral epithelium.

How this loss is achieved is not established. A simple explanation is that pressure from the erupting tooth causes local ischemia and therefore local necrosis, but other evidence indicates that this may be too facile an explanation. What is certain is that the changes taking place in this connective tissue affect the epithelia it sustains and both the reduced dental epithelium and the overlying oral epithelium begin to proliferate and migrate into the disorganized connective tissue so that eventually a solid plug of epithelium forms in advance of the erupting tooth. The central cells of this epithelial mass degenerate and form an epithelium-lined canal through which the tooth erupts without any hemorrhage. This epithelial cell mass is also involved in the formation of the dentogingival junction (see Chapter 9).

Once the tooth has broken through the

oral mucosa, it continues to erupt at the same rate until it reaches the occlusal plane and meets its antagonist. Rapid eruptive movement then ceases.

Posteruptive phase. In the posteruptive phase the tooth makes movements primarily to accommodate the growth of the jaws. The principal movement is in an axial direction. It occurs most actively between the ages of 14 and 18 and is associated with condylar growth, which separates the jaws and teeth. Although bone deposition occurs at the alveolar crest and on the socket floor (Fig. 11-7), this is not responsible for tooth movement. The same forces responsible for eruptive tooth movement achieve axial posteruptive movement, with bone deposition occurring later.

Movements are also made to compensate for occlusal and proximal wear of the tooth. It is generally assumed that the continuous deposition of cement around the apices of the roots of teeth is sufficient to compensate for occlusal wear. However, there is no evidence that this deposition of cement ac-

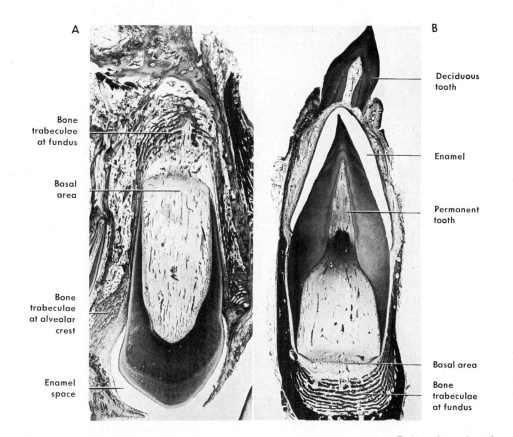

Fig. 11-7. Erupting upper deciduous canine, **A,** and lower permanent canine, **B.** Note formation of bone trabeculae at alveolar crest of deciduous canine, **A,** is a sign of rapid growth of maxilla in height. (From Kronfeld R: Dent Cosmos 74:103, 1932.)

tually moves the tooth. It is more likely that the forces causing tooth eruption are still available to bring about sufficient axial movement of the tooth to compensate for occlusal wear. The cement deposition that occurs is probably an infilling phenomenon.

Wear also takes place at the contact points between teeth, and to maintain tooth contact mesial or proximal drift takes place. Histologically this drift is seen as a selective deposition and resorption of bone on the socket walls by osteoblasts and osteoclasts respectively, and with the electron microscope collagen remodeling in both

the periodontal and transseptal ligaments is seen.

MECHANISM OF TOOTH MOVEMENT

The mechanism that brings about tooth movement is still debatable and is likely to be a combination of a number of factors. Although many possible causes have been proposed, only four merit serious consideration: (1) bone remodeling, (2) root growth, (3) vascular pressure, and (4) ligament traction. Briefly stated, the bone remodeling theory supposes that selective deposition and resorption of bone brings about eruption. The root growth theory supposes that the proliferating root impinges on a fixed case, thus converting an apically directed force into occlusal movement. The vascular pressure theory supposes that a local increase in tissue fluid pressure in the periapical region is sufficient to move the tooth. The ligament traction theory proposes that the cells and fibers of the ligament pull the tooth into occlusion.

Bone remodeling. Bone remodeling clearly is important to permit tooth movement; for instance, in animals that exhibit a genetic deficiency of osteoclasts tooth eruption is prevented. Whether the bony remodeling that occurs around teeth causes or is the effect of tooth movement is not known, and both circumstances may apply. If the tooth germ is removed experimentally and the dental follicle left intact, an eruptive pathway forms in the overlying bone. Further, if a silicone replica is substituted for the tooth germ, it also erupts. On the other hand, if the dental follicle is removed, no eruptive pathway forms. These experiments establish the absolute requirement for a dental follicle to achieve bony remodeling and tooth eruption, for it is the follicle that provides the source for new bone-forming cells and the conduit for osteoclasts derived from monocytes through its vascular supply. Other studies on bone remodeling have indicated that control may reside with the bone-lining cells, the osteoblasts. It is proposed that these cells, under hormonal influence, secrete collagenase and other proteolytic enzymes to remove the osteoid layer. In so doing these cells round up and expose the newly denuded mineralized bone surface, providing the stimulus to attract osteoclasts to the site.

Root formation. At first glance it would seem that root formation is the obvious cause of eruptive tooth movement. Root formation follows crown formation and involves cellular proliferation and formation of new tissue that must be accommodated by either movement of the crown of the tooth or resorption of bone at the base of its socket. It is the former that actually that occurs, but if occlusal movement is prevented, resorption of bone occurs at the base of the socket. This is an important point, for it illustrates that if root formation is to result in an eruptive force, the apical growth of the root needs to be translated into occlusal movement and requires the presence of a fixed base. No such fixed base exists. The bone at the base of the socket cannot act as a fixed base because pressure on bone results in its resorption. Advocates of the root growth theory of tooth eruption postulated the existence of a ligament, the cushion-hammock ligament, straddling the base of the socket from one bony wall to the other like a sling. Its function was to provide a fixed base for the growing root to react against. But the structure described as the cushion-hammock ligament is the pulp-delineating membrane that runs across the apex of the tooth and has no bony insertion. It cannot act as a fixed base. Clinical observations also indicate that root formation cannot be responsible for eruptive tooth movement. For instance, some teeth move a distance greater than the length of their roots, and eruptive movement can occur after completion of root formation. Finally, experimental resection preventing further root formation does not stop eruptive tooth movement. Yet, as is discussed later, root formation may be a necessary prerequisite for eruption.

Vascular pressure. It is known that teeth move in synchrony with the arterial pulse, so local volume changes can produce limited tooth movement. Ground substance can swell by up to 50% with the addition of water, and a differential pressure sufficient to cause tooth movement between the tissues below and above an erupting tooth has been reported in the dog. Again, whether such pressures are the prime movers of teeth is debatable because surgical excision of the root, and therefore the local vasculature, does not prevent tooth eruption.

Periodontal ligament traction. There is a good deal of evidence that the eruptive force resides in the dental follicle–periodontal ligament complex. Experiments delineating the role of the follicle, from which incidentally the periodontal ligament forms, have already been presented in the section dealing with bony remodeling. Experiments on the continuously erupting rodent incisor, designed to eliminate the effects of root growth and vascular supply, also show that, so long as periodontal tissue is available, tooth movement occurs. Drugs that interrupt the proper formation of collagen in the ligament also interfere with eruption.

Tissue culture experiments have shown that ligament fibroblasts are able to contract a collagen-gel, which in turn brings about movement of a disk of root tissue attached to that gel. Thus there is no doubt that periodontal ligament fibroblasts have the ability to contract and transmit a contractile force to the extracellular environment and in particular to the collagen fiber bundles in vitro. All the morphologic features exist in vivo to permit similar movement. Thus the fibroblasts possess contractile filaments, are in contact with one another to permit summation of contractile forces, and exhibit fibronexuses by which such forces can be transmitted to the collagen fiber bundles. These not only remodel but are also inclined at the correct angle to bring about eruptive movement. This angulation of the ligament fiber bundles is a prerequisite for tooth movement, and the orientation is believed to be established by the developing root, creating flow lines in the gel-like dental follicle. A simple analogy of the above is the sailor (fibroblast) pulling on a rope (collagen) attached to a sail (tooth). To move the sail the sailor must remain stationary and pull on the rope (contraction) and coil it on the deck (collagen remodeling).

In summary, eruptive movement could be brought about by a combination of events involving a force initiated by the fibroblast. This force is transmitted to the extracellular compartment via fibronexuses and to collagen fiber bundles, which, aligned in an appropriate inclination brought about by root formation, bring about tooth movement. These fiber bundles must have the ability to remodel for eruption to continue, and interference with this ability affects the process. The removal of bone to create the eruptive pathway is also dictated by the tissues surrounding the tooth.

Posteruptive tooth movement. In posteruptive tooth movement the mechanisms for moving the tooth axially during eruption are most likely also used to compensate for occlusal wear. Mesial, or proximal, drift involves a combination of two separate forces resulting from occlusal contact of teeth and contraction of the transseptal ligaments between teeth. When the jaws are clenched, bringing teeth into contact, force is generated in a mesial direction because of the summation of cuspal planes and because many teeth have a mesial inclination. This can be demonstrated in a number of ways. When opposing teeth are removed, the rate of mesial drift is slowed but not eliminated. Selective grinding of cuspal slopes can either enhance or counter the effect of occlusal force, and when this is done, the rate of mesial drift is respectively enhanced or decreased but again not eliminated. These observations indicate that although an anterior component of occlusal force is responsible for mesial drift, it is not solely responsible.

Running between teeth across the alveolar process is the transseptal ligament, and there is evidence that this ligament has a key role in maintaining tooth position. For example, if a tooth is bisected, the two halves move away from each other, but if the transseptal ligament is previously removed, this separation does not occur. A simple but elegant experiment demonstrates that mesial drift is indeed multifactorial. By disking away the approximal contacts, room is made to permit mesial drift, and the teeth begin to move to reestablish contact. If teeth are ground out of occlusal contact, however, the rate of drift is slowed. The conclusion must be that mesial drift is achieved by contraction of transseptal fibers and enhanced by occlusal forces.

CLINICAL CONSIDERATIONS

From all that has been written so far in this chapter it should be evident that the principal supporting tissues of the tooth, the periodontal ligament and the bone of

Table 5. Chronology of human dentition

Tooth	Formation of enamel matrix and dentin begins	Amount of enamel matrix formed at birth	Enamel completed	Emergence into oral cavity	Root completed
Primary dentition					
Maxillary					
Central incisor	14 wk in utero	Five sixths	1½ mo	7½ mo	1½ yr
Lateral incisor	16 wk in utero	Two thirds	2½ mo	9 mo	2 yr
Canine	17 wk in utero	One third	9 mo	18 mo	3¼ yr
First molar	12-15 wk in utero	Cusps united	6 mo	14 mo	2½ yr
Second molar	12-19 wk in utero	Cusp tips still isolated	11 mo	24 mo	3 yr
Mandibular					
Central incisor	18 wk in utero	Three fifths	2½ mo	6 mo	1½ yr
Lateral incisor	18 wk in utero	Three fifths	3 mo	7 mo	1½ yr
Canine	20 wk in utero	One third	9 mo	16 mo	3¼ yr
First molar	12-15 wk in utero	Cusps united	5½ mo	12 mo	2¼ yr
Second molar	12-18 wk in utero	Cusp tips still isolated	10 mo	20 mo	3 yr
Permanent dentition					
Maxillary					
Central incisor	3-4 mo			7-8 yr	10 yr
Lateral incisor	10-12 mo			8-9 yr	11 yr
Canine	4-5 mo			11-12 yr	13-15 yr
First premolar	1½-1¾ yr			10-12 yr	12-13 yr
Second premolar	2-2¼ yr			10-12 yr	12-14 yr
First molar	At birth	Sometimes a trace		6-7 yr	9-10 yr
Second molar	2½-3 yr			12-13 yr	14-16 yr
Third molar	7-9 yr			17-21 yr	18-25 yr.
Mandibular					
Central incisor	3-4 mo		4-5 yr	6-7 yr	9 yr
Lateral incisor	3-4 mo		4-5 yr	7-8 yr	10 yr
Canine	4-5 mo		6-7 yr	9-10 yr	12-14 yr
First premolar	1¾-2 yr		5-6 yr	10-12 yr	12-13 yr
Second premolar	2¼-2½ yr		6-7 yr	11-12 yr	13-14 yr
First molar	At birth	Sometimes a trace	2½-3 yr	6-7 yr	9-10 yr
Second molar	2½-3 yr		7-8 yr	11-13 yr	14-15 yr
Third molar	8-10 yr.		12-16 yr	17-21 yr	18-25 yr

From Logan WHG and Kronfeld R: J Am Dent Assoc 20:379, 1933, slightly modified by McCall and Schour.

the jaw, possess a remarkable "plasticity" that enables the tooth to react either favorably or unfavorably to its immediate environment. This plasticity of the supporting tissues is used by the orthodontist to achieve a favorable clinical response. By applying forces to the tooth and by relying on the biologic responses of bone and periodontal ligament, malalignment of teeth can often be corrected.

Table 5 gives the time of tooth emergence (in whites); one should note that there is considerable variation in these times. However, only teeth emerging significantly outside these ranges should be considered as abnormal and indicative of some fault in eruptive movement. By far the greatest number of aberrations in eruption times are delayed eruptive movements. Premature eruption of teeth occurs infrequently. Sometimes infants are born with "erupted" lower central incisors, but this is an example of gross maldevelopment. Such teeth need to be extracted as soon as possible because they prevent suckling. Premature loss of a deciduous tooth without closure of the gap may lead to early eruption of its successor. Far more common, however, is the occurrence of delayed or retarded eruption. This may be caused by either local or systemic factors. Systemic factors include nutritional, genetic, and endocrine deficiencies. Local factors include such situations as loss of a deciduous tooth and drifting of opposing teeth to block the eruptive pathway. Severe trauma may eliminate the dental follicle, and hence periodontal ligament formation is prevented. When this happens, the bone of the jaw fuses with tooth, a condition known as ankylosis, and eruption is not possible. Eruption may also be delayed by an increased density of fibrous tissue over the erupting tooth or the development of an eruption cyst from remnants of the dental lamina.

Whites exhibit an evolutionary trend to a diminution in the size of the jaws. This trend has not been accompanied by a corresponding decrease in the size of the teeth, and as a result crowding is a common occurrence. The third molars are the last teeth to erupt, and frequently all the available space has been used. As a result these teeth become impacted. Canines are also often impacted because of their late eruption time. Finally, it has been shown that the moment a tooth breaks through the oral epithelium, an acute inflammatory response occurs in the connective tissue adjacent to the tooth. This is seen even in the germ-free animals and is seen in varying degrees around all teeth throughout life. Clinically, as teeth break through the oral mucosa, there is often some pain, slight fever, and general malaise, all signs of an inflammatory process. In infants these symptoms are popularly called "teething."

REFERENCES

Beertsen W, Everts V, and van den Hoof A: Fine structure of fibroblasts in the periodontal ligament of the rat incisor and their possible role in tooth eruption, Arch Oral Biol 19:1087, 1974.

Bellows CF, Melcher AH, and Aubin JE: Contraction and organization of collagen gels by cells cultured from periodontal ligament, gingiva and bone suggest functional differences between cell types, J Cell Sci 50:299, 1981.

Bellows CF, Melcher AH, and Aubin JE: An invitro model for tooth eruption utilizing periodontal ligament fibroblasts and collagen lattices, Arch Oral Biol 28:715, 1983.

Berkovitz BKB: The effect of root transection and partial root resection on the unimpeded eruption rate of the rat incisor, Arch Oral Biol 16:1033, 1971.

Berkovitz BKB: The healing process in the incisor tooth socket of the rat following root resection and exfoliation, Arch Oral Biol 16:1045, 1971.

Berkovitz BKB: The effect of preventing eruption on the proliferative basal tissues of the rat lower incisor, Arch Oral Biol 17:1279, 1972.

Berkovitz BKB: Mechanisms of tooth eruption. In Lavelle CLB, editor: Applied physiology of the mouth, Bristol, England, 1975. John Wright and Sons Ltd.

Berkovitz BKB and Thomas NR: Unimpeded eruption in the root resected lower incisor of the rat with a preliminary note on root transection, Arch Oral Biol 14:771, 1969.

Brash JC: The growth of the alveolar bone and its relation to the movements of the teeth, including eruption, Int J Orthod 14:196, 283, 398, 487, 494, 1928.

Brodie AG: The growth of alveolar bone and the eruption of the teeth, Oral Surg 1:342, 1948.

Bryer LW: An experimental evaluation of physiology of tooth eruption, Int Dent J 7:432, 1957.

Cahill DR: Eruption pathway formation in the presence of experimental tooth impaction in puppies, Anat Rec 164:67, 1969.

Cahill DR: The histology and rate of tooth eruption with and without temporary impaction in the dog, Anat Rec 166:225, 1970.

Cahill DR: Histological changes in the bony crypt and gubernacular canal of erupting permanent premolars during deciduous premolar exfoliation in beagles, J Dent Res 53:786, 1974.

Cahill DR and Marks SC Jr: Tooth eruption: evidence for the central role of the dental follicle, J Oral Pathol 9:189, 1980.

Cahill DR and Marks SC Jr: Chronology and histology of exfoliation and eruption of mandibular premolars in dogs, J Morphol 171:213, 1982.

Carollo DA, Hoffman RL, and Brodie AG: Histology and function of the dental gubernacular cord, Angle Orthod 41:300, 1971.

Garant PR, Moon IC, and Cullen MR: Attachment of periodontal ligament fibroblasts to the extracellular matrix in the squirrel monkey, J Periodont Res 17:70, 1982.

Gowgiel JM: Eruption of irradiation-produced rootless teeth in monkeys, J Dent Res 40:538, 1961.

Herzberg F and Schour I: Effects of the removal of pulp and Hertwig's sheath on the eruption of incisors in the albino rat, J Dent Res 20:264, 1941.

Jenkins GN: The physiology of the mouth, ed 3, Oxford, 1966, Blackwell Scientific Publications Ltd.

Logan WHG and Kronfeld R: Development of the human jaws and surrounding structures from birth to the age of fifteen years, J Am Dent Assoc 20:379, 1933.

Magnusson B: Tissue changes during molar tooth eruption, Trans R Sch Dent Stockholm 13:1, 1968.

Main JHP: A histological survey of the hammock ligament, Arch Oral Biol 10:343, 1965.

Main JHP and Adams D: Experiments on the rat incisor into the cellular proliferation and blood pressure theories of tooth eruption, Arch Oral Biol 11:163, 1966.

Manson JD: Bone changes associated with tooth eruption. In The mechanisms of tooth support, a symposium, Oxford, 6-8 July, 1965, Bristol, England, 1967, John Wright & Sons, Ltd.

Marks SC Jr, Cahill DR, and Wise GE: The cytology of the dental follicle and adjacent alveolar bone during tooth eruption, Am J Anat 168:277, 1983.

Marks SC and Cahill DR: Experimental study in the dog of the nonactive role of the tooth in the eruptive process, Arch Oral Biol 29:311, 1984.

Marks SC Jr and Cahill DR: Ultrastructure of alveolar bone during tooth eruption in the dog, Am J Anat 177:427-438, 1986.

Minkoff R, Stevens CJ, and Karon JM: Autoradiography of protein turnover in subcrestal versus supracrestal fiber tracts of the developing mouse periodontium, Arch Oral Biol 26:1069, 1981.

Moss JP and Picton DCA: Mesial drift of teeth in adult monkeys (*Macaca irus*) when forces from the cheeks and tongue had been eliminated, Arch Oral Biol 15:979, 1970.

Moxham BJ and Berkovitz BKB: The periodontal ligament and physiological tooth movements. In Berkovitz BKB, Moxham BJ, and Newman HN, editors: The periodontal ligament in health and disease, Elmsford, NY, 1982, Pergamon Press, Inc.

Orban B: Growth and movement of the tooth germs and teeth, J Am Dent Assoc 15:1004, 1928.

Sicher H: Tooth eruption: the axial movement of continuously growing teeth, J Dent Res 21:201, 1942.

Sicher H: Tooth eruption: the axial movement of teeth with limited growth, J Dent Res 21:395, 1942.

Sicher H and Weinmann JP: Bone growth and physiological tooth movement, Am J Orthod 30:109, 1944.

Shore RC, Berkovitz BKB, and Moxham BJ: Intercellular contracts between fibroblasts in the periodontal connective tissues of the rat, J Anat 133(1):67, 1981.

Smith RG: A clinical study into the rate of eruption of some human permanent teeth, Arch Oral Biol 25:675, 1980.

Taylor AC and Butcher EO: The regulation of eruption rate in the incisor teeth of the white rat, J Exp Zool 117:165, 1951.

Ten Cate AR: The mechanism of tooth eruption. In Melcher AH and Bowen WH, editors: The biology of the periodontium, New York, 1969, Academic Press, Inc.

Ten Cate AR: Physiological resorption of connective tissue associated with tooth eruption. An electron microscope study, J Periodont Res 6:168, 1971.

Ten Cate AR: Morphological studies of fibrocytes in connective tissue undergoing rapid remodelling, J Anat 112:401, 1972.

Thomas NR: The properties of collagen in the periodontium of an erupting tooth. In The mechanisms
of tooth support, a symposium, Oxford, 6-8 July,
1965, Bristol, England, 1967, John Wright & Sons,
Ltd.

Thomas NR: The effect of inhibition of collagen maturation on eruption in rats, J Dent Res 44:1159,
1969.

Weinmann JP: Bone changes related to eruption of
the teeth, Angle Orthod 11:83, 1941.

Wise GE, Marks SC Jr, and Cahill DR: Ultrastructural
features of the dental follicle associated with formation of the tooth eruption pathway in the dog, J Oral
Pathol 14:15-26, 1985.

Yimaz RS, Darling A, and Levers BGH: Mesial drift of
human teeth assessed from ankylosed deciduous
molars, Arch Oral Biol 25:127, 1980.

12
SHEDDING OF DECIDUOUS TEETH

DEFINITION
PATTERN OF SHEDDING
HISTOLOGY OF SHEDDING
MECHANISM OF RESORPTION AND SHEDDING

CLINICAL CONSIDERATIONS
Remnants of deciduous teeth
Retained deciduous teeth
Submerged deciduous teeth

DEFINITION

The human dentition, like those of most mammals, consists of two generations. The first generation is known as the deciduous (primary) dentition and the second as the permanent (secondary) dentition. The necessity for two dentitions exists because infant jaws are small and the size and number of teeth they can support is limited. Since teeth, once formed, cannot increase in size, a second dentition, consisting of larger and more teeth, is required for the larger jaws of the adult. The physiologic process resulting in the elimination of the deciduous dentition is called *shedding* or *exfoliation.*

PATTERN OF SHEDDING

The shedding of deciduous teeth is the result of progressive resorption of the roots of teeth and their supporting tissue, the periodontal ligament. Most attention has been paid to the removal of the dental hard tissues, which is accomplished by easily identified multinuclear cells in every way similar to osteoclasts (Fig. 12-1). In general, the pressure generated by the growing and erupting permanent tooth dictates the pattern of deciduous tooth resorption. At first this pressure is directed against the

root surface of the deciduous tooth itself (Fig. 12-2). Because of the developmental position of the permanent incisor and canine tooth germs and their subsequent physiologic movement in an occlusal and

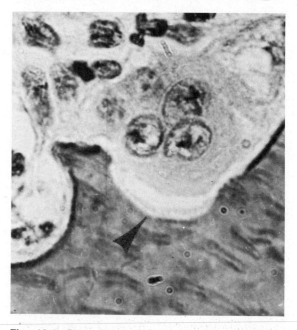

Fig. 12-1. Photomicrograph of odontoclast resorbing dentin. Note ruffled border *(arrow)* where odontoclast is in contact with dentin. (From Furseth R: Arch Oral Biol 13:417, 1968.)

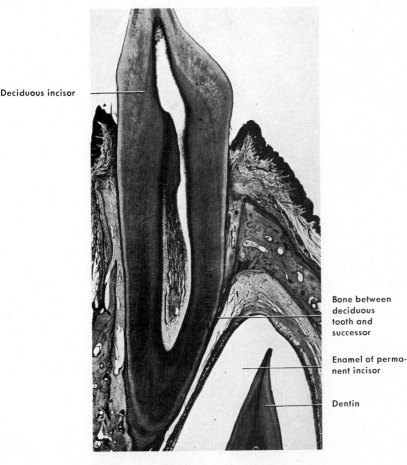

Deciduous incisor

Bone between
deciduous
tooth and
successor

Enamel of perma-
nent incisor

Dentin

Fig. 12-2. Thin lamella of bone separates permanent tooth germ from its predecessor.

vestibular direction, resorption of the roots of the deciduous incisors and canines begins on their lingual surfaces (Fig. 12-3). Later, these developing tooth germs occupy a position directly apical to the deciduous tooth, which permits them to erupt in the position formerly occupied by the deciduous tooth (Fig. 12-4). Frequently, however, and especially in the case of the permanent mandibular incisors, this apical positioning of the tooth germs does not occur, and the permanent tooth erupts lingual to the still functioning deciduous tooth (Fig. 12-5).

Resorption of the roots of deciduous molars often first begins on their inner surfaces because the early developing bicuspids are found between them (Fig. 12-6). This resorption occurs long before the deciduous molars are shed and reflects the expansion of their growing permanent successors. However, as a result of the continued growth of the jaws and occlusal movement of the deciduous molars, the successional tooth germs come to lie apical to the deciduous molars (Fig. 12-7). This change in position provides the growing bicuspids with adequate space for their con-

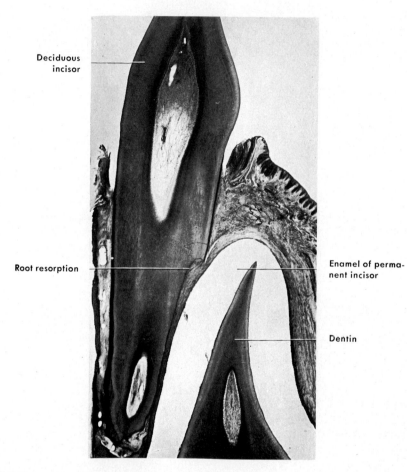

Deciduous incisor

Root resorption

Enamel of permanent incisor

Dentin

Fig. 12-3. Resorption of lingual aspect of root of deciduous incisor caused by pressure of erupting successor.

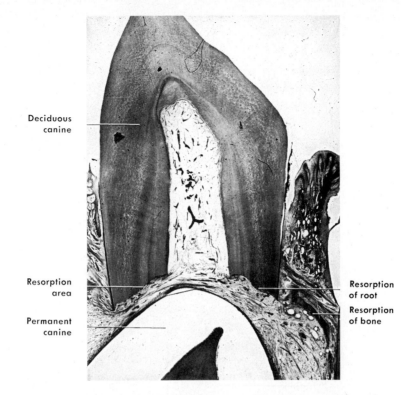

Deciduous canine

Resorption area

Permanent canine

Resorption of root

Resorption of bone

Fig. 12-4. Resorption of root of deciduous canine. Note apical position of permanent successor. (From Kronfeld R: Dent Cosmos 74:103, 1932.)

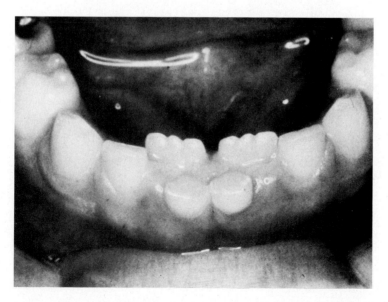

Fig. 12-5. Dentition of 6-year-old child showing how permanent incisors frequently erupt lingually to deciduous incisors before latter teeth are shed.

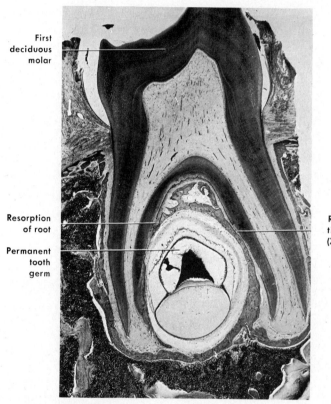

First
deciduous
molar

Resorption
of root

Permanent
tooth
germ

Repaired resorp-
tion of dentin
(X)

Fig. 12-6. Germ of lower first permanent premolar between roots of first deciduous molar. Repair of previously resorbed dentin has occurred at X. (See also Figs. 12-16 and 12-17.)

First
deciduous
molar

Traumatic
changes

First
permanent
premolar

Second
deciduous
molar

Traumatic
changes in
periodontal
ligament
(X)

Second
permanent
premolar

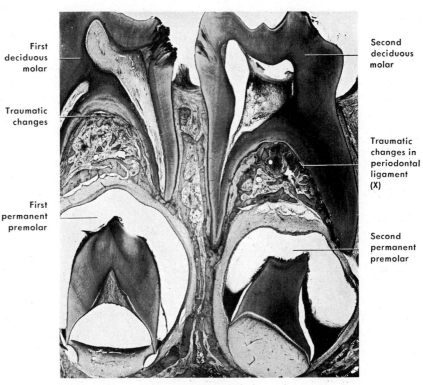

Fig. 12-7. Germs of permanent premolars below roots of deciduous molars.

tinued development and also relieves the pressure on the roots of the overlying deciduous molars. The areas of early resorption are repaired by the deposition of a cementum-like tissue. When the bicuspids begin to erupt, resorption of the deciduous molars is again initiated and this time continues until the roots are completely lost and the tooth is shed (Fig. 12-8). The bicuspids thus erupt in the position of deciduous molars.

HISTOLOGY OF SHEDDING

The cells responsible for the removal of dental hard tissue are identical to osteoclasts, the highly specialized cells responsible for the removal of bone, and are called odontoclasts.

Odontoclasts are readily identifiable in the light microscope as large, multinucleated cells occupying resorption bays on the surface of a dental hard tissue. Their cytoplasm is vacuolated, and the surface of the

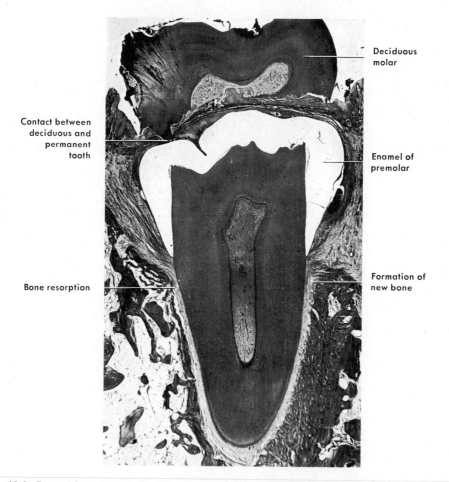

Contact between deciduous and permanent tooth

Bone resorption

Deciduous molar

Enamel of premolar

Formation of new bone

Fig. 12-8. Roots of primary molar completely resorbed. Dentin of primary tooth in contact with enamel of premolar. Resorption of bone on one side and formation of new bone on opposite side of premolar caused by transmitted eccentric pressure to premolar. (From Grimmer EA: J Dent Res 18:267, 1939.)

cell adjacent to the resorbing hard tissue forms a "ruffled" border (Fig. 12-1). The ruffled border is resolved with the electron microscope (Fig. 12-9) as an extensive folding of the cell membrane into a series of invaginations 2 to 3 μm deep, with mineral crystallites within the depths of the invaginations. Peripheral to the ruffled border is a clear zone (Fig. 12-10) in which the cytoplasm is devoid or organelles but rich in filaments consisting of the contractile pro-

teins actin and myosin. The clear zone represents the attachment apparatus of the odontoclast. The cytoplasm of the odontoclast is characterized by an exceptionally high content of mitochondria and many vacuoles, which are especially concentrated adjacent to the ruffled border. Acid phosphatase activity occurs within these vacuoles (Fig. 12-11).

Odontoclasts are able to resorb all the dental hard tissues, including, on occa-

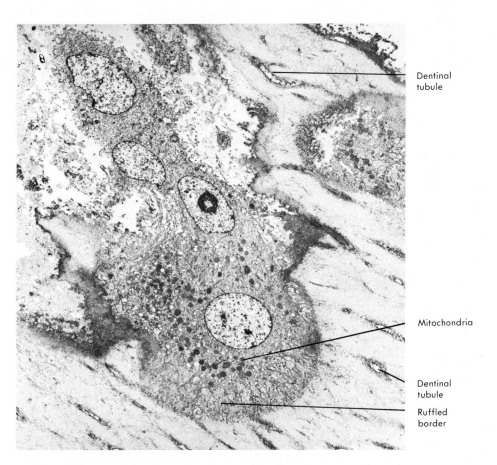

Dentinal tubule

Mitochondria

Dentinal tubule

Ruffled border

Fig. 12-9. Multinucleated odontoclast displays ruffled border that is well adapted to resorption lacuna in root dentin. Dense mitochondria are aggregated toward "resorptive" (lower) pole of cell, and most of the cytoplasm is highly vacuolated. Dentinal tubules are visible in oblique section (×3000.) (From Freilich LS: J Dent Res 50:1047, 1971.)

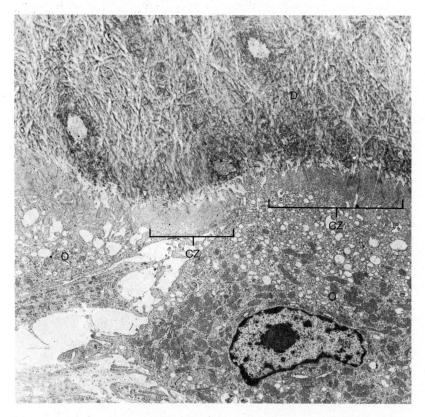

Fig. 12-10. Peripheral aspect of two odontoclasts *(o)* resorbing dentin *(d)* illustrating clear zone *(cz)* thought to be associated with attachment.

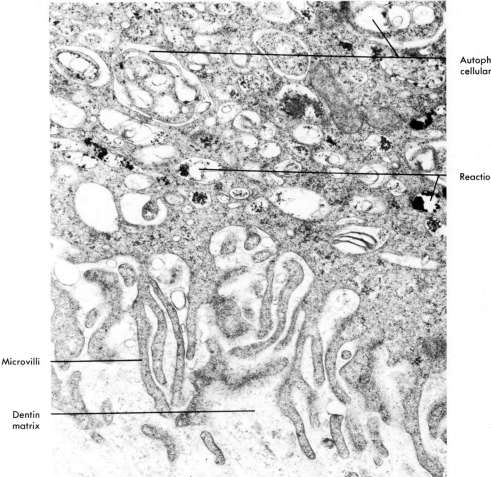

Autophagocytosed
cellular material

Reaction product

Microvilli

Dentin
matrix

Fig. 12-11. Interface between odontoclast ruffled border region (indicated by irregular microvilli) and disintegrated dentin matrix of root surface underoing resorption. Numerous membrane-bound vacuoles in odontoclast cytoplasm show varied contents, including autophagocytosed cellular material and dense patches of reaction product, indicating acid phosphatase activity. (×40,000.) (From Freilich LS: J Dent Res 50:1047, 1971.)

sions, enamel. When dentin is being resorbed, the presence of the tubules provides a pathway for the easy extension of odontoclast processes (Fig. 12-12). Odontoclasts probably have the same origin as osteoclasts. The monocyte, circulating in the blood, originally gives rise to all the different tissue macrophages, including the osteoclast, but what is not certain is whether osteoclasts are further formed from mainly resident tissue macrophages or continuously from circulating monocytes.

Debate also exists concerning the distribution of odontoclasts during tooth resorption. Odontoclasts are most commonly found on surfaces of the roots in relation to the advancing permanent tooth. However, they have also been described in the root canals and pulp chambers of resorbing teeth lying against the predentin surface.

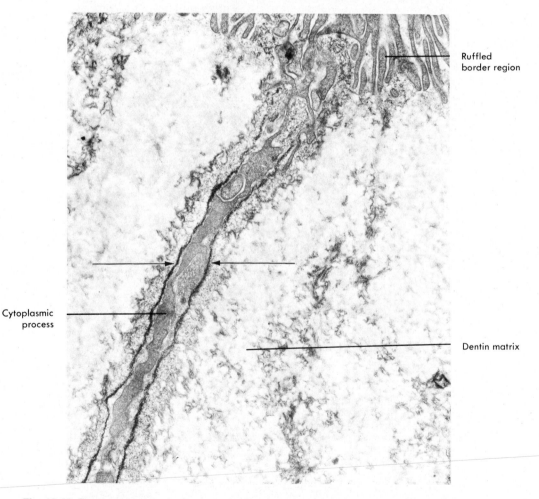

Ruffled border region

Cytoplasmic process

Dentin matrix

Fig. 12-12. Electron micrograph showing cytoplasmic process emanating from ruffled border region of odontoclast and occupying dentinal tubule. Dentin matrix occupies bulk of field. (×25,000.) (From Freilich LS: J Dent Res 50:1047, 1971.)

Although their location in the pulp chamber has been disputed, the most likely reason is that different patterns of resorption exist for different teeth. For example, single-rooted teeth are usually shed before root resorption is complete (Fig. 12-13); therefore odontoclasts are not found within the pulp chambers of these teeth, and the odontoblast layer remains intact. In molars, however, the roots are usually completely

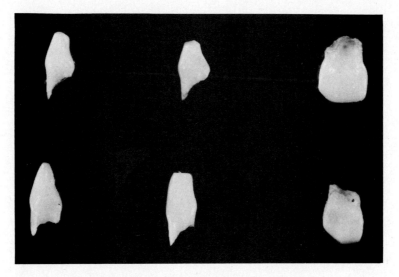

Fig. 12-13. Random selection of exfoliated deciduous incisor and canine teeth showing that considerable amount of root dentin remains at time of exfoliation.

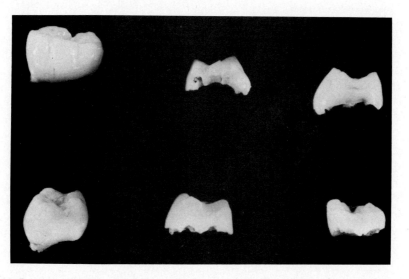

Fig. 12-14. Random selection of exfoliated deciduous molars showing that total loss of roots usually occurs before these teeth are shed. This photograph also shows occurrence of enamel resorption.

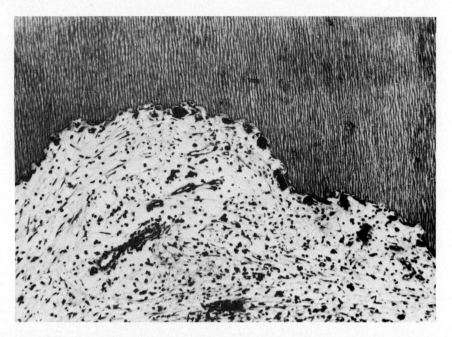

Fig. 12-15. Osteoclastic resorption in surface of coronal dentin of deciduous first molar. Odontoblast layer is absent and numerous odontoblasts can be seen lining pulp chamber. (From Weatherell JA and Hargreaves JA: Arch Oral Biol 11:749, 1966.)

resorbed and the crown is also partially resorbed, before exfoliation. When this happens (Fig. 12-14), the odontoblast layer is replaced by odontoclasts (Fig. 12-15), which resorb both primary and secondary dentin (Fig. 12-16). Sometimes all the dentin is removed, and the vascular connective tissue is visible beneath the translucent cap of enamel.

The process of tooth resorption is not continuous since there are periods of rest and repair; however, in the long term, resorption predominates over repair. Repair is achieved by cells resembling cementoblasts that lay down a dense collagenous matrix in which spotty mineralization occurs. The final repair tissue resembles cellular cementum but is less mineralized (Figs. 12-17 and 12-18).

MECHANISM OF RESORPTION AND SHEDDING

The mechanisms involved in bringing about tooth resorption and exfoliation are not yet fully understood. It seems clear that pressure from the erupting successional tooth plays a key role because the odontoclasts appear at predicted sites of pressure.

How the odontoclast actually resorbs dental hard tissue is not known. In the case of bone resorption it is thought the osteoblasts must first degrade the osteoid, thereby exposing mineralized bone to which osteoclasts can attach. The same may also hold for dentin resorption because predentin is claimed to prevent the resorption of dentin; therefore the odontoblast may have a role to play in this regard.

Whatever the preliminary steps in hard-

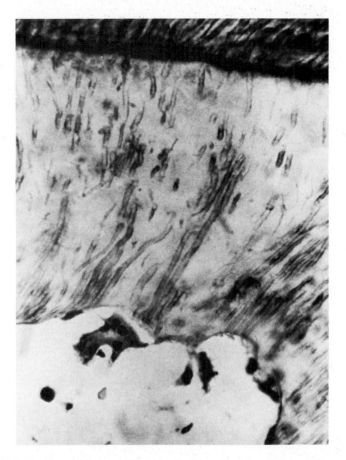

Fig. 12-16. Odontoclasts resorbing secondary dentin. (From Weatherell JA and Hargreaves JA: Arch Oral Biol 11:749, 1966.)

tissue resorption, it is clear that the odontoclast attaches to the hard-tissue surface peripherally through the clear zone, thereby creating a sealed space lined by the ruffled border of the cell. In this way a microenvironment results. The membrane of the ruffled border acts as a proton pump, adding hydrogen ions to the extracellular environment and acidifying it so that mineral dissolution occurs. Primary lysosomes secrete their enzymatic contents into the same environment to degrade the organic matrix.

Although pressure obviously has a key role in initiating tooth resorption, other factors are also involved. It is a common clinical observation that when a successional tooth germ is missing, shedding of the deciduous tooth is delayed. Also, experimental removal of a permanent tooth germ delays, but does not prevent, shedding of its deciduous predecessor. The forces of mastication applied to the deciduous tooth are also capable of initiating the resorption. As an individual grows, the muscles of mastication increase in size and exert forces on the deciduous tooth greater than its periodontal ligament can withstand. This leads to trauma to the ligament and the initiation

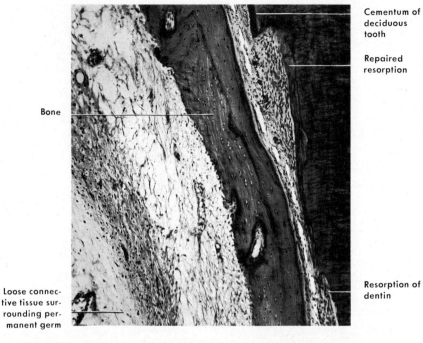

Cementum of
deciduous
tooth

Repaired
resorption

Bone

Resorption of
dentin

Loose connec-
tive tissue sur-
rounding per-
manent germ

Fig. 12-17. High magnification of repaired resorption from area X of Fig. 12-6.

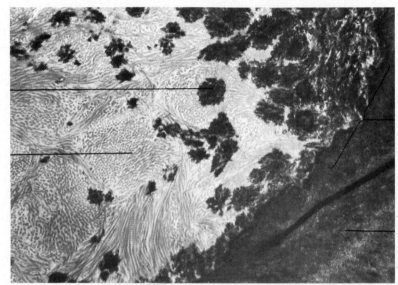

Calcific
globule

Electron-dense
reversal line

Precementum

Cementum

Fig. 12-18. Electron micrograph of resorption lacunae where repair of cementum is taking place. Newly deposited repair tissue is not as electron dense as underlying cementum. Note electron-dense reversal line and calcific globules in precementum. (From Furseth R: Arch Oral Biol 13:417, 1968.)

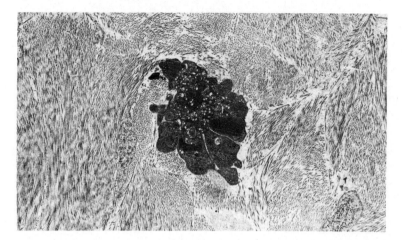

Fig. 12-19. Apoptotic cell death in periodontal ligament fibroblast of shedding tooth. (From Ten Cate AR: Oral histology, development, structure, and function, St. Louis, 1989, The CV Mosby Co.)

of resorption. That this is so has been established experimentally by placing a splint bridge into the mouth of an experimental animal in such a way as to protect the deciduous tooth from occlusal stress. When this is done, resorption of the deciduous tooth is halted and repair takes place. In practice a combination of both factors likely determines the rate of resorption. As resorption of the roots initiated by pressure of the underlying tooth occurs, there is a progressive loss of surface area for attachment of the periodontal ligament fiber bundles. This weakening of tooth support occurs because it has to withstand increasingly greater occlusal forces generated by the growing muscles of mastication.

Although the resorption of the dental hard tissues has been studied extensively, much less is known about the resorption of the dental soft tissues, the pulp and the periodontal ligament. In the case of the periodontal ligament it has been demonstrated that apoptotic cell death is involved (Fig. 12-19). This form of cell death involves shrinkage of the cells so that they can be phagocytosed by neighboring cells. Apoptotic cell death is a normal feature of embryogenesis and is programmed so that cells die at specific times to permit orderly development. The occurrence of apoptotic cell death in the resorbing periodontal ligament, together with the observation that in monozygotic twins the eruption pattern is largely (80%) determined by genetic factors, suggests that shedding is a programmed developmental event influenced by local factors.

CLINICAL CONSIDERATIONS

Remnants of deciduous teeth. Sometimes parts of the roots of deciduous teeth are not in the path of erupting permanent teeth and may escape resorption. Such remnants, consisting of dentin and cementum, may remain embedded in the jaw for a considerable time. They are most frequently found in association with the permanent premolars, especially in the region of the lower second premolars (Fig. 12-20). The reason is that the roots of the lower second deciduous molar are strongly curved or diver-

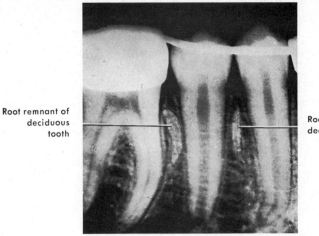

Root remnant of deciduous tooth   Root remnant of deciduous tooth

Fig. 12-20. Remnants of roots of deciduous molar embedded in interdental septa. (Courtesy Dr. G.M. Fitzgerald, University of California.)

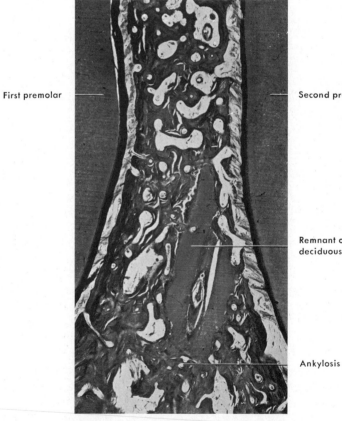

First premolar   Second premolar

Remnant of deciduous root

Ankylosis

Fig. 12-21. Remnant of deciduous tooth embedded in and ankylosed to the bone. (From Schoenbauer F: Z Stomatol 29:892, 1931.)

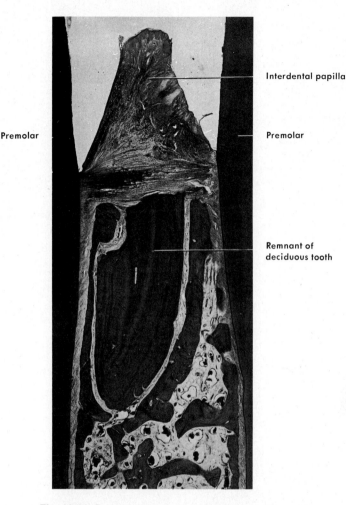

Premolar

Interdental papilla

Premolar

Remnant of
deciduous tooth

Fig. 12-22. Remnant of deciduous tooth at alveolar crest.

gent. The mesiodistal diameter of the second premolars is much smaller than the
greatest distance between the roots of the
deciduous molar. Root remnants may later
be found deep in the bone, completely surrounded by and ankylosed to the bone
(Fig. 12-21). Frequently they are cased in
heavy layers of cellular cementum. When
they are close to the surface of the jaw (Fig.
12-22), they may ultimately be exfoliated.
Progressive resorption of the root remnants

and replacement by bone may cause the
disappearance of these remnants.

Retained deciduous teeth. Deciduous teeth
may be retained for a long time beyond
their usual shedding schedule. Such teeth
are usually without permanent successors,
or their successors are impacted. They are
invariably out of function. Retained deciduous teeth are most often the upper lateral
incisor (Fig. 12-23, *A*), less frequently the
second permanent premolar, especially in

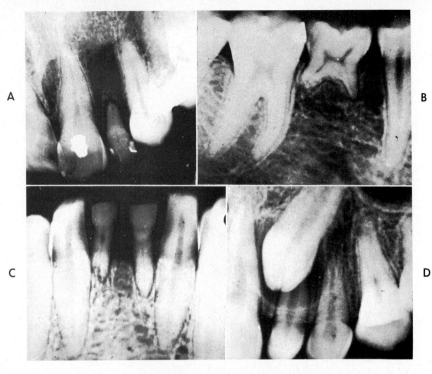

Fig. 12-23. Roentgenograms of retained deciduous teeth. **A,** Upper permanent lateral incisor missing, and deciduous tooth retained (age 56 years). **B,** Lower second premolar missing and deciduous molar retained. Roots partly resorbed. **C,** Permanent lower central incisors missing and deciduous teeth retained. **D,** Upper permanent canine embedded and deciduous canine retained. (**A** and **B** courtesy Dr. M.K. Hine, Indiana University. **C** and **D** courtesy Dr. Rowe Smith, Texarkana, Tex.)

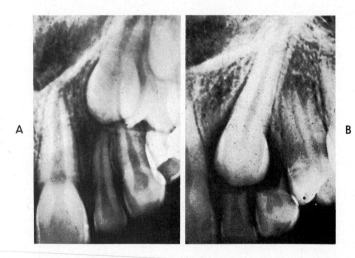

Fig. 12-24. Upper permanent lateral incisor missing. Deciduous lateral incisor and deciduous canine are resorbed because of pressure of erupting permanent canine. **A,** At 11 years of age. **B,** At 13 years of age.

the mandible (Fig. 12-23, *B*), and rarely the lower central incisor (Fig. 12-23, *C*). If a permanent tooth is ankylosed or impacted, its deciduous predecessor may also be retained (Fig. 12-23, *D*). This is most frequently seen with the deciduous and permanent canine teeth.

If the permanent lateral incisor is missing, the deciduous tooth is often resorbed under the pressure of the erupting permanent canine. This resorption may be simultaneous with that of the deciduous canine (Fig. 12-24). Sometimes the permanent canine causes resorption of the deciduous lateral incisor only and erupts in its place. In such cases the deciduous canine may be retained distally to the permanent canine. A supernumerary tooth or an adontogenic tumor may occasionally prevent the eruption of one or more of the permanent teeth. In such cases ankylosis of the deciduous tooth may occur.

Submerged deciduous teeth. Trauma may result in damage to either the dental follicle or the developing periodontal ligament. If this happens, the eruption of the tooth ceases, and it becomes ankylosed to the bone of the jaw. Because of continued eruption of neighboring teeth and increased height of the alveolar bone, the ankylosed tooth may be either "shortened" (Fig. 12-25) or submerged in the alveolar bone. Submerged deciduous teeth prevent the eruption of their permanent successors or force them from their position. Submerged deciduous teeth should therefore be removed as soon as possible.

REFERENCES

Boyde A and Lester KS: Electron microscopy of resorbing surfaces of dental hard tissues, Z Zellforsch 83:538, 1967.

Freilich LS: Ultrastructure and acid phosphatase cytochemistry of odontoclasts: effect of parathyroid extract, J Dent Res 50:1047, 1971.

Furseth R: The resorption processes of human deciduous teeth studied by light microscopy, microradiography and electron microscopy, Arch Oral Biol 13:417, 1968.

Kronfeld R: The resorption of the roots of deciduous teeth, Dent Cosmos 74:103, 1932.

Morita H, Yamashiya H, Shimizu M, et al.: The collagenolytic activity during root resorption of bovine deciduous tooth, Arch Oral Biol 15:503, 1970.

Owen M: Histogenesis of bone cells, Calcif Tissue Res 25:205, 1978.

Ten Cate AR and Anderson RD: An ultrastructural study of tooth resorption in the kitten, J Dent Res 65:1087, 1986.

Weatherell JA and Hargreaves JA: Effect of resorption on the fluoride content of human deciduous dentine, Arch Oral Biol 11:749, 1966.

Westin G: Über Zahndurchbruch and Zahnwechsel, Z Minkrosk Anat Forsch 51:393, 1942.

Yaeger JA and Kraucunas E: Fine structure of the resorptive cells in the teeth of frogs, Anat Rec 164:1, 1969.

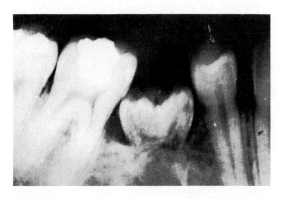

Fig. 12-25. Submerging deciduous lower second molar. Second premolar missing. (Courtesy Dr. M.K. Hine, Indiana University.)

13

TEMPOROMANDIBULAR JOINT

GROSS ANATOMY

DEVELOPMENT OF THE JOINT

HISTOLOGY
  Bony structure

Articular fibrous covering
Articular disk
Synovial membrane
CLINICAL CONSIDERATIONS

GROSS ANATOMY

The temporomandibular joint (TMJ) on each side of the head is formed by the articulation between the articular eminence and the anterior part of the glenoid fossa of the temporal bone above and the condylar head of the mandible below (Fig. 13-1 and Fig. 13-2, *A* and *B*).

Like most diarthrodial synovial joints, the TMJ contains a fibrous disk that is interposed between the articular surfaces and functions as a shock absorber (Fig. 13-1, *B*). It is an oval, fibrous, avascular, noninnervated plate that is firmly attached to the medial and lateral poles of the condyle by medial and lateral collateral ligaments (Fig. 13-1, *A*). The disk is biconcave in sagittal section, with a thin intermediate zone, a thick anterior band, and a thick posterior band.

The anterior band continues into loose fibroelastic connective tissue, which is avascular and innervateed, known as the anterior foot extension or anterior ligament. The latter attaches to the ascending slope of the articular eminence and becomes contiguous with the anterior capsule laterally and the superior head of the lateral pterygoid muscle medially (see Fig. 13-2, *A*). Some fibers of the superior head of the lat-

eral pterygoid muscle attach to the anterior band. The posterior band is continuous with a loose connective tissue rich in elastic fibers called the bilaminar zone, which is highly vascular and highly innervated. The superior stratum, or lamina, of the bilaminar zone attaches to the posterior wall of the glenoid fossa and the squamotympanic suture, and the inferior stratum attaches to the posterior aspect of the mandibular condyle.

The joint capsule is a fibroelastic sac that attaches to the ascending slope of the articular eminence anteriorly and to the lips of the squamotympanic fissure posteriorly. Between these two attachments it is attached to the margins of the glenoid fossa superiorly and to the neck of the condyle inferiorly.

The posterior capsule is highly vascular and sometimes is called pis vasculosa. Parotid gland tissue is usually found in the posterior portion of the glenoid fossa between the posterior capsule of the joint and the postglenoid tubercle. The lateral aspect of the capsule is strengthened by the temporomandibular ligament. The anterior surface of the capsule, unlike the other surfaces, is usually ill defined. The inner sur-

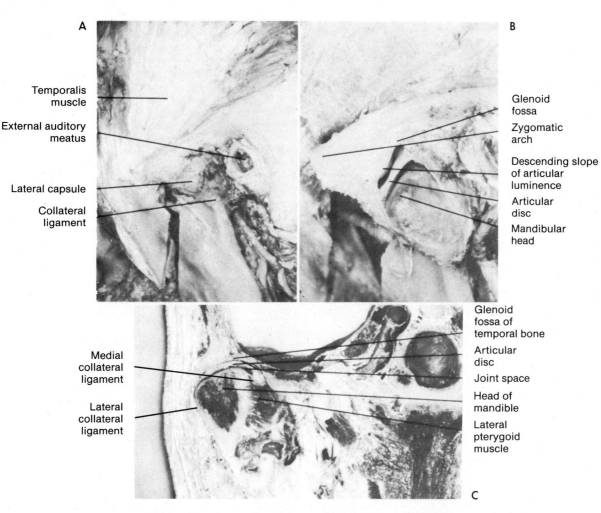

Fig. 13-1. A, Lateral view of temporomandibular joint with capsule and lateral collateral ligament in situ. **B,** Sagittal section through temporomandibular joint. **C,** Frontal section of head through condyle of mandible. (Courtesy Dr. F.R. Suarez, Georgetown University, Washington, D.C.)

face of the capsule is smooth and glistening because of the presence of a synovial membrane lining. The latter does not extend over the articular surfaces of the disk, the articular eminence, or the condyle.

The disk divides the joint space into two compartments: a lower one between the condyle and the disk (condylodiskal) and an upper one between the disk and the

temporal bone (temporodiskal). The disk acts as a third bone and provides a movable articulation for the condyle. In the lower joint space rotational movement about an axis through the heads of the condyles permits opening of the jaws; this is designated as a hinge movement. In the upper joint space, because of the firm attachment of the disk to the lateral and medial poles of the condle and the contraction of the inferior head of the lateral pterygoid muscle, a translatory movement occurs as the disks and the condyles traverse anteriorly along the descending slopes of the articular eminences to produce an anterior and inferior movement of the mandible. In a healthy joint the condyle, a disk, and temporal components are contiguous with each other during all movements, and the superior and inferior joint spaces are reduced to the thickness of a synovial film except for small pockets or recesses at the most anterior, posterior, medial, and lateral limits of the joint spaces (see Fig. 13-2, A).

Except for the avascular disk, the joint

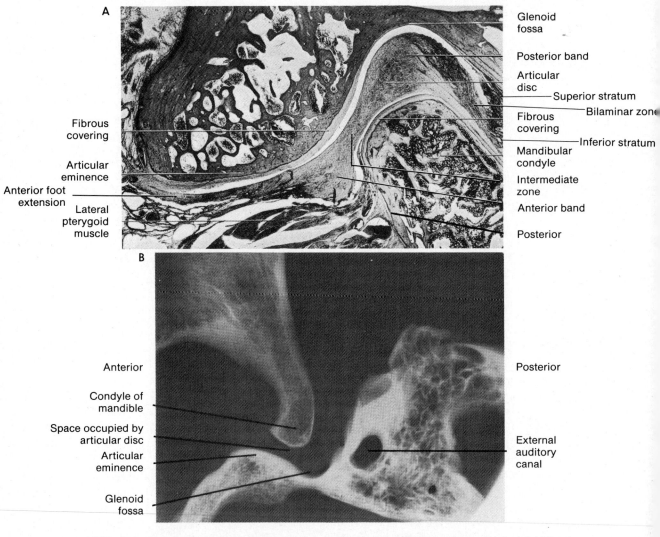

Fig. 13-2. **A,** Sagittal section through temporomandibular joint. **B,** Temporomandibular joint lateral radiograph showing condyle of mandible, articular eminence and glenoid fossa.

tissues are innervated by branches of the auriculotemporal branch of the mandibular nerve of the fifth cranial or trigeminal nerve. Proprioceptor fibers from the joint are carried by masseteric nerves and perhaps other muscular branches of the mandibular nerve.

The articular supply to the joint is through branches of the maxillary and superficial temporal arteries. Large venules are consistently seen close to the anterior ligament of the disk, the bilaminar zone, and the posterior capsule. The details of the anatomy and physiology of the macrocirculation and microcirculation of this important joint need further study.

DEVELOPMENT OF THE JOINT

At approximately 10 weeks the components of the fetus' future joint become evident in the mesenchyme between the condylar cartilage of the mandible and the developing temporal bone. Two slitlike joint cavities and an intervening disk make their appearance in this region at 12 weeks. The mesenchyme around the joint begins to form the fibrous joint capsule. Very little is known about the significance of newly forming muscles in joint formation.

The developing superior head of the lateral pterygoid muscle attaches to the anterior portion of the fetal disk. The disk also continues posteriorly through the petrotympanic fissure and attaches to the malleus of the middle ear. This connection is usually obliterated by the growth of the lips of the petrotympanic fissure and does not exist in the adult joint.

HISTOLOGY

Bony structures. The condyle of the mandible is composed of cancellous bone covered by a thin layer of compact bone (see Fig. 13-2, *A*). The trabeculae are grouped in such a way that they radiate from the neck of the mandible and reach the cortex at right angles, thus giving maximal strength to the condyle. The large marrow spaces decrease in size with progressing age as a result of noticeable thickening of the trabeculae. The red marrow in the condyle is of the myeloid or cellular type. In older individuals it is sometimes replaced by fatty marrow.

During the period of growth a layer of hyaline catilage lies underneath the fibrous covering of the condyle. This cartilaginous plate grows by apposition from the deepest layers of the covering connective tissue. At the same time its deep surface is replaced by bone (Fig. 13-3). Remnants of this cartilage may persist into old age (Fig. 13-4). Unlike metaphyseal primary cartilage of long bones, the hyaline cartilage of the condyle is not organized in parallel rows of cells at the interface between the forming bone and the cartilage. Therefore the cartilage is usually referred to as secondary cartilage.

In addition to the appositional subperiosteal mandibular bone growth, the growth of the secondary cartilage and its replacement with bone contribute to the downward and forward growth of the mandible. This process can be stimulated internally by growth hormone or externally by mechanical forces such as the use of functional appliances designed for this purpose by orthodontists.

The roof of the glenoid fossa (see Fig. 13-2) consists of a thin, compact layer of bone. The articular eminence is composed of spongy bone covered with a thin layer of compact bone. Areas of chondroid bone are commonly seen in the articular eminence, and in rare cases islands of hyaline cartilage are found.

Articular fibrous covering. The condyle and the articular eminence are covered by a rather thick layer of fibroelastic tissue

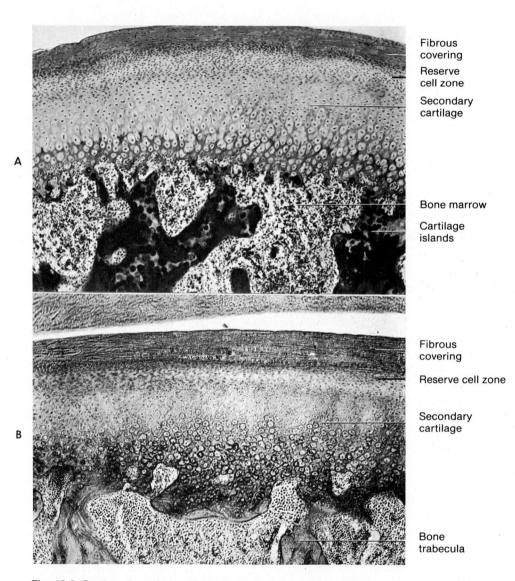

A

B

Fibrous
covering

Reserve
cell zone

Secondary
cartilage

Bone marrow

Cartilage
islands

Fibrous
covering

Reserve cell zone

Secondary
cartilage

Bone
trabecula

Fig. 13-3. Sections through mandibular head. **A,** Newborn infant. **B,** Young adult. Note transitional zone (also known as reserve cell zone) between fibrous covering and cartilage, characteristic for appositional growth of cartilage.

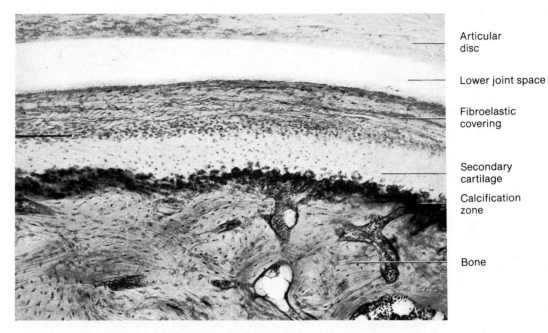

Articular
disc

Lower joint space

Fibroelastic
covering

Reserve cell
zone

Secondary
cartilage

Calcification
zone

Bone

Fig. 13-4. Higher magnification of part of mandibular condyle shown in Fig. 13-2, *A.*

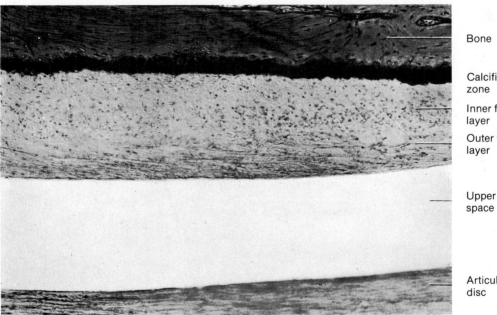

Bone

Calcification
zone

Inner fibrous
layer

Outer fibrous
layer

Upper joint
space

Articular
disc

Fig. 13-5. Higher magnification of articular tubercle shown in Fig. 13-2, *A.*

containing fibroblasts and a variable number of chondrocytes. The fibrous covering of the mandibular condyle is of fairly even thickness (see Fig. 13-4). Its superficial layers consist of a network of strong collagenous fibers. Chondrocytes may be present and have a tendency to increase in number with age. They can be recognized by their thin capsule, which stains heavily with basic dyes. The deepest layer of the fibrocartilage is rich in small undifferentiated cells as long as growing hyaline cartilage is present in the condyle. It contains only a few thin collagenous fibers. In this zone,

called the reserve cell zone, appositional growth of the hyaline cartilage of the condyle takes place (see Fig. 13-3).

The fibrous layer covering the articulating surface of the temporal bone (Fig. 13-5) is thin in the articular fossa and thickens rapidly on the posterior slope of the articular eminence (see Fig. 13-2, *A*). In this region the fibrous tissue shows a definite arrangement in two layers, with a small transitional zone between them. The two layers are characterized by the different courses of the constituent fibrous bundles. In the inner zone the fibers are at right an-

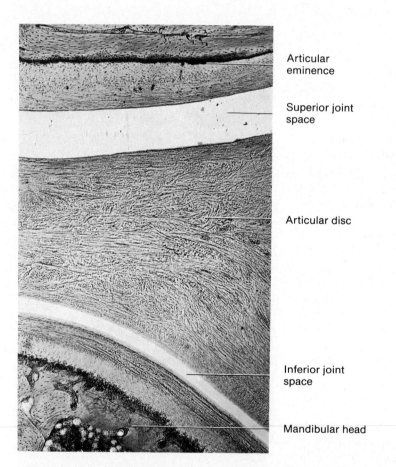

Articular eminence

Superior joint space

Articular disc

Inferior joint space

Mandibular head

Fig. 13-6. Higher magnification of articular disc shown in Fig. 13-2, *A*.

gles to the bony surface. In the outer zone they run parallel to that surface. As in the fibrous covering of the mandibular condyle, a variable number of chondrocytes are found in the tissue on the temporal surface. In adults the deepest layer shows a thin zone of calcification.

No continuous cellular lining is on the free surface of the fibrocartilage. Only isolated fibroblasts are situated on the surface itself. They are characterized by the formation of long, flat cytoplasmic processes.

Articular disk. In young individuals the articular disk is composed of dense fibrous tissue. The interlacing fibers are straight and tightly packed (Fig. 13-6). Elastic fibers are found only in relatively small numbers. The fibroblasts in the disk are elongated and send flat cytoplasmic processes into the interstices between the adjacent bundles (Fig. 13-7).

With advancing age and in areas of the disk subjected to excessive mechanical stress, some cells appear rounded and arranged in pairs similar to chondroid cells. Chondrocytes, with typical territorial matrices that stain heavily with basic dyes, can be observed in the articular disk of many species, including humans (Fig. 13-8). The presence of chondrocytes may increase the resistance and resilience of the fibrous tissue.

The fibrous tissue covering the articular eminence, the mandibular condyle, and the large central area of the disk, is devoid of blood vessels and nerves and thus has limited reparative ability.

Synovial membrane. As in other synovial joints, the articular capsule is lined with a synovial membrane that folds to form synovial villi. Synovial villi project into the joint spaces (see Fig. 13-8). The synovial membrane consists of internal cells, which do not form a continuous layer but show gaps between the cells, and the subintimal

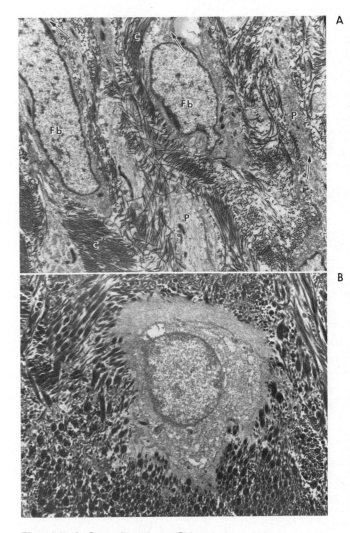

Fig. 13-7. A, Some fibroblasts *(Fb)* and elongated processes *(P)* of other fibroblasts are seen. Note rich RER *(arrows)* and surrounding type I collagen *(C)*. Monkey disc. **B,** Chondrocyte with distinct territorial matrix. Monkey disc. (**A,** ×6,500; **B,** ×8,000.) (Courtesy Dr. M. Sharawy, Medical College of Georgia, Augusta, Ga.)

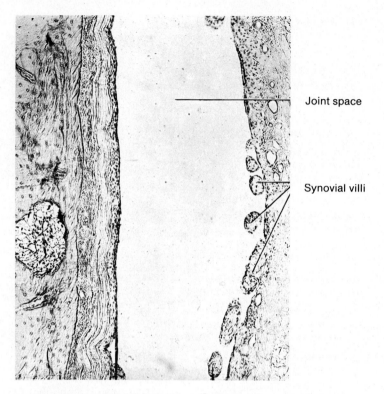

Joint space

Synovial villi

Fig. 13-8. Synovial villi lining capsule of temporomandibular joint.

connective tissue layer, rich in blood capillaries. The intimal cells are of three types. The first is rich in rough endoplasmic reticulum (RER) and is called the fibroblast-like, or B, cell. It is sometimes called a secretory S-cell (Fig. 13-9, *A* and *B*). The second type is rich in Golgi complex and lysosomes and contains little or no RER. It is called the macrophage-like, or A, cell. The third type has a cellular morphology between cell types A and B.

A small amount of a clear, straw-colored viscous fluid (synovial fluid) is found in the articular spaces. It is a lubricant and also a nutrient fluid for the avascular tissues covering the condyle and the articular eminence and for the disk. It is elaborated by diffusion from the rich capillary network of the synovial membrane that is augmented by mucin, possibly secreted by the synovial cells.

CLINICAL CONSIDERATIONS

The thinness of the bone in the articular fossa is responsible for fractures if the mandibular head is driven into the fossa by a heavy blow. In such cases injuries of the dura mater and the brain have been reported.

The finer structure of the bone and its fibrocartilaginous covering depends on mechanical influences. A change in force or direction of stress, especially after loss of posterior teeth, may cause structural changes. These changes may include fibrillation (separation between collagen bun-

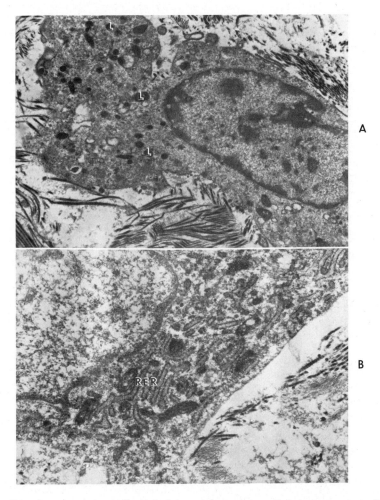

Fig. 13-9. A, Type A or macrophage-like cell of synovial membrane. Note near absence of RER and presence of numerous lysosomes *(L)*. Although not shown here, these cells often have a distinct Golgi complex. Monkey synovial membrane. **B,** Type B cell of synovial membrane. Note the presence of well-developed RER in contact to type-A cell. Monkey synovium. (**A,** ×9,375; **B,** ×21,8975.) (Courtesy Dr. M. Sharawy, Medical College of Georgia, Augusta, Ga.)

dles) of the fibrous covering of the articulating surfaces and of the disk. Abnormal functional activity may also produce injury to the articular bones. Compensation and partial repair may be accomplished by the development of cartilage on the condylar surface and in the disk. In severe trauma the articular bone is destroyed, and cartilage and new bone develop in the marrow spaces and at the periphery of the condyle. When this occurs, the function of the joint is severely impaired.

Normally, in the open position of the mandible the interincisal distance is approximately 48 mm in males and 45.5 mm in females. In approximately 18% of the population the mandible deviates on opening, and in almost 86% of this group deviation is to the left. In approximately 35% of the population the TMJ produces sounds during opening movements. The joint has palpable irregularities and produces popping and clicking noises. However, use of a stethoscope reveals that approximately 65% of TMJs produce some kind of sound. This feature by itself, especially if not a sign of disease and may not require treatment.

The term *myofacial pain dysfunction syndrome* is used to indicate a dysfunction of the TMJ. It is characterized by (1) masticatory muscle tenderness (most frequently, the lateral pterygoid and then, in order, the temporalis, medial pterygoid, and masseter), (2) limited opening of the mandible (<37 mm), and (3) joint sounds. This symptom complex is seen more often in females than in males. Its cause is usually spasm of the masticatory muscles. Since the condition may be related to stress, treatment should be as conservative as possible.

Dislocation of the TMJ may take place without the impact of an external force. The dislocation of the jaw is usually bilateral, and the displacement is anterior. When the mouth is opened unusually wide during yawning, the head of the mandible may slip forward into the infratemporal fossa, causing articular dislocation of the joint.

Recently diagnostic techniques such as computerized tomography (CT) and magnetic resonance imaging (MRI), which permit the visualization of the TMJ disks in patients, are being applied increasingly in the diagnosis of internal disk dislocation or derangement. The disk, for reasons not yet determined, becomes displaced anteromedially and creates one or more of the following signs and symptoms: pain, clicking, limitation of jaw movement, deviation of the jaw or opening, and locking. If the condition remains untreated, it could lead to osteoarthrosis.

Diagnosis of cases of the TMJ disk perforation is also on the increase, partly because of the use of arthroscopic, MRI, and arthrographic techniques in the investigation of TMJ diseases. Recently research has shown that experimentally produced disk perforation in rhesus monkeys leads to secondary osteoarthrosis. Consequently, treatment of human disk perforation will require more serious consideration than it receives at present.

REFERENCES

Bauer W: Anatomische and mikroskopische Untersuchungen über das Kiefergelenk (Anatomical and microscopic investigations on the temporomandibular joint), Z Stomatol 30:1136, 1932.

Bauer WH: Osteo-arthritis deformans of the temporomandibular joint, Am J Pathol 17:129, 1941.

Bernick S: The vascular and nerve supply to the temporomandibular joint of the rat, Oral Surg 15:488, 1962.

Breitner C: Bone changes resulting from experimental orthodontic treatment, Am J Orthod 26:521, 1940.

Cabrini R and Erausquin J: La articulación temporo-maxilar de la rata (Temporomandibular joint of the rat), Rev Odont Buenos Aires, 29:385, 1941.

Choukas NC and Sicher H: The structure of the temporo-mandibular joint, Oral Surg 13:1263, 1960.

Cohen DW: The vascularity of the articular disc of the temporo-mandibular joint, Alpha Omegan, Sept. 1955.

Cowdry EV: Special cytology, ed 2, New York, 1932, Paul B Hoeber, Med Book Div of Harper & Brothers.

Gross A and Gale EN: A prevalence study of the clinical signs associated with mandibular dysfunction, J Am Dent Assoc 107:932, 1983.

Heffez L, Maffe MF, and Langer B: Double-contrast arthrography of the temporomandibular joint: role of direct sagittal CT imaging, Oral Surg 65:511-514, 1988.

Helms CA, Gillespy T III, Sims RE, et al.: Magnetic resonance imaging of internal derangement of the temporomandibular joint, Radiol Clin North Am 24:189-192, 1986.

Helmy ES, Bays RA, and Sharawy M: Osteoarthrosis of the temporomandibular joint following experimental disc perforation in *Macaca fascicularis*, J Oral Maxillofac Surg 46:979-990, 1988.

Kawamura Y: Recent concepts of physiology of mastication, Adv Oral Biol 1:102, 1964.

Kreutziger KL and Mahan PE: Temporomandibular degenerative joint disease. Part I. Anatomy, pathophysiology and clinical description, Oral Surg 40:165, 1975.

Kreutziger KL and Mahan PE: Temporomandibular degenerative joint disease. Part II. Diagnostic procedure and comprehensive management, Oral Surg 40:297, 1975.

Lipke DP et al.: An Electromyographic study of the human lateral pterygoid muscle, J Dent Res 56 (special issue B: B230), 1977 (abstract no 713).

McLeran JH et al.: A Cinefluorographic analysis of the temporomandibular joint, J Am Dent Assoc 75:1394, 1967.

McNamara JA: The independent functions of the two heads of the lateral pterygoid muscle, Am J Anat 138:197, 1973.

Mathews MP and Moffett BC: Histologic maturation and initial aging of the human temporomandibular joint, J Dent Res 53 (special issue: 246), 1974 (abstract no 765).

Moffett B: The morphogenesis of the temporomandibular joint, Am J Orthod 52401, 1966.

Payne GS: The effect of intermaxillary elastic force on the temporomandibular articulation in the growing macaque monkey, Am J Orthod 60:491, 1971.

Radin EL et al.: Response of joints to impact loading III. Relationships between trabecular microfractures and cartilage degeneration, J Biomech 6:51, 1973.

Ramfjord SP and Ash MM: Occlusion, Philadelphia, 1966, WB Saunders Co.

Rees LA: Structure and function of the mandibular joint, Br Dent J 96:6, 1954.

Sarnat BG: The temporomandibular joint, ed 2, Springfield, Ill, 1964, Charles C Thomas, Publisher.

Schaffer J: Die Stützgewebe (Supporting tissues). In von Möllendorff W, editor: Handbunch der mikroskopischen Anatomie des Menschen, Berlin, 1930, Julius Springer Verlag, vol 2, pt 2.

Shapiro HH and Truex RC: The temporomandibular joint and the auditory function, J Am Dent Assoc 30:1147, 1943.

Sicher H: Some aspects of the anatomy and pathology of the temporomandibular articulation, NY State Dent J 14:451, 1948.

Sicher H: Temporomandibular articulation in mandibular overclosure, J Am Dent Assoc 36:131, 1948.

Sicher H: Positions and movements of the mandible, J Am Dent Assoc 48:620, 1954.

Sicher H: Structural and functional basis for disorders of the temporomandibular articulation, J Oral Surg 13:275, 1955.

Steinhardt G: Die Beansprunchung der Gelenkflächen bei verschiedenen Bissarten (Investigations on the stresses in the mandibular articulation and their structural consequences), Deutsch Zahnheilk Vortr 91:1, 1934.

Strauss F et al.: The Architecture of the disk of the human temporomandibular joint, Helv Odont Acta 4:1, 1960.

Thilander B: Innervation of the temporomandibular joint capsule in man, tr Roy Schools Den Stockholm Umea 7:1,1961.

Toller PA: Osteoarthrosis of the mandibular condyle, Brit Dent J 134:223, 1973.

Toller PA: Opaque arthrography of the temporomandibular joint, Int J Oral Surg 3:17, 1974.

Yavelow I and Arnold GS: Temporomandibular joint clicking, Oral Surg 32:708, 1971.

14
MAXILLARY SINUS

DEFINITION
HISTORICAL REVIEW
DEVELOPMENTAL ASPECTS
DEVELOPMENTAL ANOMALIES

STRUCTURE AND VARIATIONS
MICROSCOPIC FEATURES
FUNCTIONAL IMPORTANCE
CLINICAL CONSIDERATIONS

DEFINITION

The maxillary sinus is the pneumatic space that is lodged inside the body of the maxilla and that communicates with the environment by way of the middle nasal meatus and the nasal vestibule.

HISTORICAL REVIEW

A publication entitled *Eighteen Hundred Years of Controversy: The Paranasal Sinuses* (Blanton and Biggs, 1969) reflects quite accurately the present confused state of knowledge about the pneumatic cavities. The maxillary sinus, more than any other of these cavities, has been subjected to peculiar interpretations throughout history. As early as the second century, Galen (AD 130-201) made the first known descriptive remarks about the adult maxillary sinus. In the following centuries many prominent scientists (Leonardo da Vinci, 1452-1519; Berengar, 1507-1527; Massa, 1542; Vesalius, 1542; Fallopius, 1600; Veslingius, 1637; Spigelius, 1645; Highmore, 1651; Schneider, 1655; Bartholinus, 1658; Morgagni, 1723; Boerhaave, 1735; and Haller, 1763—cited by Blanton and Biggs) contributed to the everincreasing knowledge of the structure and function of the paranasal cavities.

Despite historical uncertainty about the specific contribution of each of these researchers, it is widely accepted that Highmore was the first to describe in detail the morphology of the maxillary sinus and to advance the idea of pneumatization by the sinuses. In later centuries the interest of investigators focused on the mechanism of pneumatizing processes and the functional significance of the paranasal sinuses as a whole, in addition to the structural, dimensional, sexual, racial, environmental, and developmental diversity among the sinuses.

DEVELOPMENTAL ASPECTS

The initial development of the maxillary sinus follows a number of morphogenic events in the differentiation of the nasal cavity in early gestation (about 32 mm crown-rump length [CRL] in an embryo). First, the horizontal shift of palatal shelves and subsequent fusion of the shelves with one another and with the nasal septum separate the secondary oral cavity from two secondary nasal chambers (see Chapter 1). This modification presumably influences further expansion of the lateral nasal wall in that the wall begins to fold; thus three nasal conchae and three subjacent meatuses arise. The inferior and superior meatuses remain as shallow depressions along the lateral nasal wall for approximately the first half of the intrauterine life; the middle meatus expands immediately into the lateral nasal wall. Because the cartilaginous skeleton of the lateral nasal capsule is already established, expansion of the middle meatus proceeds primarily in an inferior direction, occupying progressively more of the future maxillary body (Fig. 14-1).

The maxillary sinus thus established in the embryo of about 32 mm CRL expands vertically into the primordium of the maxil-

lary body and reaches a diameter of 1 mm in the 50 mm CRL fetus (at this time the first glandular primordia from the maxillary sinus epithelium are apparent), 3.5 mm in the 160 mm CRL fetus, and 7.5 mm in the 250 mm CRL fetus (Vidić). In the perinatal period the human maxillary sinus measures about 7 to 16 mm (standard deviation [SD] 2.64) in the anteroposterior direction, 2 to 13 mm (SD 1.52) in the superoinferior direction, and 1 to 7 mm (SD 1.18) in the mediolateral direction (Cullen and Vidić). According to Shaeffer these diameters increase to 15, 6, and 5.5 mm, respectively, at

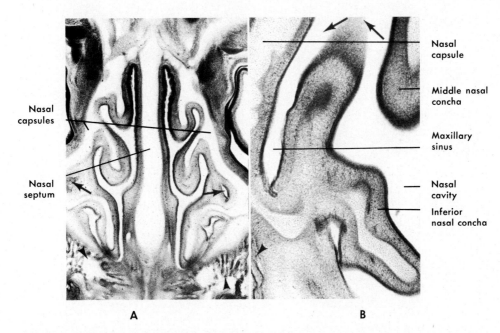

A   B

Fig. 14-1. A, This coronal section of a human fetal head (60 mm CRL) demonstrates both nasal cavities bordered by nasal septum medially, three conchae and subjacent meatuses laterally, and palate, which already shows extensive centers of ossification inferiorly *(arrowheads at bottom).* Lateral to conchae and continuous with their cartilaginous skeletons is nasal capsule. Developing maxillary sinuses on both sides of midline are indicated by arrows. (Hematoxylin and eosin stain; ×27.) **B,** This coronal section demonstrates nasal cavity, maxillary sinus, and inferior and middle nasal conchae in a 69 mm CRL fetus. Sinus grows into maxilla in an inferior direction parallel to plane of cartilaginous nasal capsule. Skeleton of both conchae is cartilaginous, while in maxilla several centers of ossification *(arrowhead)* are present. Communication between middle nasal meatus and maxillary sinus is indicated by arrows. (Hematoxylin and eosin stain; ×67.5.) **(A,** No. 1183; **B,** No. 4291; courtesy Dr. Ronan O'Rahilly, Carnegie Laboratories of Embryology, Davis, Calif.)

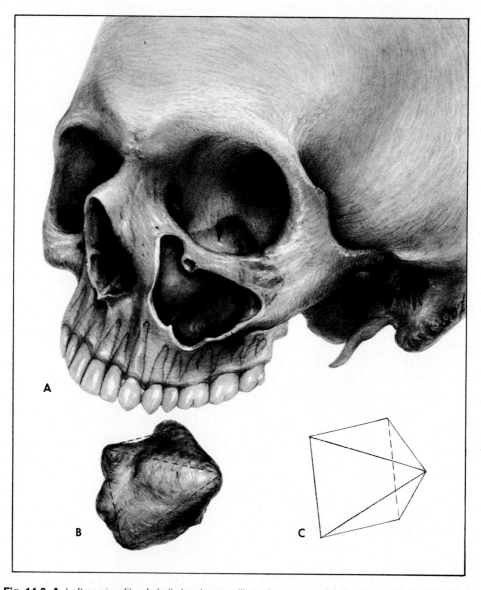

Fig. 14-2. A, Left semiprofile of skull showing maxillary sinus opened through anterior wall. Outline of superior, posterior, and inferior walls of sinus are respectively indicated in relation to floor of orbit *(upper arrowhead),* infratemporal surface of maxilla *(middle arrowhead),* and alveolar and zygomatic processes of maxilla *(lower arrowhead).* Basal wall separates space of sinus from nasal cavity. **B** and **C,** Polysulfate rubber cast of maxillary sinus about 10 ml in volume and an idealized geometric form of sinus, respectively. For convenience of visualizing the presumed pyramidal form of the sinus the orientation is the same for the sinus in situ, **A;** the cast of the sinus, **B;** and for closest geometric form to the sinus, **C.** (Courtesy Mr. and Mrs. B.F. Melloni, Department of Medical-Dental Communications, Georgetown University, Washington, D.C.)

the age of 1 year, to 31.5, 19, and 19.5 mm at the age of 15 years, and to 34, 33, and 23 mm in the adult. Although the exact time at which the human maxillary sinus attains its definite size is not known, the sinus appears to expand and modify in form until the time of eruption of all permanent teeth.

DEVELOPMENTAL ANOMALIES

Agenesis (complete absence), aplasia, and hypoplasia (altered development or underdevelopment) of the maxillary sinus occurs either alone or in association with other anomalies, for example, choanal atresia, cleft palate, high palate, septal deformity, absence of a concha, mandibulofacial dysostosis, malformation of the external nose, and the pathologic conditions of the nasal cavity as a whole (Gouzy et al., Rosenberger, Schürch, Blair et al., Mocellin, Fatin, Eckel and Beisser, and Blumenstein). The supernumerary maxillary sinus, on the other hand, is the occurrence of two completely separated sinuses on the same side. This condition is most likely initiated by outpocketing of the nasal mucosa into the primordium of the maxillary body from two points either in the middle nasal meatus or in the middle and superior or middle and inferior nasal meatuses, respectively. Consequently, the result is two permanently separated ostia of the sinus.

STRUCTURE AND VARIATIONS

The maxillary sinus is subject to a great extent of variation in shape, size, and mode of developmental pattern. It is inconceivable therefore to propose any structural description that would satisy the majority of human maxillary sinuses. Usually, however, the sinus is described as a four-sided pyramid, the base of which is facing medially toward the nasal cavity and the apex of which is pointed laterally toward the body of the zygomatic bone (Fig. 14-2). The four

sides are related to the surface of the maxilla in the following manner: (1) anterior, to the facial surface of the body; (2) inferior, to the alveolar and zygomatic processes; (3) superior, to the orbital surface; and (4) posterior, to the infratemporal surface. The four sides of the sinus, which are usually distant from one another medially, converge laterally and meet at an obtuse angle. The identity of each of the four sides is somewhat difficult to discern, and the transition of the surface from one side to the other is usually poorly defined. Thus it is apparent that the comparison of the sinus space to a geometrically well-defined body is of pedagogic value only.

The base of the sinus, which is the thinnest of all the walls, presents a perforation, the ostium, at the level of the middle nasal meatus (Fig. 14-3). In some individuals, in addition to the main ostium, two or many more accessory ostia connect the sinus with the middle nasal meatus. In 5.5% of instances the main ostium is located within the anterior third of the hiatus semilunaris, in 11% within the middle third, and 71.7% within the posterior third; in 11.3% the ostium is found outside and in a posterior position to the hiatus semilunaris. The accessory ostia are found in 23% of these instances in the middle nasal meatus (Van Alyea) and occur rarely in the inferior nasal meatus (Delaney and Morse).

In the course of development the maxillary sinus often pneumatizes the maxilla beyond the boundaries of the maxillary body. Some of the processes of the maxilla consequently become invaded by the air space. These expansions, referred to as the *recesses*, are found in the alveolar process (50% of all instances), zygomatic process (41.5% of all instances), frontal process (40.5% of all instances), and palatine process (1.75% of all instances) of the maxilla (Hajniš et al.). The occurrence of the zygo-

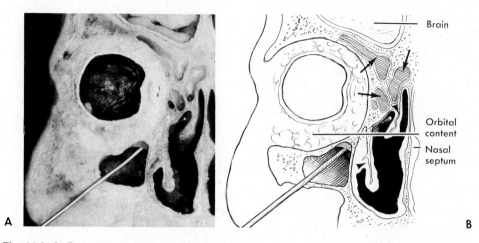

Fig. 14-3. A, Coronal section of adult female face was made approximately 7 mm anterior to ostium of maxillary sinus. **B,** Drawing made from **A** (proportion, 1:1). Probe indicates ostium, or communication between upper part of sinus lumen and middle nasal meatus. Several ethmoidal air cells *(arrows),* middle and inferior conchae *(two arrowheads),* orbital content, nasal septum, and frontal lobe of brain are also indicated. (**A,** Frontal section courtesy Dr. F.R. Suarez, Georgetown University, Washington, D.C. **B,** courtesy Mr. and Mrs. B.F. Melloni, Department of Medical-Dental Communications, Georgetown University, Washington, D.C.)

matic recess usually brings the superior alveolar neurovascular bundles into proximity with the space of the sinus. The frontal recess invades and sometimes surrounds the content of the infraorbital canal, whereas the alveolopalatine recesses reduce the amount of the bone between the dental apices and the sinus space. The latter development most often pneumatizes the floor of the sinus adjacent to the roots of the first molar (Fig. 14-4) and less often to the roots of the second premolar, first premolar, and second molar, in that order of frequency (Osmont et al.). The fully developed alveolar recess is characterized by three depressions separated by two incomplete bony septa. The anterior depression, or fossa, corresponds to the original site of premolar buds, the middle to the molar buds, and the posterior to the third molar bud (Perović).

MICROSCOPIC FEATURES

Three microscopically distinct layers surround the space of the maxillary sinus: the epithelial layer, the basal lamina, and the subepithelial layer, including the periostium (Figs. 14-5 and 14-6). The epithelium, which is pseudostratified, columnar, and ciliated, is derived from the olfactory epithelium of the middle nasal meatus and therefore undergoes the same pattern of differentiation as does the respiratory segment of the nasal epithelium proper. The most numerous cellular type in the maxillary sinus epithelium is the columnar ciliated cell. In addition, there are basal cells, columnar nonciliated cells, and mucus-producing, secretory goblet cells (Figs. 14-6 and 14-7). A ciliated cell encloses the nucleus and an electron-lucent cytoplasm with numerous mitochondria and enzyme-containing organelles. The basal bodies,

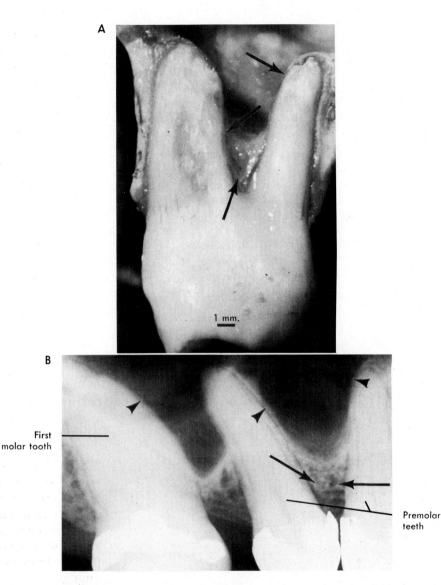

Fig. 14-4. A demonstrates in a coronal section made immediately mesial to upper first molar tooth the gross relationships of the vestibular (left) and palatine (right) roots with floor of maxillary sinus. Amount of bone *(arrows)* interposed between roots and the space of the sinus is reduced at certain levels to a thin lamina. **B,** Lateral radiograph of both right upper premolar and first molar teeth. Maxillary sinus expands, in this instance, deep into alveolar process *(arrows)* between each two of the indicated teeth. Bony lamina separating dental roots from sinus *(arrowheads)* is extremely thin at certain levels. (**B** courtesy Dr. Donald Reynolds, Georgetown University, Washington, D.C.)

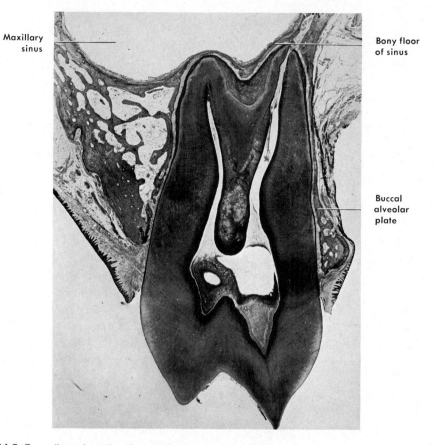

Maxillary sinus

Bony floor of sinus

Buccal alveolar plate

Fig. 14-5. Buccolingual section through first upper premolar. Apex is separated from sinus by thin plate of bone.

which serve as the attachment of the ciliary microtubules to the cell, are characteristic of the apical segment of the cell. The cilia are typically composed of 9 + 1 pairs of microtubules, and they provide the motile apparatus to the sinus epithelium (Satir). By way of ciliary beating, the mucous blanket lining the epithelial surface moves generally from the sinus interior toward the nasal cavity.

The goblet cell displays all of the characteristic features of a secretory cell. In its basal segment the cell is occupied by, in addition to the nucleus, the cytocavitary network consisting of the rough and smooth endoplasmic reticulum and the Golgi apparatus, all of which are involved in the synthesis of the secretory mucosubstances. From the Golgi apparatus the zymogenic granules transport the mucopolysaccharides toward the cellular apex and finally release this material onto the epithelial surface by exocytosis (Fig. 14-8). In addition to the epithelial secretion, the surface of the sinus is provided with a mixed secretory product (serous secretion, consisting primarily of water with small amounts of neutral nonspecific lipids, pro-

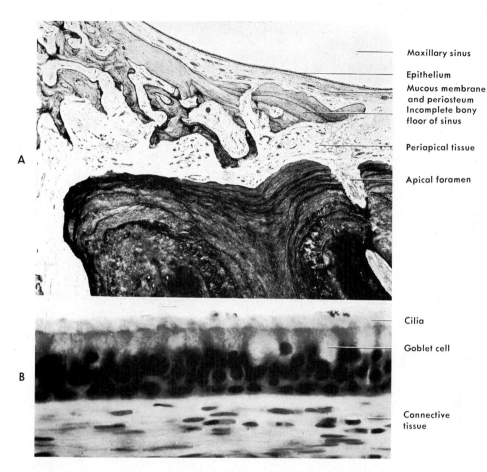

Maxillary sinus

Epithelium
Mucous membrane
and periosteum
Incomplete bony
floor of sinus

Periapical tissue

Apical foramen

Cilia

Goblet cell

Connective
tissue

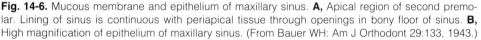

Fig. 14-6. Mucous membrane and epithelium of maxillary sinus. **A,** Apical region of second premolar. Lining of sinus is continuous with periapical tissue through openings in bony floor of sinus. **B,** High magnification of epithelium of maxillary sinus. (From Bauer WH: Am J Orthodont 29:133, 1943.)

teins, and carbohydrates, and mucous secretion, consisting of compound glycoproteins or mucopolysaccharides or both) from the subepithelial glands (Fig. 14-9). These are located in the subepithelial layer of the sinus and reach the sinus lumen by way of excretory ducts (Fig. 14-10) after the ducts have pierced the basal lamina.

On the basis of histochemical differentiation and fine structural characteristics (Vidić and Tandler) it is evident that the acini of subepithelial glands contain in varying proportions two types of secretory cells, serous and mucous. The serous cell is stained with ninhydrin-Schiff and sudan black B procedures and encloses an electron-dense, homogeneous secretory material. The mucous cell reacts positively with the alcian blue 8GX procedure for acid sialomucin or sulfomucin or both and produces an electron-lucent, heterogeneous secretory material. The myoepithelial cells

Text continued on p. 430.

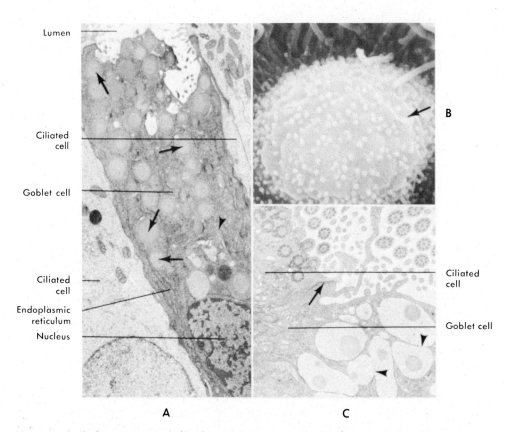

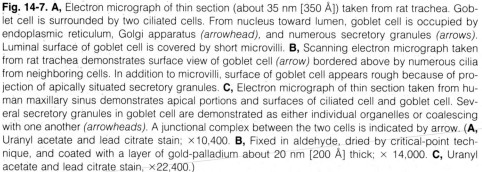

Fig. 14-7. A, Electron micrograph of thin section (about 35 nm [350 Å]) taken from rat trachea. Goblet cell is surrounded by two ciliated cells. From nucleus toward lumen, goblet cell is occupied by endoplasmic reticulum, Golgi apparatus *(arrowhead),* and numerous secretory granules *(arrows).* Luminal surface of goblet cell is covered by short microvilli. **B,** Scanning electron micrograph taken from rat trachea demonstrates surface view of goblet cell *(arrow)* bordered above by numerous cilia from neighboring cells. In addition to microvilli, surface of goblet cell appears rough because of projection of apically situated secretory granules. **C,** Electron micrograph of thin section taken from human maxillary sinus demonstrates apical portions and surfaces of ciliated cell and goblet cell. Several secretory granules in goblet cell are demonstrated as either individual organelles or coalescing with one another *(arrowheads).* A junctional complex between the two cells is indicated by arrow. (**A,** Uranyl acetate and lead citrate stain; ×10,400. **B,** Fixed in aldehyde, dried by critical-point technique, and coated with a layer of gold-palladium about 20 nm [200 Å] thick; × 14,000. **C,** Uranyl acetate and lead citrate stain, ×22,400.)

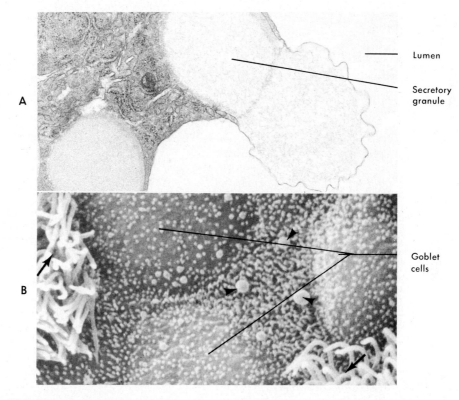

A ·

B ·

Lumen

Secretory
granule

Goblet
cells

Fig. 14-8. Secretory material from goblet cell is released into lumen by exocytosis. **A,** Electron micrograph of thin section taken from rat trachea shows a secretory granule in process of extrusion from cell into lumen. **B,** Scanning electron micrograph taken from rat trachea shows several goblet cells and parts of two ciliated cells *(arrows)*. Arrowheads indicate surface projection of secretory granules in process of extrusion from cell into lumen. (**A,** Uranyl acetate and lead citrate stain; ×48,000. **B,** Fixed in aldehydes, dried by critical-point technique, and coated with a layer of gold-palladium about 20 nm [200 Å] thick; ×11,600.)

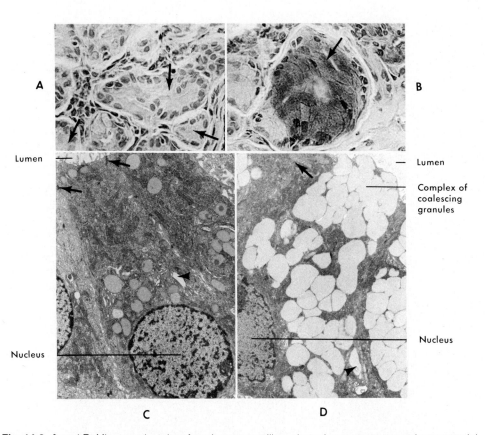

A

B

Lumen

Lumen

Complex of
coalescing
granules

Nucleus

Nucleus

C

D

Fig. 14-9. A and **B,** Micrographs taken from human maxillary sinus demonstrate several serous acini (see arrows in **A**) and mucous acinus (see arrow in **B**). Note positive reaction of secretory material with alcian blue in mucous acinus and no reaction in serous gland. **C** and **D,** Electron micrographs illustrate respectively a thin section of several serous and mucous secretory cells taken from human submucosal maxillary gland. In both representative cells, from nucleus toward acinar lumen, cytoplasm is occupied by endoplasmic reticulum, mitochondria, secretory granules, and Golgi apparatus *(arrowheads)*. Note difference in electron opacity between the two types of secretory granules. Serous granules are separated from one another by respective membranes, while mucous granules frequently coalesce among them. (Note the complex of coalescing granules.) Junctional complexes between cells in both illustrations are indicated by arrows. (**A,** Alcian blue and fast red procedure; ×1900 for serous acini and ×2000 for mucous acinus. **B,** Uranyl acetate and lead citrate stain; ×7200 for serous gland and ×6750 for mucous gland.)

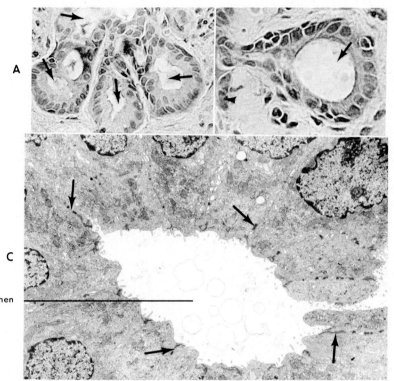

Fig. 14-10. A and **B,** Micrographs represent excretory ducts of maxillary gland taken from human maxillary sinus. Ductal cells, from cuboid to columnar in shape, surround lumen *(arrows),* which measures in these instances up to 12.5 μm in radius. **B,** Duct is demonstrated in a close apposition to epithelium of sinus *(arrowhead).* **C,** Thin section of several cells lining lumen of excretory duct from human maxillary gland. In addition to nucleus, these cells contain endoplasmic reticulum, Golgi apparatus, numerous mitochondria, lipid droplets, and occasional lysosomes. *Arrows,* Many junctional complexes between ductal cells. (**A** and **B,** Alcian blue and fast red procedure; **C,** uranyl acetate and lead citrate stain; **A** to **C,** ×1600, ×2400, ×6900.)

(Fig. 14-11) surround the acini composed of either both secretory cells or a pure population of cells of either secretory type.

The secretion from these glands, like that of the other exocrine glands, is controlled by both divisions of the autonomic nervous system (Fig. 14-11). The autonomic axons, together with general sensory components, are supplied to the maxillary sinus from the maxillary nerve complex. Numerous nonmyelinated and fewer myelinated axons are readily observable in the subepithelial layer of the sinus (Fig. 14-12). They are related here to the blood capillaries, fibroblasts, fibrocytes, collagen bundles, and other connective tissue elements.

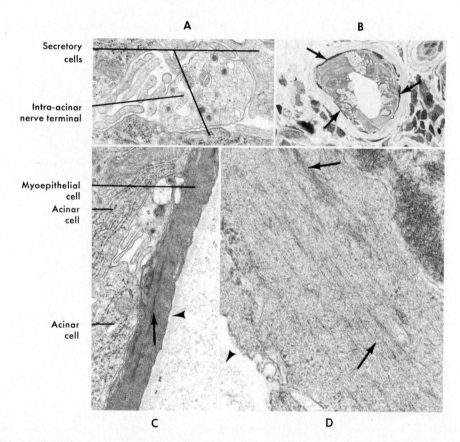

Fig. 14-11. A, Electron micrograph of intra-acinar nerve terminal in juxtaposition to two secretory cells taken from human maxillary gland. Note, in addition to mitochondria, two populations of small vesicles, dense and translucent, inside nerve terminal. **B,** Thin section (0.5 μm) of several mucous and ductal cells from human maxillary gland. Periphery of this acinus is surrounded by dark-appearing myoepithelial cells *(arrows)*. **C** and **D** illustrate relationship between acinar cells and myoepithelial cell and numerous bundles of filaments *(arrows)* that occupy most of the cytoplasm of the myoepithelial cells, respectively. In both instances basement lamina adjacent to myoepithelial cell is indicated by arrowhead. (**A, C,** and **D,** Uranyl acetate and lead citrate stain; **B,** toluidine blue stain; **A** to **D,** ×37,500, ×1600, ×27,000, ×96,000.)

FUNCTIONAL IMPORTANCE

Very little is known about the participation of the paranasal sinuses in the functioning of either the nasal cavity or the respiratory system as a whole. This is partially because of the relative inaccessibility of the sinuses to the systemic functional studies and because of the great variation in size of sinuses and their relationship to and communication with the nasal cavity. It is not surprising then that the theories of the functional importance of the sinuses range from no importance on the one hand to a multitude of involvements on the other hand.

The sinus is regarded by some as an accessory space to the nasal cavity, occurring only as a result of an inadequate process of ossification (Negus). In contrast, others report the functional contributions of the maxillary sinus in many aspects of olfactory and respiratory physiology. In individuals in whom the maxillary ostium is large enough and conveniently situated in the

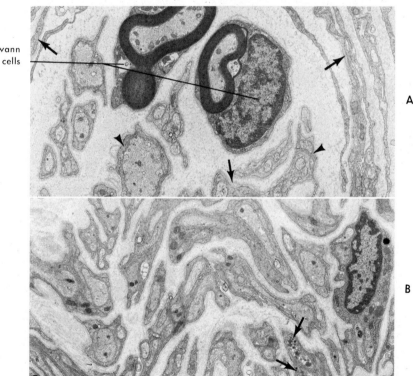

Fig. 14-12. A, Electron micrograph of two myelinated and several nonmyelinated axons in mucoperiosteal layer of human maxillary sinus. Schwann cells *(labeled and at arrowheads)* are intimately related to axons, which contain individual mitochondria and microtubules or microfilaments cut in different planes. *Arrows,* Connective tissue elements surrounding either individual axon or entire nerve. **B,** Nonmyelinated axons isolated from human mucoperiosteal layer of maxillary sinus. Most of them contain the same organelles as in **A.** However, some *(arrows)* are occupied by dense or translucent vesicles. (**A** and **B,** Uranyl acetate and lead citrate stain; **A,** ×11,200; **B,** ×19,200.)

hiatus semilunaris the air pressure in the sinus fluctuates from ±0.7 to ±4 mm of water between the nasal expiration and inspiration (Lamm and Schaffrath). This dependence of the pressure in the sinus on the wave of respiration is, however, less probable in instances of either the small maxillary ostium or the ostium hidden in the depth of the hiatus semilunaris. On the basis of the same two conditions related to the structure and topography of the ostium some suggested functions attributed to the sinus by Koertvelyessy, Allen, Döderlein, Latkowski, and Doiteau (humidification and warming of inspired air and contribution to the olfaction, for instance) are subject to controversy. However, it is possible that if air is arrested in the sinus for a certain time, it quickly reaches body temperature and thus protects the internal structures, particularly the brain, against exposure to cold air (Koertvelyessy, Allen, Latkowski, and Maurer). The other contributions by paranasal cavities to the resonance of voice, lightening of the skull weight (Merideth, Nemours), enhancement of faciocranial resistance to mechanical shock, and the production of bactericidal lysozyme to the nasal cavity are reviewed in detail by Latkowski and by Blanton and Biggs.

CLINICAL CONSIDERATIONS

The section on developmental anomalies discusses several modifications of genetic and other origins in the developmental pathways of the maxillary sinus (agenesia, aplasia, hypoplasia, and supernumerary sinus). Some other criteria that correlate the extent of pneumatization by sinuses with the general dysfunctions of the endocrine system are by now developed. In the case of pituitary giantism, for example, all sinuses assume a much larger volume than in healthy individuals of the same geographic

environment (Püschel and Schlosshauer). It is also known that in some congenital infections such as by spirochetes in congenital syphilis the pneumatic processes are greatly suppressed, resulting in small sinuses (Richter).

In most respects the pathogenic relationship of the maxillary sinus to the orodental complexes is the result of topographic arrangement and of the functional and systemic association between the two territories. The transfer of a pathologic condition from the sinus to the orodental apparatus, or vice versa, is achieved either by mechanical connections or by way of the blood or lymphatic pathways. Since the upper first molar tooth is most often closest to the floor of the maxillary sinus, surgical manipulation on this tooth is most likely to break through the partitioning bony lamina and thus to establish an oroantral fistula (2.19% of all such fistulas are caused by first molars, 2.01% by second molars). If untreated, the lumen of such fistulas might epithelialize and permanently connect the maxillary space with the oral cavity. A similar condition might arise as a result of either a molar or a premolar radicular cyst, granuloma, or abscess. Hypercementosis of root apices and subsequent extraction of the affected tooth may also lead to a perforation. It is necessary therefore to consider on a radiograph the relationship between any such premolar or molar tooth with the floor of the maxillary sinus prior to surgical intervention.

The chronic infections of the mucoperiosteal layer of the sinus, on the other hand, might involve superior alveolar nerves if these nerves are closely related to the sinus and cause the neuralgia that mimics possible dental origin (Osmont, Jars, and Ged). In this instance the diagnosis must be based on a careful inspection of all the upper teeth as well as of the maxillary sinus to differentiate cause and eventual result of this condition. The neuralgia of the maxillary nerve (tic douloureux) could also have an etiologic origin in the superior dental apparatus or the mucoperiosteal layer of the sinus or both. For the diagnosis and treatment of this condition, it is most important to determine precisely the causal focus. Because of overlap of innervated territories and close topographic relationships between the teeth and the sinus, however, the causal focus is often difficult to assess.

The pathogenic association of the sinus with the orodental system, or vice versa, is based, in addition to a close topographic relationship, on an extensive vascular connection between these two regions by the superior alveolar vessels. As a consequence of this vascular arrangement, nonspecific bacterial sinusitis may be followed by some oral manifestations. Also the infections caused by the streptococci, staphylococci, pneumococci, or the virus of the common cold are likely to spread from either of the two regions to involve the other one. Finally, malignant lesions (e.g., adenocarcinoma, squamous cell carcinoma, osteosarcoma, fibrosarcoma, lymphosarcoma) of the maxillary sinus may produce their primary manifestation in the maxillary teeth. This may consist of pain, loosening, supraeruption, or bleeding in their gingival tissue.

REFERENCES

Allen BC: Applied anatomy of paranasal sinuses, J Am Osteopath Assoc 60:978, 1961.

Ardouin P: Étude embryologique du développement du sinus maxillaire, Rev Laryngol Otol Rhinol (Bord) 79:834, 1958.

Blair VP, Brown JB, and Byars LT: Observations on sinus abnormalities in congenital total and hemiabsence of the nose, Ann Otol Rhinol Laryngol 46:592, 1937.

Blanton PL and Biggs NL: Eighteen hundred years of controversy: the paranasal sinuses, Am J Anat 124:135, 1969.

Blumenstein G: Die Entwicklung der Kieferhöhlen bei Rachenmandelhyperplasie, Nasenrachenfibrom, Choanalatresia und Dysostosis mandibulofacialis im Vergleich zur normalen Entwicklung, Hals-Nasen-Ohrenklinik der Westfälischen Wilhelms Universität (Thesis), Münster, Germany, 1963.

Cheraskin E: Diagnostic stomatology: a clinical pathologic approach, New York, 1961, McGraw-Hill Book Co.

Colby RA, Kerr DA, and Robinson HBG: Color atlas of oral pathology, Philadelphia, 1961, JB Lippincott Co.

Cullen RL and Vidić B: The dimensions and shape of the human maxillary sinus in the perinatal period, Acta Anat 83:411, 1972.

Delaney AJ and Morse HR: Inferior meatal accessory ostia: report of a case, Ann Otol Rhinol Laryngol 60:635, 1951.

Döderlein W: Experimentelle Untersuchungen zur Physiologie der Nasen und Mundatmung und über die physiologische Bedeutung der Nasennebenhöhlen, Z Hals-Nasen-u Ohrenheilk 30:459, 1932.

Doiteau R: Contribution à l'étude de la physiologie des sinus de la face: renouvellement de l'air intrasinusien échanges gazeux permuqueux, Rev Laryngol Otol Rhinol (Bord) 77:900, 1956.

Eckel W and Beisser D: Untersuchungen zur Frage eines Einflusses der Gaumenspaltbildung auf die Kieferhöhlengrösse, Z Laryngol Rhinol Otol 40:23, 1961.

Fatin M: A rare case of congenital malformation: total absence of half the nose, probably supporting the theory of bilateral nasal origin, J Egypt Med Assoc 38(8):470, 1955.

Gouzy J, Voilgue G, and Jakubowicz B: A propos de deux cas d'agénésie du sinus maxillaire, J Fr Otorhinolaryngol 17:579, 1968.

Hajiniš K, Kustra T, Farkaš LG, et al.: Sinus maxillaris, Z Morph Anthropol 59:185, 1967.

Koertvelyessy T: Relationships between the frontal sinus and climatic conditions: a skeletal approach to cold adaptation, Am J Phys Anthropol 37:161, 1972.

Lamm H and Schaffrath H: Druckmessungen im gesunden Sinus maxillaris bei verschiedenen Atmungstypen, Z Laryngol Rhinol Otol 46:172, 1967.

Latkowski B: Poglady na znaczenie zatok bocznych nosa, Pol Tyg Lek 19:1206, 1964.

Maurer R: Zur Physiologie der Schädelpneumatisation, Arch Ohren-Nasen-u Kelhkopfheilk 163:471, 1953.

Merideth HW: The paranasal sinuses, Rocky Mt Med J 49:343, 1952.

Mocellin L: Um caso de pan-agenesia dos seios paranasais, Rev Bras Cirurg 48(4):283, 1964.

Negus V: The function of the paranasal sinuses, AMA Arch Otolaryngol 66:430, 1957.

Nemours PR: A comparison of the accessory nasal sinuses of man with those of the lower vertebrates, Trans Am Laryngol Otol Rhinol Soc 37:195, 1931.

Osmont J, Jars G, and Ged S: Anatomie chirurgicale du sinus maxillaire, Rev Odontostomatol Midi Fr 25:50, 1967.

Perović D: Medicinska Enciklopedija, vol 6, Zagreb, 1962, Naklada Leksikografskog Zavoda FNRJ

Püschel L and Schlosshauer B: Ueber den Einfluss des somatotropen and androgenen Hormons auf die Pneumatisation, Arch Ohren-Nasen-u Kehlkopfheilk 167:595, 1955.

Richter H: Ueber exogene Einflüsse auf die Entwicklung der Nasennebenhöhlen, Arch Ohren-Naseu-U Kehlkopfheilk 143:251, 1937.

Rosenberger HC: Does sinus infection affect sinus growth? Laryngoscope 55:62, 1945.

Satir P: How cilia move, Sci Am 231:45, 1974.

Schaeffer JP: The nose, paranasal sinuses, nasolacrimal passageways, and olfactory organ in man, Philadelphia, 1920, P Blakiston's Son & Co.

Schaeffer JP: The anatomy of the paranasal sinuses in children, Arch Otolaryngol 15:657, 1932.

Schaeffer JP: The clinical anatomy and development of the paranasal sinuses, Penn Med J 65:395, 1935.

Schürch O: Ueber die Beziehungen der Grössenvariationen der Highmorshöhle zum individuellen Schädelbau und deren praktische Bedeutung für die Therapie der Kieferhöhleneiterungen, Arch Laryngol Rhinol 18:229, 1906.

Scopp IW: Oral medicine: a clinical approach with basic science correlation, ed 2, St. Louis, 1973, The CV Mosby Co.

Terracol J and Ardouin P: Anatomie des fosses nasales et des cavités annexes, Paris, 1965, Librairie Maloine SA

Van Alyea OE: The ostium maxillare, Arch Otolaryngol 24:553, 1936.

Vidić B: The morphogenesis of the lateral nasal wall in the early prenatal life of man, Am J Anat 130:121, 1971.

Vidić B and Tandler B: Ultrastructure of the secretory cells of the submucosal glands in the human maxillary sinus, J Morphol 150:167, 1976.

15

HISTOCHEMISTRY OF ORAL TISSUES

Histochemical techniques are based on precise chemical rationales for their ability to identify or stain different biochemical substances. These techniques necessitate using more stringent precautions to preserve the chemical integrity of the tissues than, perhaps, are required in a biochemical or an immunochemical assay. Also, histochemical techniques provide in situ information that cannot be obtained with biochemical methods. Application of immunobiologic principles in the histochemical localization of specific proteins, glycoproteins, or proteoglycans allows detection of a host of biologic molecules that play important roles in normal tissues during de-velopment and in different pathologic conditions. Numerous innovative techniques promoting localization of different chemical residues or components of a large molecule are also available for histochemical application. A case in point is the use of plant lectins as histochemical probes in the characterization of sugar moieties within glycoprotein molecules. Use of these probes has generated much more specific and meaningful in situ information than could be obtained from biochemical assays of total tissue homogenate pools.

In situ hybridization is the latest histochemical technique that permits identification of a gene (DNA nucleotide sequence) or gene product (messenger RNA [mRNA]) on a tissue section. The technique draws on the principles and methods of modern molecular biology and genetics wherein synthetic nucleotide probes, complementary DNA (cDNA) probes, or mRNA probes are prepared and allowed to hybridize corresponding/complementary molecular sites in a tissue section. Tissue sections are protected from DNA/RNA degradation, and their proteins and lipids are removed before hybridization. Since the probes are generally radiolabeled with ^{32}P, ^{3}H, or ^{35}S, the loci of hybridization are visualized by standard autoradiographic procedures. To affirm that the hybridized probe (i.e., mRNA) is an appropriate substrate for translation, mRNA can be translated in vitro to its protein product. This protein product can then be analyzed with the appropriate monoclonal antibody, using standard immunohistochemical techniques. In situ hybridization and the immunohistochemical methods thus complement each other, enhance ultimate specificity, and make for perhaps some of the most powerful investigative and diagnostic tools in biology and medicine.

Most histochemical techniques have generally been used for qualitative analysis of chemical substances in cells and tissues. However, many sophisticated techniques are available for quantitative analysis of histochemical reactions. They include use

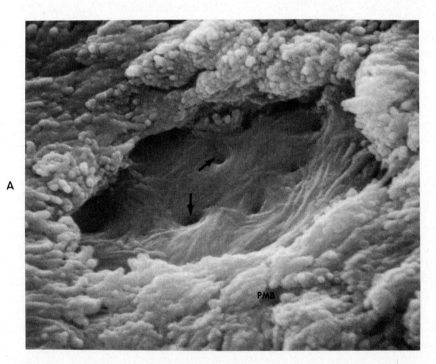

Fig. 15-1. Scanning electron micrographs of cancellous bone in deorganified dog mandible. A metallic implant was surgically inserted subperiosteally in previously edentulatized mandible and was kept in place for 24 months prior to removal of bone sample for microscopic analysis. **A,** A forming osteocytic lacuna with openings of canaliculi *(arrows)* visible on its inside while the newly deposited perilacunar mineral matrix *(PMB)* is seen roofing over and around it. (×7000.)

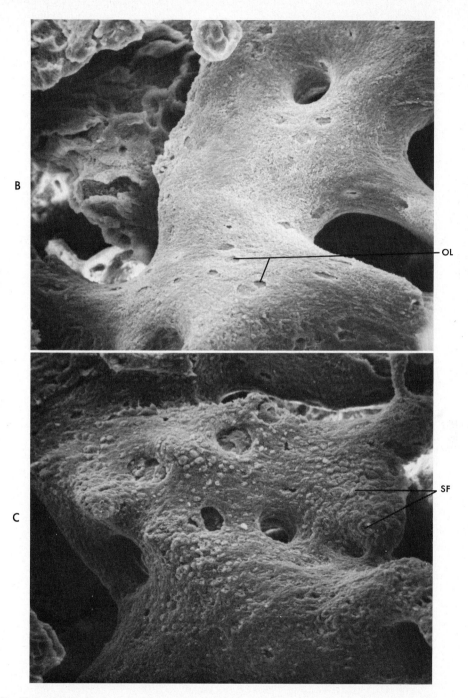

Fig. 15-1, cont'd. B, A typical bone trabeculum revealing several developing osteocytic lacunae *(OL)* on its forming surface. (×280.) **C,** An atypical bone trabeculum, which reveals a rough surface studded with fully or partially mineralized Sharpey fibers *(SF).* (×280.) (From Russell TE and Kapur SP: J Oral Implantol 7:415, 1977.)

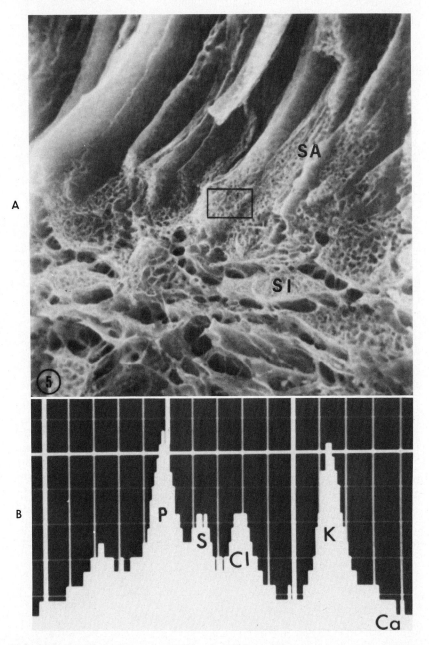

Fig. 15-2. A, Scanning electron microscopic view of freeze-fractured surface ot secretory ameloblasts *(SA)* and stratum intermedium *(SI)* from developing rat molar tooth. (×2700.) Rectangular area marks proximal region of an ameloblast that was bombarded with electrons in order to obtain an electron probe spectrum, **B,** for an analysis of its mineral content. **B,** X-ray spectrum for this site reveals notable peaks for phosphorus *(P),* potassium *(K),* sulfur *(S),* and chloride *(Cl)* in order of descending heights. No significant calcium *(Ca)* peak is evident. (From Reith EJ and Boyde A: Histochemistry 55:17, 1978.)

of the original microphotocell counter, double-beam recording microdensitometry, and more recently the scanning and integrating microdensitometry. This latter method has been used successfully by Chayen in measuring lysosomal membrane permeability and by Stuart and Simpson in measuring the activity of dehydrogenase enzymes in single cells from bone marrow biopsies of normal and leukemic patients. Phillips and co-workers have done a quantitative analysis of total mineral content in bone by combining microradiography and microdensitometry using a scanning autodensidater attachment.

Many new techniques, not precisely histochemical, are frequently used by histochemists in making qualitative as well as quantitative analysis of tissue substances, particularly mineral elements. These include x-ray and interference microscopy for measuring the dry mass of a biologic substance or a reaction product, x-ray diffraction, x-ray spectrophotometry, and electron probe microanalysis. Recently, scanning electron microscopy (SEM) has come to occupy an important place in dental research. SEM has been used in the study of bone morphology and in the analysis of changes in bone architecture induced by the presence of surgically inserted metallic implants (Fig. 15-1). Neiders and co-workers have made conjunctive use of SEM with an electron probe attachment for obtaining a visual surface texture image of tooth cementum analyzed for its mineral content. Reith and Boyde have also used an electron probe with SEM in a study of calcium transport across ameloblasts in the enamel organ (Fig. 15-2). Techniques of polarized light and x-ray analysis have been used for the study of enamel. Phosphorescence

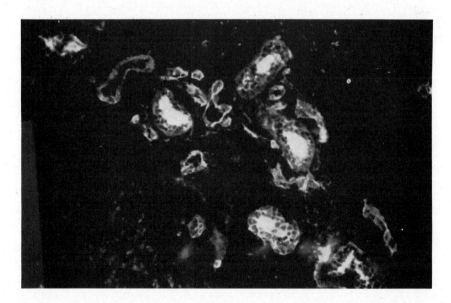

Fig. 15-3. Submaxillary gland secreting mucus in which the A antigen is demonstrated by immunofluorescence using rabbit anti-A serum and goat antirabbit serum: fluorescein. Human fetus, 8 cm crown-rump length. This secretion and mucus-borne antigen persist throughout life. (Courtesy Dr. A.E. Szulman, Pittsburgh.)

emitted as a result of tetracycline binding to mineralized tissues has been demonstrated in bone, dentin, and enamel at liquid nitrogen temperatures. Laser spectroscopy has also been used for qualitative and quantitative microanalysis of inorganic components of calcified tissues. Immunohistochemical techniques using fluorescein tags have been applied to the study of oral tissues (Fig. 15-3).

Light microscopic histochemical techniques have been increasingly adapted for use in electron microscopic histochemistry. The visualization of carbohydrates, specific proteins, and phosphatases are some examples of such adaptive use (Fig. 15-4).

Radioautographic techniques play a vital role in histochemistry because of their ability to elucidate the uptake of chemical substances by the metabolic pathways of dif-

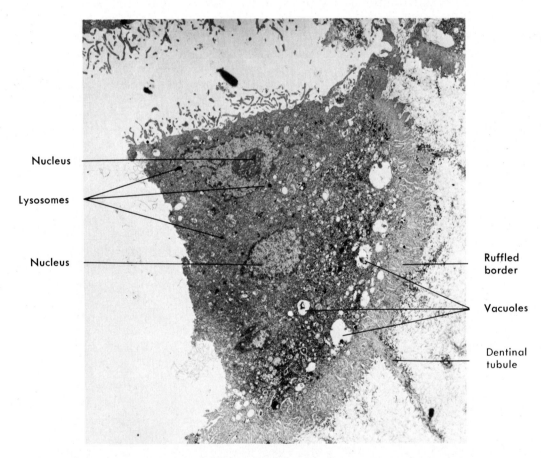

Fig. 15-4. Electron micrograph of odontoclast from mongrel-puppy primary tooth undergoing resorption. Notice acid phosphatase reaction product in form of a black precipitate along dentinal tubule, ruffled border, vacuoles, and in lysosomes. (Glutaraldehyde fixation, Gomori's metal substitution method; ×6250.) (From Freilich LS: A morphological and histological study of the cells associated with physiological root resorption in human and canine primary teeth, doctoral dissertation, Washington, DC, 1972, Georgetown University.)

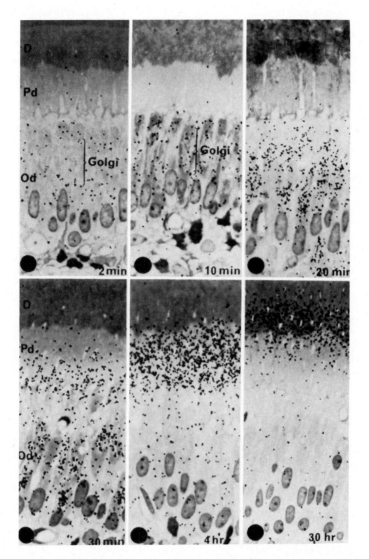

Fig. 15-5. Light microscopic radioautographs illustrate path of ^{3}H-proline (injected into a young rat) over odontoblasts, *OD;* predentin, *PD;* and dentin, *D,* at growing end of incisor tooth. Notice that silver grains representing path of ^{3}H-proline appear first in granular endoplasmic reticulum at 2 minutes and subsequently at 10 and 20 minutes in Golgi region of odontoblasts. Thirty minutes after injection silver grains start appearing in odontoblastic processes and predentin, whereas at 4 hours entire radioactivity is located in predentin. Thirty hours after injection, dentin is completely labeled with ^{3}H-proline, now incorporated into collagen fibrils of dental matrix. (×1000.) (From Weinstock M and Leblond CP: J Cell Biol 60:92, 1974.)

ferent tissues and by different regions of the cytoplasm (Figs. 15-5 and 15-6). Tissue sections taken from animals injected with a radioisotope are covered with a photographic film or emulsion and left in the dark. Radio waves emitted by the isotope hit the silver halides of the film, and these tracks are later developed by processing of the slide or the metal grid like a photographic film. The radioisotope appears as dark granules in the light microscope and as linear tracks of the radio waves in the electron microscopic autoradiographs.

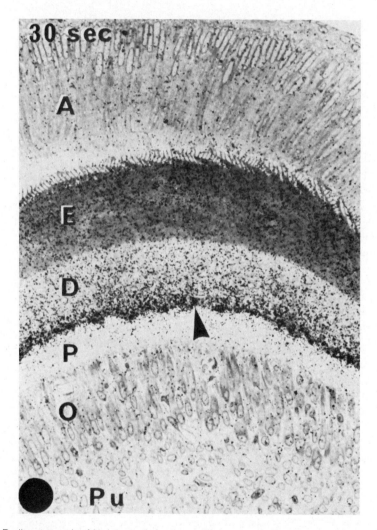

Fig. 15-6. Radioautograph of incisor tooth (undecalcified cross section) at its growing end in young rat killed 30 seconds after intravenous injection of ^{45}Ca. *A*, Ameloblasts; *E*, enamel; *D*, dentin; *P*, predentin; *O*, odontoblasts; *Pu*, pulp. Notice that ^{45}Ca is immediately incorporated into dentin over predentin-dentin junction at arrow. Some ^{45}Ca activity in form of few grains is seen in odontoblasts and predentin. (×250.) (From Munhoz COG and Leblond CP: Calcif Tissue Res 15:221, 1974.)

STRUCTURE AND CHEMICAL COMPOSITION OF ORAL TISSUES

Oral structures are primarily composed of connective tissue and epithelial linings and associated glands. An understanding of these structures and their chemical composition is important in the consideration of biologic problems related to oral health. Significant chemical constituents of these tissues are proteoglycans, glycoproteins, mucins, and enzymes.

Connective tissue

Connective tissue is derived from the mesenchyme and consists of various types of cells and fibers that are embedded in an amorphous, semigel, colloidal ground substance. The connective tissue ground substance is primarily composed of proteoglycans and glycoproteins. Proteoglycans are large molecules formed of a protein core to which a large number of glycosaminoglycan (GAG) chains composed of repeating disaccharide units are attached. The GAGs may be unsulfated (hyaluronic acid) or sulfated (chondroitin sulfates, keratan sulfates, and heparan sulfates). Heparin, a highly sulfated GAG, is secreted by connective tissue mast cells. Hyaluronic acid is synthesized as a very large, free, nonsulfated GAG that does not require a protein core and differs from chondroitin sulfates in having acetylglucosamines instead of acetylgalactosamines as its constituents. Hyaluronic acid binds proteoglycan molecules along its length to form large proteoglycan polymers. The numbers and types of GAGs attached to the protein core in a proteoglycan molecule, as well as the polymeric state of proteoglycans, determine the viscosity of the amorphous ground substance. Hyaluronic acid predominates in the loose connective tissues and, because of its high capacity to bind water, is primarily responsible for transport and diffusion of metabolic substances across tissues. Bacterial infections may occur as a result of the hydrolytic action of the bacterial enzyme hyaluronidase on the polymeric integrity of hyaluronic acid. Chondroitin sulfates predominate in the cartilage proteoglycans and are primarily responsible for the supportive and somewhat plastic texture of this tissue. Chondroitin sulfates constitute 1% of the total bone tissue, whereas only 0.5% is present in dentin. Other organic components of bone are approximately 93% type I collagen and 5% noncollagenous proteins, including phosphoproteins, glycoproteins, osteocalcin (Gla protein), and osteonectin.

Glycoproteins present in the connective tissue ground substance are protein macromolecules, which contain fewer associated carbohydrate moieties than are present in the proteoglycans. Also, carbohydrates are not present in the form of regular repeating units. Several glycoproteins secreted into the connective tissue by epithelial cells and fibroblasts have been identified in the last few years. Of them, the most well known and characterized are (1) *fibronectin* (secreted by fibroblasts, smooth muscle cells, and various other cell types); (2) *laminin* (secreted by epithelial cells and present in all basement membranes); (3) *chondronectin* (secreted by chondrocytes); and (4) *osteonectin* (secreted by osteoblasts). All of these glycoproteins promote attachment of cells to their extracellular collagen matrices and therefore not only maintain normal cell morphology but also control cell function.

Both proteoglycans and glycoproteins in connective tissues undergo alterations in various pathologic states. During inflammation or in early stages of wound healing there is a histochemically detectable increase in both glycoproteins and proteoglycans. However, as wound healing progresses, there is a gradual decline in the levels of both substances until normal levels are restored. Levels of fibronectin and its cell membrane receptors are known to undergo a decline in certain forms of cancer. These reduced levels are correlated with the altered or transformed behavior of the cancer cells. Some investigators have suggested that metastatic cancer cells preferentially bind to type IV collagen via laminin, both being components of the basement membranes. In contrast, it has been suggested that nonmalignant tumor cells do not use laminin for attachment.

Fibroblasts are the most common cell type in the connective tissues. They are responsible for the elaboration of glycoproteins such as fibronectin and proteoglycans that form the amorphous ground substance. They also elaborate the fibrous components of the ground substance, including different types of collagen (especially types I and III), reticular fibers, and elastic fibers.

Current biochemical, histochemical, and ultrastructural evidence suggests that collagen is initially synthesized as much larger preprocollagen polypeptide chains. The prepeptide component is removed during or shortly after translocation in the rough endoplasmic reticulum. Posttranslational changes include hydroxylation of proline and lysine residues, glycosilation of hydroxylysine residues, formation of disulfide bonds between adjacent chains, and the formation of the characteristic triple helix. Procollagen is secreted on the cell surface where the propeptide sequence is deleted by a specific protease. This is immediately followed by the formation of the collagen microfibrils. The microfibrils serve as a template for initiation and extension of the polymerization and the accretion of more newly secreted monomeric tropocollagen into collagen fibrils. Hydroxylation steps are facilitated by vitamin C and are essential for providing conformation and stability

to the triple helix. Deficiency of vitamin C results in the loss of molecular stability, resulting in the formation of abnormal, immature collagen and consequent collagen diseases.

The newly elaborated collagen fibrils, formed during development or in wound healing, are equivalent to reticular fibers in their electron microscopic structure. Both of these fibers stain positively for glycoproteins with silver stains and the periodic acid–Schiff (PAS) method. These reactions indicate the presence of a considerable packing of glycoprotein between aligned microfibrils of tropocollagen macromolecules.

Elastic fibers are elaborated by fibroblasts and also possibly by smooth muscle cells in the walls of blood vessels. They are composed of a protein component characterized by the presence of the amino acids desmocine and isodesmocine and glycosaminoglycans. Unlike collagen and reticular fibers, elastic fibers are not considered to be important constituents of the fully repaired tissues. Elastic fibers are stained by aldehyde fuchsin, resorcin fuchsin, and specifically by the dye orcein in histologic preparations. A fluorescent staining method, using tetraphenylporphine sulfonate in combination with silver or gold, has been developed by Albert and Fleischer for electron microscopic visualization of elastic fibers.

Besides fibroblasts, other cellular elements of connective tissue are macrophages, which scavenge on tissue debris; mast cells, which are rich in the highly sulfated proteoglycan heparin (an anticoagulant) and histamine (a vasodilator); and plasma cells, which elaborate immunoglobulins.

Epithelial tissues and derivatives

Salivary glands elaborate the so-called mucins or mucoids. The definition of these substances is exclusively chemical from the biochemical standpoint, but from a histochemical point of view this definition is in part based on color reactions. Histochemical detection of mucins is generally based on their glycosaminoglycan content, which affects certain staining reactions. The acidic nature is attributable to the presence of glucuronic acid, sulfate, or sialic acids. Histochemical observations show that a number of acid mucins lack sulfate esters. Histochemical characteristics of the oral epithelium, the epithelial components of the tooth germ, and the salivary glands are considered in another section of this chapter.

Several histochemical studies have been made on the structural proteins of the salivary gland leukocytes or the so-called salivary corpuscles. Histochemical techniques are also being used in oral exfoliative cytology for the detection of oral cancer. Identification of lung carcinoma by analysis of normal and abnormal cells present in sputum is used clinically.

Enzymes

Histochemistry has enabled histologists to demonstrate the actual sites of cellular enzymatic activity. The topographic distribution of enzymes may be ascertained by the quantitative microchemical techniques developed by the Linderstrøm-Lang group or by techniques that result in the formation of visible reaction products in tissue sections. The latter approach is widely used in histochemical demonstration of enzymes.

The most frequently studied enzymes in oral tissues are those related to the transfer of phosphate esters (specific and nonspecific phosphatases) in the organic matrix of bone, dentin, and enamel (alkaline phosphatase) and to resorption of bone and of dentin (acid phosphatase). Oxidases and dehydrogenases, reflecting the metabolic activity of different tissues in oral structures, have also been studied extensively. Esterases, generally associated with the hydrolysis of carboxylic acid esters of alcohol, have been studied in salivary glands and in the taste buds. More recently, studies on lysosomal sulfatase and on adenyl cyclase involved in the formation of cyclic adenosine monophosphate (cAMP) have been reported.

HISTOCHEMICAL TECHNIQUES
Fixation procedures

For histochemical study, a tissue block must be preserved in such a way that it causes minimal changes in the reactivity of the cytoplasmic and extracellular macromolecules, for example, enzymes, structural proteins, protein-carbohydrate complexes, lipids, and nucleic acids. This is accomplished by using optimum osmotic conditions, cold temperatures, controlled pH of the fixing solutions, and the minimum possible exposure to the fixative.

Formaldehyde is considered to be one of the ideal fixatives, especially for enzymes and other proteins. This is because of its ability to react with major reactive groups of proteins to form polymeric or macromolecular networks, without affecting their native reactivity to histochemical procedures. Formaldehyde has a preservative effect on lipids by altering their relationship with the proteins. Use of electrolytes such as calcium or cadmium in formaldehyde or chromation of tissue blocks subsequent to fixation prevents dissolution of phospholipids. Formaldehyde is generally used as a 10% solution buffered to pH 7 at cold temperatures in the range of 0° to 4° C.

Acrolein and glutaraldehyde are other frequently used aldehydes, with the latter being routinely used for electron microscopy. Conjunctive use of colloids such as sucrose, ficoll, polyvinylpyrrolidone, and dextrans in the fixing solutions is often made to prevent osmotic rupture of cell organelles. This helps to improve the in situ localization of the histochemical reactions.

Other fixatives used for the study of glycogen, glycoproteins, proteoglycans, and nucleic acids are frequently mixtures of many chemical ingredients. *Rossman's fluid,* used for visualization of glycogen, glycoproteins, and proteoglycans, contains formaldehyde, alcohol, picric acid, and acetic acid. *Carnoy's mixture,* used for histochemical staining of nucleic acids, is composed of ethyl alcohol, acetic acid, and chloroform. Alcohol denatures proteins without causing irreversible chemical changes in the active groups but, being a poor fixative, is used in combination with acetic acid and chloroform. *Feulgen's reaction,* used for visualizing DNA, requires acid hydrolysis of the DNA polymers to expose the deoxyribose sugar residues of DNA molecules. The aldehyde groups thus exposed (on the deoxyribose sugar residues) are then chemically reacted with leucofuchsin (Schiff's reagent) to form a reddish purple reaction product.

Some enzyme systems such as cytochrome oxidases are highly labile and therefore cannot be preserved by chemical fixation. Visualization of such enzymes is performed on fresh frozen (cryostat) sections. However, to prevent diffusion and to preserve the in vivo status of the tissue macromolecules, one must fix the tissue blocks by a freeze-drying procedure. Tissues are frozen rapidly at very low temperatures, usually in liquid nitrogen, and then placed in a refrigerated vacuum chamber where ice, formed in the tissues, is removed by sublimation, that is, by direct transformation into vapor without going through a liquid phase. After dehydration in vacuum, tissue blocks are embedded in paraffin and sectioned routinely with a mi-

crotome. Freeze-dried tissues exhibit optimal enzyme activity, show excellent histologic characteristics, and do not show any shrinkage artifacts that are seen with routine fixation. Besides oxidative enzymes, freeze-drying is used for visualization of other enzyme systems, for example, phosphatases and dehydrogenases, and also for the precise localization of otherwise diffusible inorganic ions.

Techniques of freeze-fracture and freeze-etching have been devised for use in electron microscopy to avoid use of chemicals in tissue preparation. This technique has enabled biologists to obtain excellent three-dimensional images of the surfaces of various cell membranes not previously observed.

Histochemical study of teeth and bone requires careful fixation and controlled decalcification procedures. Simultaneous fixation and decalcification with formaldehyde or glutaraldehyde and ethylenediaminetetraacetate acid (EDTA) have been successfully used in the study of teeth and bone for light and electron microscopic histochemistry. Decalcified ground sections have also been used in histochemical studies of teeth and bone. Techniques have been developed for sectioning freeze-dried, undecalcified tissues. Gray and Opdyke have described a saw for the preparation of 10 to 50 μm sections of undecalcified tissues. Such sectioning has been used for histochemical studies of dental decay. Study of bone has been considerably enhanced by the process of deorganification (deproteinization). Swedlow and colleagues and Kapur and Russell have studied bone architecture with SEM to great advantage after deorganification with concentrated hydrazine.

Specific histochemical methods

Histochemical techniques primarily used in the study of oral tissues may be categorized as (1) glycogen, glycoprotein, and proteoglycan methods; (2) protein and lipid methods; and (3) enzyme methods. They are all characterized by a direct staining reaction or by the formation of an insoluble dye or precipitate at the reactive sites.

Glycogen, glycoproteins, and proteoglycans. The best-known and most frequently used technique for detection of carbohydrate groupings is the periodic acid–Schiff (PAS) technique. The chemical basis of this method lies in the fact that periodic acid oxidizes the glycol groups to aldehydes and these in turn are revealed as a reddish-purple dye product on treatment with leucofuchsin (Schiff reagent). Use of fluorescent reagent anthracene-9-carboxyaldehyde carbohydrazone as a substitute for Schiff reagent has been made by Cotelli and Livingston. Treatment of tissue sections with amylase prior to oxidation removes glycogen from the tissues, and this is reflected in a reduced Schiff reaction product. A comparison of the amylase-digested and -undigested sections is used in estimating the amounts of glycogen or other carbohydrate-protein molecules. Electron microscopic visualization of carbohydrates has been achieved, among other techniques, by use of phosphotungstic acid and lead citrate after oxidation with periodic acid. The periodate–thiocarbohydrazide–silver proteinate method of Theiry shows high specificity for glycol containing glycoconjugates at the electron microscopic level.

Proteoglycans are well demonstrated by thiazine dyes such as toluidine blue, azure A, and Alcian blue. Toluidine blue produces a metachromatic reaction ranging from a purple to a red reaction product. This change of color (metachromasia) from the original (orthochromatic) blue color of the monomeric form of toluidine blue reflects the extent of polymerization of the dye molecules as they tag onto the anionic residues on the glycosaminoglycans mole-

cule. Thus heparin present in the mast cell granules and chondroitin sulfates present in the intercellular ground substance of the cartilage or developing bone give an intense red metachromasia, demonstrating the highly acidic or sulfated nature of these proteoglycans. Alcian blue staining has been used to considerable advantage in characterizing the specific types of acid-radicals present within proteoglycans. When used at pH 2 to 2.8, Alcian blue stains weakly acid-sulfated proteoglycans. However, when it is used at pH 1 to 1.2, Alcian blue binds to highly sulfated proteoglycans. By incubating tissue sections in the enzyme sialidase prior to staining with Alcian blue, distinction can be made between sialidase-resistant and sialidase-non-resistant molecules.

Several techniques are available for the localization of proteoglycans or sulfated glycoconjugates at the electron microscopic level. The high-iron diamine thiocarbohydrazide–silver proteinate (HID-TCH-SP) method of Spicer provides high specificity for sulfated glycoconjugates. This method excludes reaction with carboxyl and phosphate groups. Several cationic dyes, including ruthenium red, silver tetraphenylporphine sulfonate, Alcian blue, bismuth nitrate, and cuprolinic blue, have been used successfully by several investigators in localizing proteoglycans in oral tissue.

A new histochemical method is now available for staining hyaluronic acid using a biotynilated hyaluronic acid-binding complex, prepared by extraction from cartilage proteoglycans, as a probe. Subsequent to incubation of the formaldehyde-fixed tissue sections with this probe, sections are incubated in peroxidase-conjugated strepavidin; then this complex is visualized by its binding to 3 amino-9-ethyl carbazole, which acts as a peroxidase substrate.

Specific plant lectins have been used in the identification or characterization of specific carbohydrate moieties within a glycoprotein molecule in the study of carbohydrate histochemistry. Fluorescein dyes or horseradish peroxidase techniques are used as tags for the visualization of lectin binding sites on carbohydrate moieties within a glycoprotein molecule. Electron microscopic localization of sugar moieties in the glycoprotein molecules has been made by using ferritin and horseradish peroxidase as lectin tags.

Proteins and lipids. Histochemistry of proteins is based on classic reactions of protein chemistry involving various amino acid groups, that is, amino, imino, carboxyl, disulfide, and sulfhydryl groups. Reagents such as dinitrofluorbenzene, ninhydrin, or ferric ferricyanide are utilized to give insoluble colored reaction products.

Histochemical study of lipids frequently implies use of frozen or freeze-dried sections. Total lipids are studied by using fat colorant dyes such as Sudan dyes. Chromation of formol-calcium–fixed tissues and their subsequent staining with Sudan black has been used for the identification of phospholipids. Extraction procedures with various lipid solvents are considered essential to accompany most histochemical staining procedures for lipids.

Enzymes. The enzyme techniques utilize many different principles. Some of the criteria used in deciding the application of a technique are related to avoidance of inhibition by the substrate and insolubility of the primary reaction product and its immediate coupling to the capture reagent to prevent diffusion and false localization of enzyme activity.

The Gomori method for phosphatases uses phosphoric esters of glycerol, glucose, or adenosine. The enzymatically liberated phosphate ion is converted into an insoluble salt, which can be visualized by polarized light or phase contrast, or the salt can be transformed into a cobalt or lead compound, which is black. Riboflavin 5′-phosphate has been used as substrate, which at the site of phosphatase activity results in the formation of a fluorescent precipitate. Electron microscopic demonstration of phosphatase is also based, with some modification, on Gomori's original method of metal substitution. A technique using ruthenium red has demonstrated acid phosphatase in electron microscopic studies.

Another procedure used for demonstration of phosphatases is the simultaneously coupling azo dye technique. It uses a naphthol phosphate or other type of ester. The enzymatically released naphthol is coupled in situ with a diazonium salt to form an insoluble colored reaction product. With regard to the original Gomori glycerophosphate technique, it has been shown that the calcium phosphate formed may diffuse and give false localization. Because of this and other considerations in calcified tissues, the azo dye techniques are better suited for the study of phosphatases in teeth and bones. Sophisticated substrates for use with azo dye techniques have been developed. They facilitate precise microscopic localization of alkaline and acid phosphatases as well as esterases. Aminopeptidases can also be detected by an azo dye method.

Immunohistochemistry. Precise localization of specific biologic molecules in different intracellular compartments, on cell surfaces, or in extracellular matrices is made possible by the application of some basic principles of immunochemistry. The immunohistochemical techniques are based on the premise that protein-based antigens or immunogens bind avidly to their specific antibodies. Antibodies to specific antigens can be prepared by injecting the known antigen into an animal to provoke an immune response. This response results in the production of antibody immunoglobins, and these can be isolated from the serum of the injected animal.

When a solution containing an antibody or an antiserum is directly applied to a tissue section containing the antigen, the antibody binds specifically to that antigen. This antigen-antibody complex is subsequently attached to a second antibody, which is conjugated either to a fluorescent dye, such as rhodamine or (FITC) fluorescien isothiocynate or to an enzymeconjugated to its antibody, such as peroxidase-antiperoxidase (PAP). The antigen-antibody complexes bound to a fluorescent dye are examined in a fluorescence microscope. The antigenic sites fluoresce against a dark background and are immediately photographed on high speed film. The enzyme-bound antigen-antibody complexes are further developed histochemically by exposure to an enzyme substrate. This results in the development of a dark brown to a black color, which allows examination of the antigenic sites by light or electron microscopy. Ferritin and colloidal gold are also frequently used as heavy metal markers for the antigen-antibody complexes because of their electron density and also because of their specific particle size.

HISTOCHEMISTRY OF ORAL HARD TISSUES
Carbohydrates and protein

The PAS method is used more than any other in studying the ground substance of teeth and bones. Under specific conditions, this method is believed to demonstrate the carbohydrate moiety as well as the glycoprotein complexes. The ground substance of normal mature bone and dentin exhibits little or no reactivity with the PAS technique (Fig. 15-7). However, developing or resorbing bone and dentin stain intensely with PAS. Newly formed bone and dentin

are also rich in PAS-reactive carbohydrates. In addition to glycogen and glycoproteins, the mineralizing zone of developing bone and dentin matrix is also rich in chondroitin sulfate. Sulfated glycoconjugates accumulate in predentin and are either removed or masked to staining in the dentin.

Interglobular, less-calcified dentin exhibits a distinct PAS reaction (Fig. 15-7) as does abnormally and poorly calcified dentin matrix in dentinogenesis imperfecta and in odontomas.

Enamel matrix is essentially nonreactive with the PAS method. However, enamel lamellae are intensely stained in ground sections (Fig. 15-8). In some areas the rod interprismatic substance exhibits some reactivity. Use of HID-TCH-SP staining, combined with use of testicular hyaluronidase, heparinitase, and chondroitinase ABC, has revealed that sulfated glycoconjugates present in Golgi vesicles of ameloblasts and on the surface layer of developing enamel matrix do not contain heparan sulfate, chondroitin sulfate, and dermatan sulfate, in contradistinction to their presence in the predentin matrix and odontoblasts.

Specific protein methods identify certain amino acids or their groupings, that is, amino, carboxyl, or sulfhydryl. Only a few of these techniques have been applied in the study of teeth and bone. Of interest are the dinitrofluorobenzene (DNFB) and ninhydrin-Schiff methods. The DNFB reagent combines with α-amino groups of proteins in tissue sections to form a pale yellow complex. An intense reddish color is subsequently revealed by a reduction and diazotization technique, which results in the formation of an azo dye. The pattern of staining is essentially the same as seen with the PAS method in both normal and abnormal dentin. A modification of DNFB method wherein the final reaction product is a mer-

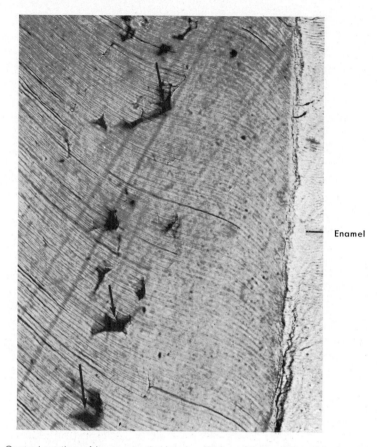

Enamel

Fig. 15-7. Ground section of human tooth showing PAS reactivity of interglobular dentin *(arrows)*. (×143.)

captide of lead or silver has been used for electron microscopic histochemistry of amino groups. The ninhydrin-Schiff method is dependent on the formation of imino groups that decompose to a keto acid to form aldehyde groups, and these are reacted with leucofuchsin (Schiff reagent) to form a final red-colored reaction product. Some of these techniques have been applied to the study of dental caries in bone and in dentin resorption.

Histochemical reactions imply a need for some specific protein groups to initiate the mineralization of predentin and osteoid. Everett and Miller have noted the absence of carboxyl and amino complexes in predentin and osteoid in contradistinction to the presence of these complexes in dentin and bone. Sulfhydryl groups are present optimally at the mineralizing front in predentin and osteoid while being present minimally in the mineralized regions of these tissues.

Immature, newly formed enamel in rats shows histochemical staining for sulfhydryls and tyrosine residues characteristic of keratin. However, these protein residues are not demonstrable in the mature enamel.

In the last few years three major classes

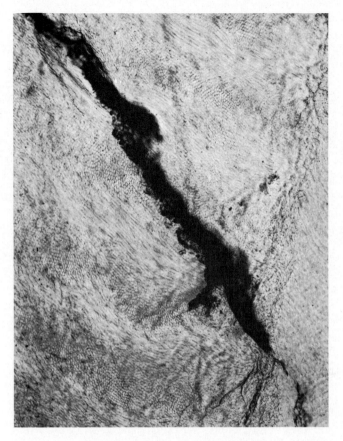

Fig. 15-8. Ground section of human enamel. Lamella stains with PAS method. (×143.)

of calcium-binding proteins have been identified in dentin and developing enamel. Phosphophoryn, a 60-70 kD phosphoprotein, has been identified by immunochemical and immunohistochemical methods in actively synthesizing odontoblasts and in dentin, particularly in the intertubular dentin. It has high affinity for calcium and type I collagen. Because of its chemical properties, phosphophoryn is considered to play a significant role in regulating the ordered deposition of hydroxyapatite crystals within the preformed dentinal matrix.

Amelogenins and enamelins, two major classes of calcium-binding proteins, are now known. This is made possible through the use of chemical and immunohistochemical techniques using monoclonal antibodies. Amelogenins secreted by the ameloblasts are relatively low-molecular-weight proteins and are of predominant proteins in the developing enamel matrix. During enamel maturation they undergo degradation and disappear at a much faster rate than enamelins do. Enamelins have very high affinity for binding apatite crystals and remain until late stages of enamel maturation.

Several immunohistochemical studies mapping distribution of basement membrane components such as type IV collagen, laminin, proteoglycans, and fibronectin during tooth development have shown close association of these proteins with different stages of cell differentiation and matrix secretion (Figs. 15-9 and 15-10). Disappearance of type III collagen and confinement of fibronectin surrounding preodontoblasts to the epitheliomesenchymal junction after the polarization of odontoblasts during tooth development are other interesting observations emphasizing the significance of these proteins in the regulation of the complex developmental changes occurring in the tooth anlage. Significance of such observations is further highlighted in certain disease states. The presence of a bluish-brown opalescence and a diminished pulpal chamber in the teeth of patients with *dentinogenesis imperfecta type II* or in *osteogenesis imperfecta* is associated with the localization of type III collagen in dentin. Type III collagen is absent in normal adult dentin.

Lipids

Biochemical studies indicate a rather low lipid content in the organic matrix of dentin. Lipids have been demonstrated by the sudanophilic reaction in the odontoblast processes and enamel rod sheaths. Sudanophilia is based on the solubility of Sudan dyes with lipids of varied description. Sudanophilia is widespread in the developing tooth, being present in the zone of mineralization and predentin and in the basal zone of the ameloblasts. These reactive zones of the predentin and ameloblasts imply a role of phospholipids in the process of mineralization of dentin and enamel matrices.

Enzyme histochemistry of hard tissue

Histochemical techniques are extremely useful in demonstrating specific enzymes

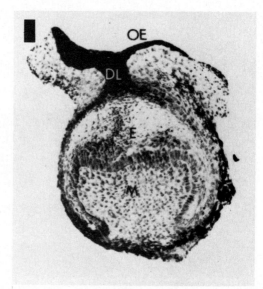

Fig. 15-9. Light micrograph of mandibular first molar of day 16 mouse embryo stained with periodic acid–Schiff *(PAS).* This section corresponds to sections shown in Fig. 5-10. Notice epithelial enamel organ *(E)* surrounds a condensation of dental papilla mesenchyme *(M).* Dental lamina *(DL)* connects tooth germ to oral epithelium *(OE).* (From Thesleff I, Barrach HJ, Foidart JM, et al.: Dev Biol 81:182, 1981.)

in specific cellular and intercellular locations in bone and teeth.

Alkaline phosphatase. Alkaline phosphatase is capable of hydrolyzing phosphoric acid esters. In hard tissues alkaline phosphatase has been implicated in the process of mineralization. However, some studies have raised doubts concerning this assumption and instead suggest that the enzyme is involved in the synthesis of organic matrix only.

Alkaline phosphatase is observed to be associated with osteogenesis and dentinogenesis (Figs. 15-11 and 15-12). The osteoblasts and odontoblasts give an intense staining reaction for the enzyme (Figs. 15-12 and 15-13). No enzyme activity is found in bone or dentin matrices per se, except in

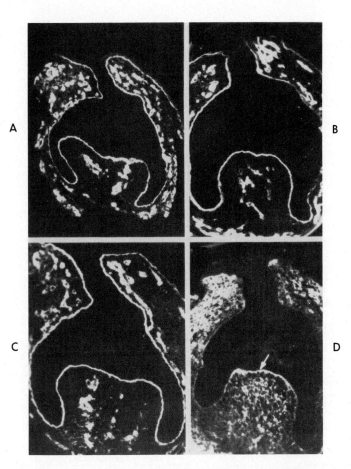

Fig. 15-10. Sections of day 16 embryonic molars stained immunohistochemically with, **A,** antibody to type IV collagen; **B,** antibody to laminin; **C,** antibody to basement membrane proteoglycan; and **D,** with antiserum to fibronectin. (see Fig. 15-9 for reference.) Linear deposits are seen in oral and dental basement membranes and in walls of blood vessels. Distributions of type IV collagen, laminin, and basement membrane proteoglycan appear identical. Immunofluorescence of fibronectin is particularly intense in dental basement membrane *(arrow)* and is prominent in mesenchyme of dental papilla. No stain is observed in enamel organ epithelial cells. (From Thesleff I, Barrach HJ, Foidart JM, et al.: Dev Biol 81:182, 1981.)

close association with the matrix-synthesizing cells. At sites of intramembranous bone development, alkaline phosphatase activity is observed in the endosteum, periosteum, and osteocytes (Table 6). Wergedal and Baylink report no enzyme activity at the actual calcification sites. However, conflicting views are reported about endochondral bone formation where the enzyme is localized in matrices and cells of the hypertrophic and provisional zones of calcification. The view that alkaline phosphatase is involved in actual calcification is also strengthened by observations in vitamin D treatment of human rickets wherein the increase in the calcification zone parallels an

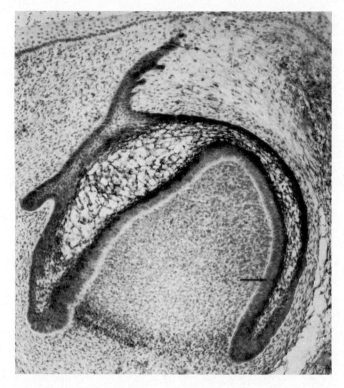

Fig. 15-11. Alkaline phosphatase reaction of tooth of monkey embryo. Ameloblastic layer *(arrow)* is nonreactive. (×87.)

Table 6. Enzyme activity of cells associated with bones and teeth*

	Alkaline phosphatase†	Acid phosphatase†	Amino-peptidase‡	Cytochrome oxidase‡	Succinic dehydrogenase‡
Bone					
Osteoblasts	++	0	+	+	+
Osteocytes	++	0	+	+	+
Osteoclasts	0	++	?	++	++
Cartilage					
Active chondrocyte	++	0	++	++	++
Resting chondrocyte	0	0	+	+	+
Hypertrophic chondro-cyte	++	0	+	+	+
Tooth					
Stellate reticulum	++	0	+	+	+
Stratum intermedium	++	0	+	+	+
Ameloblasts (molar)	0	0	0	0 or +	0
Odontoblasts	+ or ++	0	+	+	+

*0, No staining; +, less active; ++, more active.
†Freeze-dried paraffin-embedded tissues.
‡Fresh-frozen tissues.

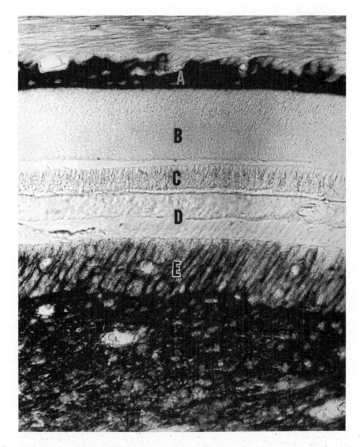

Fig. 15-12. Freeze-dried undecalcified incisor of hamster. *A,* Stratum intermedium; *B,* ameloblasts; *C,* enamel matrix; *D,* dentin matrix; *E,* odontoblasts. Note alkaline phosphatase reactivity of Korff's fibers and subjacent pulp. (×87.)

increase in serum alkaline phosphatase.

In the developing molar and incisor teeth, alkaline phosphatase is present in the stratum intermedium, the odontoblasts (Fig. 15-12) and subjacent Korff's fibers, and the ground substance. No activity is observed in the ameoloblasts (Fig. 15-12). However, in the incisors of rodents enzyme activity is present in the ameloblasts and the reduced enamel organ at the growing end of the tooth (Table 6), with the remaining ameloblasts of the incisor being unreactive, as in the molars. The existence of al-

kaline phosphatase in the dentin proper has been reported.

Adenosine triphosphatase. A Ca^{++}- and Mg^{++}-dependent adenosine triphosphatase (ATPase) has been localized at the distal and lateral cell membranes of the ruffle-ended and late transitional (preabsorptive) ameloblasts. In comparison, early transitional or smooth-ended ameloblasts show ATPase distribution along the basolateral membranes but not in the distal region. Such distribution of this enzyme is significant since it is implied to control the access

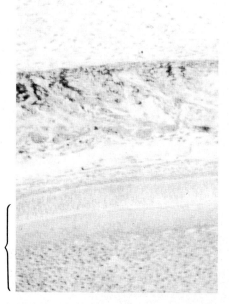

Fig. 15-13. Alkaline phosphatase *(dark areas)* in osteoblasts and acid phosphatase *(dark areas)* reaction in osteoclasts in resorbing bone adjacent to incisor tooth. *(brace)* in 3-day-old hamster. (MX naphthol phosphate and red-violet LB salt incubation for alkaline phosphatase; GR naphthol phosphate and blue BBN salt incubation for acid phosphatase, ×143.) (From Burstone MS: In Sognnaes RF, editor: Calcification in biological systems, Washington, DC, 1960, American Association for the Advancement of Science Publications, p 64.)

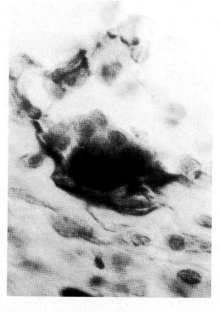

Fig. 15-14. Hamster osteoclast showing cytoplasmic acid phosphatase reaction *(dark)*, with some enzyme activity also present in resorbing bone matrix. (AS-BI naphthol phosphate and red-violet LB salt incubation. Nuclear counterstain is hematoxylin; ×750.) (From Burstone MS: In Sognnaes RF, editor: Calcification in biological systems, Washington, DC, 1960, American Association for the Advancement of Science Publications, p 64.)

of calcium to the enamel mineralizing the front.

Acid phosphatase. Acid phosphatase is less widely distributed than its alkaline counterpart (Table 6). Histochemical localization of intracellular acid phosphatase is generally more discrete than that of alkaline phosphatase because it is localized mainly in specific membrane-bound organelles, the lysosomes.

Osteoclasts in bone and odontoclasts in resorbing dentin exhibit an intense acid phosphatase activity (Figs. 15-13 and 15-14). The enzyme is localized in the part of the cytoplasm that lies apposed to the resorbing surface of bone and dentin (Figs. 15-14 and 15-15). Electron microscopic studies reveal that the enzyme is localized in the lysosomes, although activity is also seen extracellularly between the microvillus-like projections of the ruffled border (Fig. 15-4). Uptake of resorbed mineral, hydrolyzed collagen fibrils, and injected radioactive substances at the site of resorption has been observed.

Several studies imply that acid phosphatase may (in addition to its function in bone and dentin resorption) confer "calcifiability" to the organic matrix by its hydrolytic action on the protein-polysaccharide

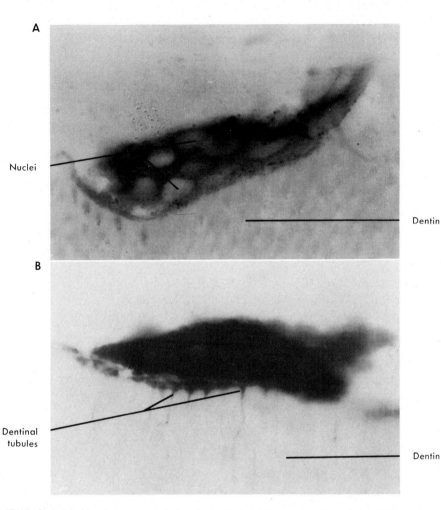

Fig. 15-15. A, Acid phosphatase activity in odontoclasts of mongrel-puppy primary tooth undergoing resorption. Notice reaction product is localized in discrete granules in cytoplasm. No reaction is seen in nuclei. **B,** Acid phosphatase activity in odontoclast and dentinal tubules of mongrel-puppy primary tooth undergoing resorption. (Alpha-naphthyl acid phosphatase and fast garnet GBC salt incubation; ×1060.) (From Freilich LS: A morphological and histological study of the cells associated with physiological root resorption in human and canine primary teeth, doctoral dissertation, Washington, DC, 1972, Georgetown University.)

granules present in the zone of mineralization.

Esterase. According to histochemical definition, esterases hydrolyze simpler fatty acid esters than do lipases, which hydrolyze complex fatty acid esters.

Most histochemical techniques for esterases do not reveal any activity in bone or dentin. However, with use of specific naphthol esters such as naphthol AS-D acetate, an intense staining reaction is observed in the calcifying matrices of bone and dentin. This reactive zone, situated in the tooth between predentin and dentin, is also sudanophilic, indicating the presence of phospholipids.

Considerable esterase activity has also been found in the cells and microorganisms associated with the formation of calculus deposits on teeth.

Aminopeptidase. Aminopeptidases are proteolytic enzymes that hydrolyze certain terminal peptide bonds. Azo dye techniques using L-leucyl-β-naphthylamide or DL-alanyl-β-naphthylamide have been developed for histochemical demonstration of this enzyme. Human osteoclasts give a strong reaction. Although no staining reaction occurs in the osteoclasts of rodents, the enzyme is demonstrated in the stratum intermedium and odontoblasts during dentinogenesis. Some staining reaction is also noticed in the periosteum, perichondrium, and chondrocytes (Table 6). It is significant that aminopeptidase has also been localized in the macrophages and certain sites associated with the breakdown of connective tissues.

Cytochrome oxidase. Cytochrome oxidase is an iron-porphyrin protein that enables cells to utilize molecular oxygen. Its histochemical localization therefore reflects the oxygen requirements of the cells and tissues and the levels of their metabolic and physiologic activity.

The original histochemical reaction, the "nadi" reaction, using α-naphthol and *N,N*-dimethyl-*p*-phenylenediamine, is considered inadequate because of the instability of the substrate solution, lipid solubility, crystallization, and fading of the reaction product—indophenol blue. New techniques using *p*-aminodiphenylamine in conjunction with *p*-methoxy-*p*-aminodiphenylamine or 8-aminotetrahydroquinoline have overcome these technical problems so that the reaction is discretely localized in the mitochondria.

Both osteoclasts and osteoblasts show oxidase activity, with the reaction being more predominant in the former. Stratum intermedium of both molars and incisors also exhibits oxidase activity (Table 6).

Succinate dehydrogenase. Succinate dehydrogenase is closely associated with cytochrome oxidase in the mitochondria. It is one of a series of citric acid cycle enzymes that catalyzes the removal of hydrogen, which in turn is removed by a hydrogen acceptor or carrier. This serves as the basis of the histochemical reaction used in demonstrating this enzyme. The enzyme present in the tissues acts on the substrate (usually sodium succinate), causing the removal of hydrogen, which is picked up by a synthetic acceptor (a tetrazolium compound) present in the incubating medium. The reduced acceptor substance, called formazan, appears as a colored reaction product.

The distribution of succinate dehydrogenase in oral hard tissues is essentially similar to that of cytochrome oxidase. The dehydrogenase activity is higher in osteoclasts than in osteoblasts. The stratum intermedium and the odontoblasts in developing teeth also reveal a positive reaction (Table 6).

Citric acid cycle in osteoblasts and osteoclasts. Besides observations on succinate dehydrogenase, studies on isocitric dehydrogenase, α-ketoglutaric dehydrogenase, and DPN-TPNH-diaphorases have also been reported. It is indicated that osteoclasts maintain a high rate of citrate and lactate production at the expense of glutamate and thereby actively promote decalcification of bone matrix and calcified cartilage.

Summary. A survey of the distribution of various enzymes associated with bone and teeth is given in Table 6. It is interesting to note that although acid phosphatase activity is associated with the osteoclasts only, distribution of other enzymes is widespread in hard oral tissues.

HISTOCHEMISTRY OF ORAL SOFT TISSUES
Polysaccharides, proteins, and mucins

Polysaccharides. The dye carmine is often used to demonstrate glycogen, but it is not as specific as the PAS method. Epithelial glycogen is known to increase during inflammation and repair. Attached human gingiva shows variation in the extent of its keratinization, and this variability is reflected in the glycogen content of the tissue. On the other hand, the nonkeratinized alveolar mucosa virtually always shows constant levels of glycogen. Animal experiments involving benign and malignant epithelial proliferations demonstrate an increase in glycogen.

Proteoglycans with chondroitin sulfate and hyaluronic acid form a major intercellular component of human gingival epithelium. The molecular conformation and relatively rapid rate of synthesis and secretion of these macromolecules in the gingiva may explain the lack of susceptibility of this material to the degradative action of specific enzymes. When oral soft tissues are stained with the metachromatic dye toluidine blue, mast cells become visible in varying numbers in the loose connective tissue, particularly along the blood vessels. The metachromatic reaction given by the cytoplasmic granules of these cells is caused by the presence of heparin—a sulfated proteoglycan. The cytoplasmic granules also contain histamine—a vasodilator that can be demonstrated by fluorescence microscopy. Mast cells are present in particularly large numbers in the tongue and in the gingiva. The lack of these cells in acute necrotizing gingivitis is significant.

Proteins and protein groups. Keratinization is one of the important characteristics of the epidermis. Although under normal circumstances it occurs only in some areas of the oral epithelium, in pathologic conditions it occurs anywhere in the mouth. The mechanism by which the cells of the malpighian layer are altered to form keratin has been only partly elucidated. The disulfide bridges present in keratin are believed to result from the oxidation of sulfhydryl groups of cysteine. Sulfhydryl groups are demonstrated histochemically by the ferric ferricyanide method in which this compound is reduced to a Prussian blue color by these protein groups. Thus the extent of the blue reaction product reflects the degree of keratinization. Attempts to demonstrate sulfhydryl groups in electron microscopy have not been completely successful. However, electron microscopic demonstration of disulfide groups, using alkaline methenamine silver, has been made.

Mucins. Salivary mucins form semiviscous protective coatings over oral mucous membranes. They are composed of high-molecular-weight carbohydrate-protein complexes. Two types of mucins are recognized by the predominant carbohydrate component in their molecules—fucomucins, rich in L-fucose, and sialomucin, rich in sialic acid. The latter is believed to confer acidity on certain types of mucins. Both of these mucins are present together in saliva, with one predominating over the other.

Histochemical techniques have been very useful in our understanding of the salivary mucins present in various salivary glands and their chemical composition. The dyes mucicarmine and mucihematen are frequently used for nonspecific staining of mucins. PAS technique is used to identify neutral mucins (Fig. 15-16). Alcian blue, toluidine blue, colloidal iron, and aldehyde fuchsin methods are used to localize the acid mucins. These techniques re-

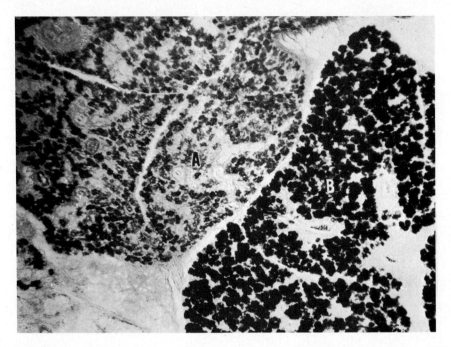

Fig. 15-16. Freeze-dried mouse submandibular gland, *A*, and sublingual gland, *B*, showing PAS reactivity of mucins. (×140.)

veal species differences in the mucins of different salivary glands.

Enzyme histochemistry

Alkaline phosphatase. Alkaline phosphatase activity in human gingiva is specifically demonstrable in the capillary endothelium of the lamina propria (Fig. 15-17). The reaction product, observed in the gingival epithelium and in the collagen fibers, seems to be a diffusion artifact.

Oral epithelium of the rat exhibits an increased alkaline phosphatase activity during the estrous cycle, correlated to phosphatase changes in the vaginal epithelium. Alkaline phosphatase is implicated in the mechanism of keratinization, although its precise role in this process is still uncertain.

The basement membranes associated with salivary gland acini exhibit high alkaline phosphatase activity. Similar activity in taste buds of several species of animals has also been reported.

Acid phosphatase. Acid phosphatase activity in human gingiva seems related to the degree of keratinization, being very high in the zone of keratinization and low in nonkeratinized regions. This pattern corresponds with that observed in the skin epidermis. Cells of the functional epithelium in the gingival sulcus have been reported by Lange and Schroeder to be rich in lysosomal enzymes in the normal healthy tissue.

Esterase. Little information is available on the esterase activity of human gingiva. Superficial layers, including the keratinizing zone, show the presence of some esterase activity.

High esterase activity is demonstrable in

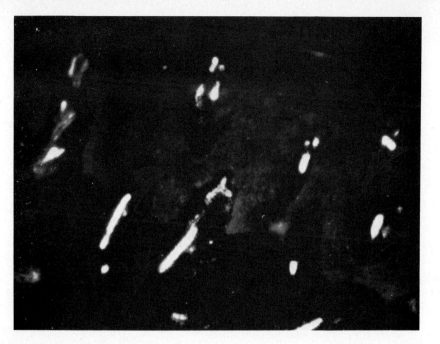

Fig. 15-17. Alkaline phosphatase activity of capillaries of lamina propria of human gingiva revealed by ultraviolet fluorescence. (×80.)

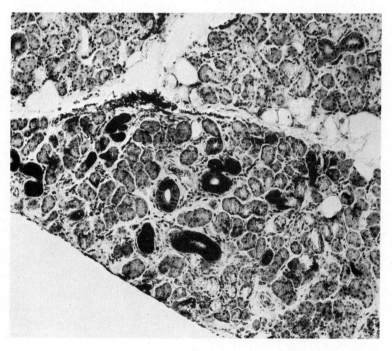

Fig. 15-18. Esterase activity of ducts of freeze-dried human parotid gland. (Nuclear counterstain; ×110.)

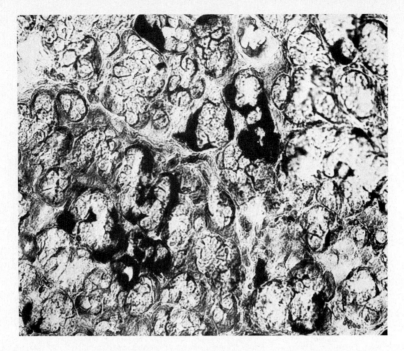

Fig. 15-19. Esterase activity of demilune cells of freeze-dried human sublingual gland. (×210.)

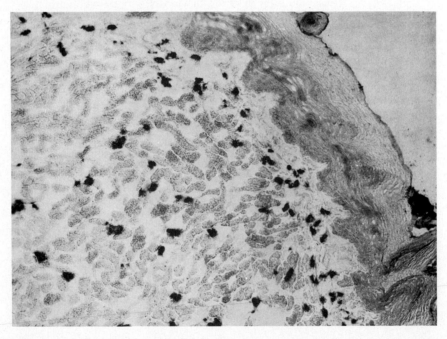

Fig. 15-20. Mast cells of rat tongue incubated with substrate solution containing naphthol AS-D chloroacetate. (×250.)

the salivary gland ducts and also in the serous demilunes of the sublingual gland (Figs. 15-18 and 15-19). Similar activity is observed in the taste buds of several animal species, and this has been implicated in gustatory discrimination. Mast cells in oral tissues also have esterase activity (Fig. 15-20).

Aminopeptidase. The activity of this enzyme in human gingiva is low and is localized primarily in the basal cell layers of the epithelium and in the underlying connective tissue. An increase in aminopeptidase activity during inflammation and in hyperplasia caused by the drug phenytoin has been reported.

Aminopeptidase is also observed in the salivary gland ducts.

β-Glucuronidase. β-Glucuronidases hydrolyze the β-glycoside linkage of glucuronides, are involved in conjugation of steroid hormones and in hydrolysis of conjugated glucuronides, and play a role in cell proliferation. The enzyme has been localized in the basal cell layers of the oral epithelium in humans and rats.

Cytochrome oxidase. Histochemical techniques demonstrate low levels of cytochrome oxidase activity in human gingiva. Specifically, this cytochrome oxidase activity is localized in the basal layers of the free and attached gingiva, crevicular epithelium, and epithelial attachment (Fig. 15-21). In chronic gingivitis a striking increase in cytochrome oxidase activity is observed in the epithelium from the free gingival groove through to the epithelial attachment. In chronic gingivitis the underlying connective tissue also shows a variable increase in oxidase activity.

Cytochrome oxidase activity is also demonstrated in the salivary glands, especially in the duct system (Fig. 15-22).

Succinate dehydrogenase and glucose 6-phosphate dehydrogenase. The distribution

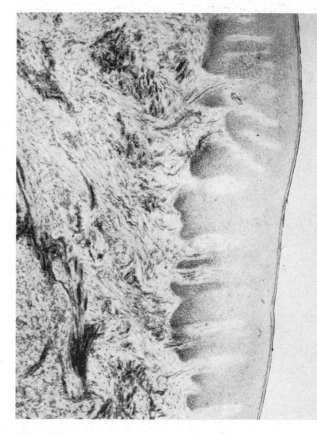

Fig. 15-21. Human attached gingiva showing cytochrome oxidase activity of basal cell layer and in connective tissue of lamina propria.

pattern of succinate dehydrogenase is similar to that of cytochrome oxidase. This dehydrogenase is observed primarily in the basal cell layers of the gingival epithelium and in the ducts of the salivary glands. Glucose 6-phosphate dehydrogenase is present in significant quantities in the human oral mucosal epithelium. The levels of this enzyme become highly elevated in malignant dysplastic lesions of the oral mucosa. Elevation of this enzyme is considered to assist in the diagnosis of oral cancers.

Angiogenic factor in inflamed gingiva. A novel human angiogenic factor, 67kD pro-

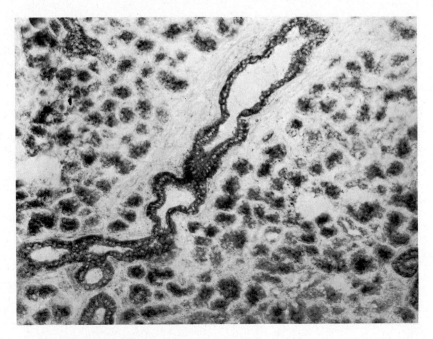

Fig. 15-22. Cytochrome oxidase activity of human parotid gland. (×143.)

tein, obtained from a melanoma cell line has been identified immunohistochemicaly in inflamed gingival tissue (using a monoclonal antibody to this protein). Specifically, the factor was localized in the macrophages. Such activity was absent in healthy gingival tissue. Similar activity has also been found in the macrophages of inflamed tissue of rheumatoid origin.

CLINICAL CONSIDERATIONS

Histochemical techniques are not only an important tool in dental research but are also frequently used in histopathologic diagnosis. Although the tissue biopsy materials are usually stained with hematoxylin and eosin, there are numerous occasions when this type of staining technique does not permit a definitive diagnosis. In a differential diagnosis of an epithelial tumor in or around the oral cavity a histochemical stain for mucin may assist the oral patholo-

gist in distinguishing a tumor of salivary gland origin from an odontogenic tumor or a tumor arising from nonglandular epithelium. Because these tumors often require different types of treatment, this distinction is of great practical importance.

A variety of fungi that infect humans contain mucopolysaccharides. The hyphae and spores of these fungi are present in the infected tissues, and their correct diagnosis can often be made only after special histochemical stains for mucin have been done. In the human oral cavity diagnosis of histoplasmosis, actino mycosis, blastomycosis, and coccidioidomycosis can often be made only after special histochemical stains.

Histochemical stains that reveal lipids are of value in correctly diagnosing tumors that arise from the fat cells (lipoma and liposarcoma). They are also an important aid in establishing the identity of vesicles that may appear in tumor cells of various benign and malignant lesions. Since cytoplasmic vesicles may represent lipid, mucin, glycogen, or intracellular edema, their true identity is sometimes important for correct diagnosis and therapy.

REFERENCES

Albert EN and Fleischer E: A new electron dense stain for elastic tissue, J Histochem Cytochem 18:697, 1970.

Argyris TS: Glycogen in the epidermis of mice painted with methylchol-anthrene, J Natl Cancer Inst 12:1159, 1952.

Baer PN and Burstone MS: Esterase activity associated with formation of deposits on teeth, Oral Surg 12:1147, 1959.

Balough K: Decalcification with versene for histochemical study of oxidative enzyme systems, J Histochem Cytochem 10:232, 1962.

Balough K: Histochemical study of oxidative enzyme systems in teeth and peridental tissues, J Dent Res 42:1457, 1963.

Baradi AF and Bourne GH: Gustatory and olfactory epithelia. In Bourne GH and Danielli JF, editors: International review of cytology, vol 2, New York, 1953, Academic Press, Inc.

Baradi AF and Bourne GH: Histochemical localization of cholinesterase in gustatory epithelia, J Histochem Cytochem 7:2, 1959.

Baradi AF and Bourne GH: New observations on alkaline glycophosphatase reaction in the papilla foliata, J Biophys Biochem Cytol 5:173, 1959.

Bernhard W and Avrameas S: Ultrastructural visualization of cellular carbohydrate components by means of concanavalin A, Exp Cell Res 64:232, 1971.

Birkedal-Hansen H: Effect of fixation on detection of carbohydrates in demineralized paraffin sections of rat jaw, Scand J Dent Res 82:99, 1974.

Bourne GH, editor: The biochemistry and physiology of bone, New York, 1956, Academic Press, Inc.

Boyde A and Reith EJ: Electron probe analysis of maturation ameloblasts of the rat incisor and calf molar, Histochemistry 55:41, 1978.

Bradfield JRG: Glycogen of the vertebrate epidermis, Nature 167:40, 1951.

Burstone MS: A cytologic study of salivary glands of the mouse tongue, J Dent Res 32:126, 1953.

Burstone MS: The ground substance of abnormal dentin, secondary dentin, and pulp calcification, J Dent Res 32:269, 1953.

Burstone MS: Esterase of the salivary glands, J Histochem Cytochem 4:130, 1956.

Burstone MS: Histochemical observations on enzymatic processes in bones and teeth, Ann NY Acad Sci 85:431, 1960.

Burstone MS: Histochemical study of cytochrome oxidase in normal and inflamed gingiva, Oral Surg 13:1501, 1960.

Burstone MS: Hydrolytic enzymes in dentinogenesis and osteogenesis. In Sognnaes RF, editor: Calcification in biological systems, Washington, DC, 1960, American Association for the Advancement of Science.

Burstone MS: Postcoupling, noncoupling and fluorescence techniques for the demonstration of alkaline phosphatase, J Natl Cancer Inst 24:1199, 1960.

Burstone MS: Enzyme histochemistry and its application in the study of neoplasms, New York, 1962, Academic Press, Inc.

Burstone MS: Enzyme histochemistry and cytochemistry. In Bourne GH, editor: Cytology and cell physiology, New York, 1964, Academic Press, Inc.

Burstone MS and Folk JE: Histochemical demonstration of aminopeptidase, J Histochem Cytochem 4:217, 1956.

Cabrini RL and Carranza FA: Histochemical distribution of acid phosphatase in human gingiva, J Periodontol, 29:34, 1958.

Cabrini RL and Carranza FA: Histochemical localization of β-glucuronidase in stratified squamous epithelium, Naturwissenschaften 22:553, 1958.

Cabrini RL and Carranza FA: Histochemical distribution of beta-glucuronidase in gingival tissues, Arch Oral Biol 2:28, 1960.

Carranza F and Cabrini RL: Mast cells in human gingiva, Oral Surg 8:1093, 1955.

Chayen J and Bitensky L: Lysosomal enzymes and inflammation with particular references to rheumatoid diseases, Ann Rheum Dis 30:522, 1971.

Chayen J, Bitensky L, and Butcher RG: Practical histochemistry, New York, 1973, John Wiley & Sons.

Cotelli DC and Livingston DC: Fluorescent reagent for the periodic acid–Schiff and Feulgen reactions for cytochemical studies, J Histochem Cytochem 24:956, 1976.

Davis LG, Dibner MD, and Battey JF: Basic methods in molecular biology, New York, 1986, Elsevier Science Publishing Co.

Eichel B: Oxidative enzymes of gingiva, Ann NY Acad Sci 85:479, 1960.

Essner E, Schrieber J, and Griewski RA: Localization of carbohydrate components in rat colon with fluoresceinated lectins, J Histochem Cytochem Cytochem 26:452, 1978.

Etzler ME and Branstrator ML: Differential localization of cell surface and secretory components in rat intestinal epithelium by use of lectins, J Cell Biol 62:329, 1974.

Evans AW, Johnson NW, and Butcher RG: A quantitative histochemical study of glucose-6-phosphate dehydrogenase activity in premalignant and malignant lesions of human oral mucosa, Histochem J 15:483, 1983.

Eveland WC: Fluorescent antibody technique in medical diagnosis, Curr Med Dig 31:351, 1964.

Everett MM and Miller WA: Histochemical studies on calcified tissues. I. Amino acid histochemistry of fetal calf and human enamel matrix, Calcif Tissue Res 14:229, 1972.

Everett MM and Miller WA: Histochemical studies on calcified tissues. II. Amino acid histochemistry of developing dentin and bone, Calcif Tissue Res 16:73, 1974.

Felton JH, Person P, and Stahl SS: Biochemical and histochemical studies of aerobic oxidative metabolism of oral tissues. II. Enzymatic dissection of gingival and tongue epithelia from connective tissues, J Dent Res 44:392, 1965.

Fisher ER: Tissue mast cells, JAMA 173:171, 1960.

Freilich LS: Ultrastructure and acid phosphatase cytochemistry of odontoclasts: effects of parathyroid extract, J Dent Res 50:1047, 1971.

Fruhbeis B, Zwadlo G, Berocker EB, et al: Immunolocalization of an angiogenic factor (HAF) in normal, inflammatory and tumor tissues, Int J Cancer 42:207, 1988.

Gersh I and Gatchpole J: The organization of ground substance and basement membrane and its significance in tissue injury, disease, and growth, Am J Anat 85:457, 1949.

Gerson S: Activity of glucose-6-phosphate dehydrogenase and acid phosphatase in nonkeratinized and keratinized oral epithelia and epidermis in rabbit, J Periodont Res 8:151, 1973.

Goldberg M and Septier D: Electron microscopic visualization of proteoglycans in rat incisor predentin and dentin with cuprolinic blue, Arch Oral Biol 28:79, 1983.

Goldman HM, Ruben MP, and Sherman D: The application of laser spectroscopy for the qualitative and quantitative analysis of the inorganic components of calcified tissues, Oral Surg 17:102, 1964.

Gray JA and Opdyke DL: A device for thin sectioning of hard tissues, J Dent Res 41:172, 1962.

Green SJ, Tarone G, and Underhill CB: Distribution of hyaluronate receptors in the adult lung, J Cell Sci 89:145, 1988.

Gregg JM: Analysis of tooth eruption and alveolar bone growth utilizing tetracycline fluorescence, J Dent Res 43 (suppl):887, 1964.

Greep RO, Fischer CJ, and Morse A: Alkaline phosphatase in odontogenesis and osteogenesis and its histochemical demonstration after demineralization, J Am Dent Assoc 36:427, 1948.

Gros D, Obrenovitch A, Challice CE, et al.: Ultrastructural visualization of cellular carbohydrate components by means of lectins on ultrathin glycol methacrylate sections, J Histochem Cytochem 25:104, 1977.

Gustafson G: The histopathology of caries of human dental enamel, Acta Odontol Scand 15:13, 1957.

Hancox NM and Boothroyd B: Structure-function relationship in the osteoclast. In Sognnaes RF, editor: Mechanism of hard tissue destruction, Washington, DC, 1963, American Association for the Advancement of Science.

Herold RC, Boyde A, Rosenbloom J, et al.: Monoclonal antibody and immunogold cytochemical localization of amelogenins in bovine secretory amelogenesis, Arch Oral Biol 32:439, 1987.

Hess WC, Lee CY, and Peckham SC: The lipid content of enamel and dentin, J Dent Res 35:273, 1956.

Hewitt AT, Klienman HK, Pennypacker JP, et al.: Identification of an attachment factor for chondrocytes, Proc Natl Acad Sci USA 77:385, 1980.

Hoerman KC and Mancewicz SA: Phosphorescence of calcified tissues, J Dent Res 43(suppl):775, 1964.

Holliday TD: Diagnostic exfoliative cytology, its value as an everyday hospital investigation, Lancet 1:488, 1963.

Kapur SP and Russell TE: Sharpey fiber bone development in surgically implanted dog mandible: a scanning electron microscopic study, Acta Anat (Basel) 102:260, 1978.

Kleinman HK: Role of cell attachment proteins in defining cell matrix interactions. In Liotta LA and Hart IR, editors: Tumor invasion and metatasis, Boston, 1982, Martinus Nijhoff Publishers.

Kogaya Y and Furuhashi K: Sulfated glycoconjugates in rat incisor secretory ameloblasts and developing enamel matrix, Calcif Tissue Int 43:307, 1988.

Lange DE and Schroeder HE: Structural localization of lysosomal enzymes in gingival sulcus cells, J Dent Res 51:272, 1972.

Larmas LA, Makinen KK, and Paunio KU: A histochemical study of arylaminopeptidases in hydantoin induced hyperplastic, healthy and inflamed human gingiva, J Periodont Res 8:21, 1973.

Lau EC, Bessem CC, Slavkin HC, et al: Amelogenin antigenic domain defined by clonal epitope selection, Calcif Tissue Int 40:231, 1987.

Laurie GW, Leblond CP, and Martin GR: Light microscopic immunolocalization of type IV collagen, laminin, heparan sulfate proteoglycan, and fibronectin in the basement membrane of a variety of rat organs, Am J Anat 167:71, 1983.

Lesot H, Osman M, and Ruch JV: Immunofluorescent localization of collagens, fibronectin, and laminin during terminal differentiation of odontoblasts, Dev Biol 82:371, 1981.

Lev R and Spicer SS: Specific staining of sulphate groups with alcian blue at low pH, J Histochem Cytochem 12:39, 1964.

Linde A, Johansson S, Jonsson R, et al.: Localization of fibronectin during dentinogenesis in rat incisor, Arch Oral Biol 27:1069, 1982.

Luft JH: Ruthenium red and violet. I. Chemistry, purification, methods of use for electron microscopy and mechanism of action, Anat Rec 171:347, 1971.

Matsuzawa T and Anderson HC: Phosphatases of epiphyseal cartilage studied by electron microscopic cytochemical methods, J Histochem Cytochem 19:801, 1971.

Matukas VJ and Krikos GA: Evidence for changes in protein-polysaccharide association with the onset of calcification in cartilage, J Cell Biol 39:43, 1968.

Millard HD: Oral exfoliative cytology as an aid to diagnosis, J Am Dent Assoc 69:547, 1964.

Mörnstad H and Sundström B: Cytochemical demonstration of adenyl cyclase in rat incisor enamel organ, Scand J Dent Res 82:146, 1974.

Munhoz CO, Cassio OG, and Leblond CP: Deposition of calcium phosphate into dentin and enamel as shown by radioautography of sections of incisor teeth following injection of ^{45}Ca into rats, Calcif Tissue Res 14:221, 1974.

Nakama T, Nakamura O, Daikuhara Y, et al.: A monoclonal antibody against dentin phosphophoryn recognizes a bone protein(s) appearing at the beginning of ossification, Calcif Tissue Int 43:263, 1988.

Nanci A, Bendayan M, and Slavkin HC: Enamel protein biosynthesis and secretion in mouse incisor secretory ameloblasts as revealed by high resolution immunocytochemistry, J Histochem Cytochem 33:1153, 1985.

Narayanan AS and Page RC: Connective tissue of the periodontium: a summary of current work, Coll Relat Res 3:33, 1983.

Neiders ME, Eick JD, Miller WA, et al.: Electron probe microanalysis of cementum and underlying dentin in young permanent tooth, J Dent Res 51:122, 1972.

Nicolson GL and Singer SJ: Ferritin conjugated plant agglutinins as specific saccharide stains for electron microscopy: application to saccharides bound to cell membranes, Proc Natl Acad Sci USA 68:942, 1971.

Ogata Y, Shimokawa H, and Sasaki S: Purification,

characterization and biosynthesis of bovine enamelins, Calcif Tissue Int 43:389, 1988.

Opdyke DL: The histochemistry of dental decay, Arch Oral Biol 7:207, 1962.

Pearse AGE: Histochemistry, theoretical and applied, vol 2, Baltimore, 1972, The Williams & Wilkins Co.

Perry MM: Identification of glycogen in thin sections of amphibian embryos, J Cell Sci 2:257, 1967.

Person P and Burnett GW: Dynamic equilibria of oral tissues. II. Cytochrome oxidase and succinoxidase activity of oral tissues, J Periodontol 26:99, 1955.

Philips FR: A short manual of respiratory cytology: a guide to the identification of carcinoma cells in the sputum, Springfield, Ill, 1964, Charles C Thomas, Publisher.

Phillips HB, Owen-Jones S, and Chandler B: Quantitative histology of bone: a computerized method for measuring the total mineral content of bone, Calcif Tissue Res 26:85, 1978.

Piez KA and Reddi AH, editors: Extracellular matrix biochemistry, New York, 1984, Elsevier Science Publishers.

Polak JM and Noorden S, editors: Immunocytochemistry: practical applications in pathology and biology, Boston, 1983, PSG/Wright Publishing Co., Inc.

Porter KR and Pappas GD: Collagen formation by fibroblasts of the chick embryo dermis, J Biophys Biochem Cytol 5:153, 1959.

Rabinowitz JL, Ruthberg M, Cohen DW, et al.: Human gingival lipids, J Periodont Res 8:381, 1973.

Rahima M, Tsay TG, Andujar M, et al.: Localization of phosphophoryn in rat incisor dentin using immunocytochemical techniques, J Histochem Cytochem 36:153, 1988.

Rasmussen H and Bordier P: They physiological and cellular basis of metabolic bone disease, Baltimore, 1974, The Williams & Wilkins Co.

Reith EJ and Boyde A: Histochemistry and electron probe analysis of secretory ameloblasts of developing molar teeth, Histochemistry 55:17, 1978.

Rovalstad GH and Calandra JC: Enzyme studies of salivary corpuscles, Dent Progr 2:21, 1961.

Russell TE and Kapur SP: Bone surfaces adjacent to a sub-periosteal implant: an SEM study, Oral Implant 7:415, 1977.

Salama AH, Zaki AE, and Eisenmann DR: Cytochemical localization of Ca2(-Mg2) adenosine triphosphatase in rat incisor ameloblasts during enamel secretion and maturation, J Histochem Cytochem 35:471, 1987.

Sandritter W and Schreiber M: Histochemie von Sputumzellen. I. Qualitative histochemische Untersuchungen, Frankfurt, Z Pathol 68:693, 1958.

Saulk JJ, Gay R, Miller EJ, et al.: Immunohistochemical localization of type III collagen in the dentin of patients with osteogenesis imperfecta and hereditary opalescent dentin, J Oral Pathol 2:210, 1980.

Schajowicz F and Cabrini RL: Histochemical studies on glycogen in normal ossification and calcification, J Bone Joint Surg 40:1081, 1958.

Shackleford JM and Klapper CE: Structure and carbohydrate histochemistry of mammalian salivary glands, Am J Anat 111:825, 1962.

Shimizu M, Glimcher MJ, Travis D, et al.: Mouse bone collagenase: isolation, partial purification, and mechanism of action, Proc Soc Exp Biol Med 130:1175, 1969.

Sognnaes RF: Mechanism of hard tissue destruction, Washington, DC, 1963, The American Association for the Advancement of Science.

Soyenkoff R, Friedman BK, and Newton M: The lipids of dental tissues: a preliminary study, J Dent Res 30:599, 1951.

Spicer SS: A correlative study of the histochemical properties of rodent acid mucopolysaccharides, J Histochem Cytochem 8:18, 1960.

Spicer SS: Histochemical differentiation of mammalian mucopolysaccharides, Ann NY Acad Sci 106:379, 1963.

Spicer SS and Warren L: The histochemistry of sialic acid containing mucoproteins, J Histochem Cytochem 8:135, 1960.

Steinman RR, Hewes CG, and Woods RW: Histochemical analysis of lesions in incipient dental caries, J Dent Res 38:592, 1959.

Stetlar-Stevenson WG and Weis A: Bovine dentin phosphophoryn: calcium ion binding properties of a high molecular weight preparation, Calcif Tissue Int 40:97, 1987.

Stoward PJ: Fixation in histochemistry, London, 1973, Chapman & Hall Ltd.

Stuart J and Simpson JS: Dehydrogenase enzyme cytochemistry of unfixed leucocytes, J Clin Pathol 23:517, 1970.

Swedlow DB, Harper RA, and Katz JL: Evolution of a new preparative technique for bone examination in the SEM. Scanning electon microscopy (part II). Proceedings of the Workshop on Biological Specimen Preparation for SEM, Chicago, 1972, IIT Research Institute.

Symons NBB: Alkaline phosphatase activity in the developing tooth of the rat, J Anat 89:238, 1955.

Symons NBB: Lipid distribution in the developing teeth of the rat, Br Dent J 105:27, 1958.

Takagi M, Parmley TR, and Denys FR: Ultrastructural localization of complex carbohydrates in odontoblasts, predentin and dentin, J Histochem Cytochem 29:747, 1981.

Takagi M, Parmley TR, Spicer SS, et al.: Ultrastructural localization of acid glycoconjugates with the low iron diamine method, J Histochem 30:471, 1982.

Terranova VP, Liotta LA, Russo RG, et al.: Role of laminin in the attachment and metastasis of murine tumor cells, Cancer Res 42:2265, 1982.

Thesleff I, Barrach HJ, Foidart JM, et al.: Changes in the distribution of type IV collagen laminin, proteoglycan, and fibronectin during mouse tooth development, Dev Biol 81:182, 1981.

Turesky S, Crowly J, and Glickman I: A histochemical study of protein-bound sulfhydryl and disulfide groups in normal and inflamed human gingiva, J Dent Res 36:255, 1957.

Turesky S, Glickman I, and Litwin T: A histochemical evaluation of normal and inflamed human gingiva, J Dent Res 30:792, 1951.

Valentino K, Eberwine JH, and Barchas JD, editors: In situ hybridization—applications in neurobiology, New York, 1987, Oxford University Press.

Van Scott EJ and Flesh P: Sulfhydryl groups and disulfide linkages in normal and pathological keratinization, Arch Derm Syph 70:141, 1954.

Veterans Administration Cooperative Study: Oral exfoliative cytology, Washington, DC, 1962, US Government Printing Office.

Walker DG: Citric acid cycle in osteoblasts and osteoclasts, Bull Johns Hopkins Hosp 108:80, 1961.

Weinmann JP, Meyer J, and Mardfin D: Occurrence and role of glycogen in the epithelium of the alveolar mucosa and of the attached gingiva, Am J Anat 104:381, 1959.

Weinstock M and Leblond CP: Synthesis, migration, and release of precursor collagen by odontoblasts as visualized by radioautography after [3H] proline administration, J Cell Biol 60:92, 1974.

Weinstock A, Weinstock M, and Leblond CP: Autoradiographic detection of 3H-glucose incorporation into glycoprotein by odontoblasts and its deposition at the site of the calcification front in dentin, Calcif Tissue Res 8:181, 1972.

Wergedal JE and Baylink DJ: Distribution of acid and alkaline phosphatase activity in undemineralized sections of the rat tibial diaphysis, J Histochem Cytochem 17:799, 1969.

Wiebkin OW and Thonard JC: Mucopolysaccharide localization in gingival epithelium. I. An autoradiographic demonstration, J Periodont Res 16:600, 1981.

Wiebkin OW and Thonard JC: Mucopolysaccharide localization in gingival epithelium: factors affecting biosynthesis of sulfated proteoglycans in organ cultures of gingival epithelium, J Periodont Res 17:629, 1982.

Wied GL, editor: Introduction to quantitative cytochemistry, New York, 1965, Academic Press, Inc.

Wisotzky J: Effects of neo-tetrazolium chloride on the phosphorescence of teeth, J Dent Res 43:659, 1964.

Wisotzky J: Effect of tetracycline on the phosphorescence of teeth, J Dent Res 51:7, 1972.

Yamada K and Shimizu S: The histochemistry of galactose residues of complex carbohydrates as studied by peroxidase labelled *Ricinus communis* agglutinin, Histochemistry 53:143, 1977.

Yoshiki S and Kurahashi Y: A light and electron microscopic study of alkaline phosphatase activity in the early stage of dentinogenesis in the young rat, Arch Oral Biol 16:1143, 1971.

Zander HAL: Distribution of phosphatase in gingival tissue, J Dent Res 20:347, 1941.

APPENDIX
PREPARATION OF SPECIMENS FOR HISTOLOGIC STUDY

PREPARATION OF SECTIONS OF PARAFFIN-EMBEDDED SPECIMENS
Obtaining the specimen
Fixation of the specimen
Dehydration of the specimen
Infiltration of the specimen with paraffin
Embedding the specimen
Cutting the sections of the specimen
Mounting the cut sections on slides
Staining the sections

PREPARATION OF SECTIONS OF PARLODION-EMBEDDED SPECIMENS
Obtaining the specimen

Fixation of the specimen
Decalcification of the specimen
Washing the specimen
Dehydration of the specimen
Infiltration of the specimen with parlodion
Embedding the specimen in parlodion
Cutting the sections of the specimen
Staining the sections

PREPARATION OF GROUND SECTIONS OF TEETH OR BONE

PREPARATION OF FROZEN SECTIONS

TYPES OF MICROSCOPY

The morphologic study of oral tissues involves the preparation of tissue sections for microscopic examination. Knowledge of various types of microscopes and related histologic techniques will assist the student in interpretation of the structure and function of oral tissues.

The fundamental methods of tissue preparation for various types of microscopy, although basically similar to those for light microscopy, show differences in specific procedures. For example, differences in the tissue preparation for electron microscopy are necessitated by the lower penetrating power of electrons compared with the light and the greater resolving power of the electron microscope. Tissues for light microscopic study must be sufficiently thin to transmit light, and its components must have sufficient contrast for the parts to be distinguishable from each other. Routine

histologic techniques involve the fixation of tissues in protoplasmic coagulating solution, dehydration in organic solvents, embedding in paraffin or plastics, and cutting of thin sections on a microtome. The sections are mounted on an appropriate supporting structure, stained, and examined under a microscope. The basic procedures are modified depending on the nature of the specimen and the type of microscope to be used for examination of structures of particular interest.

Four methods of preparation of oral tissues for microscopic examination are commonly used:

1. *Specimens may be embedded in paraffin and sectioned.* The most commonly used method of preparing soft tissues for study with an ordinary light microscope is that of embedding the specimen in paraffin and then cutting

sections 4 to 10 μm thick. The sections are mounted on microscope slides, passed through a selected series of stains, and covered with a cover glass.

2. *Specimens may be embedded in parlodion and sectioned.* Specimens containing boneor teeth require different preparation. Such specimens must be decalcified (the mineral substance removed) and usually embedded in parlodion rather than in paraffin before being sectioned on a microtome.

3. *Specimens of calcified tissue may be ground into thin sections.* Sections of undecalcified tooth or bone may be obtained by preparing a *ground section.* This is done by slicing the undecalcified specimen, which is ground down to a section of about 50 μm on a revolving stone or disk.

4. *Specimens of soft tissue may be frozen and sectioned.* When it is important that pathologic tissue specimens be examined immediately, or if the reagents used for paraffin or parlodion embedding would destroy the tissue characteristics that are to be studied, the fresh, unfixed, or fixed soft tissue may be frozen and sectioned without being embedded. Such tissue sections are usually referred to as *frozen sections.*

These four methods of specimen preparation are described in more detail.

PREPARATION OF SECTIONS OF PARAFFIN-EMBEDDED SPECIMENS

The method of preparing a specimen for sectioning by embedding it in paraffin is suitable for oral specimens such as specimens of gingiva, cheek, and tongue that contain no calcified tissue.

Obtaining the specimen. Specimens taken from humans or experimental animals must be removed carefully, without crushing, either while the animal is alive or immediately after it has been killed.

Fixation of the specimen. Immediately after removal of the specimen it must be placed in a *fixing solution.* Specimens that have not been placed in such a solution are seldom any good. There are many good fixing solutions available. Sometimes the kinds of stains subsequently to be used determine the kind of solution to be chosen. One of the most commonly used fixatives for dental tissues is 10% neutral formalin.

The purposes of fixation are to coagulate the protein, thus reducing alteration by subsequent treatment, and to make the tissues more readily permeable to the subsequent applications of reagents. The fixation period varies from several hours to several days, depending on the size and density of the specimens and on the type of fixing solution used.

After fixation in formalin, the specimen is washed overnight in running water.

Dehydration of the specimen. Since it is necessary that the specimen be completely infiltrated with the paraffin in which it is to be embedded, it must first be infiltrated with some substance that is miscible with paraffin. Paraffin and water do not mix. Therefore after being washed in running water to remove the formalin, the specimen is gradually dehydrated by being passed through a series of increasing percentages of alcohol (40%, 60%, 80%, 95%, and absolute alcohol), remaining in each dish for several hours. (The time required for each step of the process depends on the size and density of the specimen.) To ensure that the water is replaced by alcohol, two or three changes of absolute alcohol are used. Then, since paraffin and alcohol are not miscible, the specimen is passed from alcohol through two changes of xylene, which is miscible with both alcohol and paraffin.

Infiltration of the specimen with paraffin. When xylene has completely replaced the alcohol in the tissue, the specimen is ready to be infiltrated with paraffin. It is removed from the xylene and placed in a dish of melted embedding paraffin, and the dish is put into a constant-temperature oven regulated to about 60° C. (The exact temperature depends on the melting point of the paraffin used.) During the course of several hours the specimen is changed to two or three successive dishes of paraffin so that all of the xylene in the tissue is replaced by paraffin. The time in the oven depends on the size and density of the specimen; a specimen the size of a 2 or 3 mm cube may need to remain in the oven only a couple of hours, whereas a larger, firmer specimen may require 12 to 24 hours to ensure complete paraffin infiltration.

Embedding the specimen. When the specimen is completely infiltrated with paraffin, it is embedded in the center of a block of paraffin. A small paper box, perhaps a 19 mm cube for a small specimen, is filled with melted paraffin, and with warm forceps the specimen is removed from the dish of melted paraffin and placed in the center of the box of paraffin. Attention must be given here to the orientation of the specimen so that it will be cut in the plane desired for examination. A good plan is to place the surface to be cut first toward the bottom of the box. The paper box containing the paraffin and the specimen is then immersed in cool water to harden the paraffin. The hardened paraffin block is removed from the paper box and is mounted on a paraffin-coated wooden cube (about a 19 mm cube). The mounted paraffin block is trimmed with a razor blade so that there is about 3 mm of paraffin surrounding the specimen on all four sides so that the edges are parallel. The specimen is now ready to be sectioned on a microtome.

Cutting the sections of the specimen. The wooden cube to which the paraffin block is attached is clamped on a precision rotary microtome, the microtome is adjusted to cut sections of the desired thickness (usually 4 to 10 µm), and the perfectly sharpened microtome knife is clamped into place for sectioning.

Mounting the cut sections on slides. Suitable lengths of the paraffin ribbon are then mounted on prepared microscope slides. The preparation of the slides is done by the coating of clean slides with a thin film of Meyer's albumin adhesive (egg albumin and glycerin). A short length of paraffin ribbon is floated in a pan of warm water (about 45° C). A prepared slide is slipped under the ribbon and then is lifted from the water with the ribbon, which contains the tissue sections, arranged on its upper surface. The slide is placed on a constant-temperature drying table, which is regulated to about 42° C so that the sections will adhere to the slide. The slide is then allowed to dry on this table.

Staining the sections. There are innumerable tissue stains, methods of using stains, and methods of preparing tissues to receive stains. Some of the many factors that influence the choice of stains are the kind or kinds of tissue to be studied and the particular characteristics of immediate interest.

One combination of stains often used for routine microscopic study is hematoxylin and eosin, commonly known as H & E. A usual procedure for staining sections with hematoxylin and eosin follows.

The dried slides are placed vertically in glass staining trays; the trays are then passed through a series of staining dishes that contain the various reagents (Table 7).

The slides are removed one at a time from the xylene, and the sections are covered with a mounting medium and a cover glass if affixed. When the mounting me-

Table 7. Staining of sections

1. Xylene	2 min	To remove paraffin from sections
2. Xylene	2 min	To remove paraffin from sections
3. Absolute alcohol	2 min	To remove xylene
4. 95% alcohol	1 min	Approach to water
5. 80% alcohol	1 min	Approach to water
6. 60% alcohol	1 min	Approach to water
7. Distilled water	1 min	Water precedes stains dissolved in water
8. Hematoxylin (Harris's)	3-10 min	To stain nuclei
9. Distilled water	Rinse	To rinse off excess stain
10. Ammonium alum (saturated solution)	2-10 min	To differentiate; nuclei will retain stain
11. Sodium bicarbonate (saturated solution)	1-2 min	Makes stain blue
12. Distilled water	1 min	Removes $NaHCO_3$
13. 80% alcohol	1 min	Partially dehydrates
14. 95% alcohol	1 min	Alcohol precedes stains dissolved in alcohol
15. Eosin (alcohol soluble)	1-2 min	To stain cytoplasm and intercellular substance
16. 95% alcohol	Rinse, or longer	Alcohol destains eosin and should be used as long as needed
17. 95% alcohol	Rinse, or longer	To remove excess eosin
18. Absolute alcohol	1 min	To dehydrate
19. Absolute alcohol	2 min	To dehydrate
20. Xylene	2 min	To remove alcohol and clear
21. Xylene	2 min	To clear

dium has hardened, the slides are ready for examination.

PREPARATION OF SECTIONS OF PARLODION-EMBEDDED SPECIMENS

Specimens that contain bone and teeth cannot be cut with a microtome knife unless the calcified tissues are first made soft by decalcification. Furthermore, if a specimen contains any appreciable amount of bone or teeth, the decalcified specimen is better embedded in parlodion (celloidin, pyroxylin) than in paraffin. It is extremely difficult, if not impossible, to get good sections of a large mandible containing teeth in situ if the specimen is embedded in paraffin.

Let us suppose that we are to section a specimen of dog mandible bearing two premolar teeth. One method is as follows.

Obtaining the specimen. The portion of the mandible containing the two premolar teeth is separated as carefully as possible from the rest of the mandible by means of a sharp scalpel and a bone saw. Unwanted soft tissue is removed. If the area of the specimen next to the line of sawing will be seriously damaged by the saw, the specimen should be cut a little larger than needed and then trimmed to the desired size after partial decalcification. It is better to have the mandible cut into several pieces before placing it in the fixative because a smaller specimen allows quicker penetration of the fixing solution to its center. If the tooth pulp is of interest, a bur should be used to open the root apex of the teeth to permit entrance of the fixing solution into the pulp chamber. This operation must be done with care so that too much heat does not burn the pulp tissue.

Fixation of the specimen. The specimen so cut and prepared is quickly rinsed in running water and for fixation is placed immediately in about 400 ml of 10% neutral formalin. It should remain in the formalin not less than a week and preferably longer. It may be stored in formalin for a long period.

Decalcification of the specimen. When fixation is complete, the specimen is then decalcified. Decalcification may be accomplished in several ways. One way is to suspend the specimen in about 400 ml of 5% nitric acid. The acid is changed daily for 8 to 10 days, and then the specimen is tested for complete decalcification.

One way to test for complete decalcification is to pierce the hard tissue with a needle. When the needle enters the bone and tooth easily, the tissue is probably ready for further treatment.

Another way to test for complete decalcification is to determine by a precipitation test whether there is calcium present in the nitric acid in which the specimen is immersed. This is done by placing in a test tube 5 or 6 ml of the acid in which the specimen has been standing and then adding 1 ml of concentrated ammonium hydroxide and several drops of a saturated aqueous solution of ammonium oxalate. A precipitate will form if any appreciable amount of calcium is present. If a precipitate forms, the acid covering the specimen should be changed, and a couple of days later the test for complete decalcification should be repeated. If no precipitate is detected after the test tube has stood for an hour and after several additions of ammonium oxalate, it may be assumed that the specimen is almost completely decalcified. The specimen should be allowed to remain in the same acid for 48 hours longer and the test repeated.

The end point of decalcification is sometimes difficult to determine, but it is important. Specimens left in the acid too short a time are not completely decalcified and cannot be cut successfully, and specimens left in the acid too long a time do not stain well. Because of the adverse effect of prolonged exposure to acid on the staining quality of tissues, specimens should be reduced to their minimum size before decalcification is begun to keep the time necessary for acid treatment as short as possible.

Washing the specimen. When decalcification is complete, the specimen must be washed in running water for at least 24 hours to remove all of the acid.

Dehydration of the specimen. After washing, dehydration is accomplished by the placement of the specimen successively in increasing percentages of alcohol (40%, 60%, 80%, 95%, and absolute alcohol). The specimen should remain in each of the alcohols, up to and including 95%, for 24 to 48 hours, and it should then be placed in several changes of absolute alcohol over a period of 48 to 72 hours. It is necessary to remove, as much as possible, all of the water from the tissues to have good infiltration of parlodion.

From absolute alcohol the specimen is transferred to ether-alcohol (1 part anhydrous ether, 1 part absolute alcohol), because parlodion is dissolved in ether-alcohol. There should be several changes of ether-alcohol over a period of 48 to 72 hours.

Infiltration of the specimen with parlodion. Parlodion is purified nitrocellulose dissolved in ether-alcohol. From the ether-alcohol in which it has been standing, the specimen is transferred to 2% parlodion, covered tightly to prevent evaporation, and allowed to stand for a period of from 2 weeks to a month.

From 2% parlodion the specimen is transferred to increasing percentages of parlodion (4%, 6%, 10%, and 12%). The estimation of the time required for the infiltration of a specimen is a matter of experience, with the determining factors being the size of the specimen and the amount of bone and tooth material present. For the specimen of mandible being described here, the time required for complete parlodion infiltration might vary from several weeks to several months.

Embedding the specimen in parlodion. When infiltration with parlodion is complete, the specimen is embedded in the center of a block of parlodion. A glass dish with straight sidewalls and a lid is a good container to use for embedding. Some 12% parlodion is poured into the dish, and the specimen is placed in the parlodion. Then more parlodion is added so that there is about 13 mm of parlodion above the specimen, the additional amount being necessary to allow for shrinkage during hardening.

Orientation of the specimen at this point to ensure the proper plane of cutting is important. If this piece of dog mandible is to be sectioned in such a way that the premolar teeth are cut in a mesiodistal plane and the first sections are cut from the buccal surface, then the buccal surface of the mandible should be placed toward the bottom of the dish when the specimen is embedded.

The dish is now covered with a lid that fits loosely enough to permit very slow evaporation of the ether-alcohol in which the parlodion is dissolved. As the ether-alcohol evaporates, the parlodion will become solidified and will eventually acquire a consistency *somewhat* like that of hard rubber.

This process of hardening the parlodion may require 2 or 3 weeks. When the block is very firm, it is removed from the dish and placed in chloroform until it sinks. It is then transferred to several changes of 70% alcohol to remove the chloroform.

Blocks of parlodion-embedded material must never be allowed to dry out. The blocks should be stored in 70% alcohol to allow the parlodion to harden further. Blocks that are to be stored for many months or years should eventually be transferred to a mixture of 70% alcohol and glycerin for storage.

Cutting the sections of the specimen. The hardened block of the parlodion-embedded specimen is fastened with liquid parlodion to a fiber block or to a metal object holder so that it can be clamped onto the precision sliding microtome. (This is a different instrument from the rotary microtome used for cutting paraffin.) Sections are cut with a sharp microtome knife. For the specimen of dog mandible being described here, the sections may have to be cut at a thickness of as much as 15 μm. Unlike paraffin sections, these parlodion sections must be handled one at a time. As each section is cut, it is straightened out with a camel's hair brush on the top surface of the horizontally placed microtome knife and is then removed from the knife and placed flat in a dish of 70% alcohol. It must not be allowed to become dry. If it is important that the sections be kept in serial order, a square of paper should be inserted after every fourth or fifth section as they are stored in the dish of alcohol.

Staining the sections. Ordinarily the parlodion is not removed from the sections, and the sections are not mounted on slides until after staining, dehydrating, and clearing are completed. The sections are passed through the series of reagents separately or in groups of three or four, using a perforated section lifter to make the transfer.

From the 70% alcohol in which they are stored when cut, the sections may be stained with hematoxylin and eosin as follows.

Referring to Table 7, omit steps 1 to 3 and start with step 4; that is, transfer the parlodion sections from 70% to 95% alcohol. Follow each step down through step 17, which is 95% alcohol. At this point, for the absolute alcohol specified in steps 18 and 19, substitute carbolxylene (75 ml xylene plus 25 ml melted carbolic acid crystals). This substitution is made because the parlodion is slightly soluble in absolute alcohol. From carbolxylene the sections are transferred to xylene (steps 20 and 21).

The sections should not be allowed to become folded or rolled up during the staining process. When they are put into the carbolxylene, they must be flattened out carefully, because the xylene that follows will slightly harden the parlodion sections so that they cannot easily be flattened.

To mount the stained section on a slide, slip the clean side (no adhesive is used) into the dish of xylene beneath the section, lift the section onto the slide from the liquid, straightening it carefully, and quickly and firmly press it with a small piece of filter paper. The slide bearing the section is then quickly dipped back into the xylene and drained, mounting medium is flowed over the section, and a cover glass is dropped into place.

A modification of this embedding method, using acid celloidin instead of parlodion, will preserve much of the organic matrix of tooth enamel during the process of decalcification.

For variations in the hematoxylin and eosin stain and for information on the many other kinds of stains useful for both paraffin-embedded and parlodion-embedded specimens, the histology student must refer to books on microtechnique.

PREPARATION OF GROUND SECTIONS OF TEETH OR BONE

Decalcification of bone and teeth often obscures the structures. Teeth in particular are damaged because tooth enamel, being about 96% mineral substance, is usually completely destroyed by ordinary methods of decalcification. Undecalcified teeth and undecalcified bone may be studied by making thin ground sections of the specimens.

The equipment used for making ground sections includes a laboratory lathe, a coarse- and a fine-abrasive lathe wheel, a stream of water directed onto the rotating wheel and a pan beneath to catch the water, a wooden block (about a 25 mm cube), some 13 mm adhesive tape, a camel's hair brush, ether, mounting medium, microscope slides, and cover glasses.

Let us suppose that a thin ground section is to be prepared of a human mandibular molar tooth cut longitudinally in a mesiodistal plane. The coarse-abrasive lathe wheel is attached to the lathe, water is directed onto the wheel, the tooth is held securely in the fingers, and its buccal surface is applied firmly to that flat surface of the rapidly rotating wheel. The tooth is ground down nearly to the level of the desired section.

The coarse wheel is now exchanged for a fine-abrasive lathe wheel, and the cut surface of the tooth is ground again until the level of the desired section is reached.

At this point a piece of adhesive tape is wrapped around the wooden block in such a way that the sticky side of the tape is directed *outward*. The ground surface of the tooth is wiped dry and then is pressed onto the adhesive tape on one side of the wooden block. It will stick fast. With the block held securely in the fingers, the lingual surface of the tooth is applied to the coarse abrasive lathe wheel, and the tooth is ground down to a thickness of about 0.5 mm. Then the coarse wheel is again exchanged for the fine-abrasive lathe wheel, and the grinding is continued until the section is as thin as desired.

The finished ground section is soaked off

of the adhesive tape with ether and then dried for several minutes. Drying for too long will result in cracking. It is then mounted on a microscope slide. To do this, a drop of mounting medium is placed on the slide, the section is lifted with a camel's hair brush and placed on the drop, another drop of mounting medium is put on top of the section, and a cover glass is affixed for microscopic study.

The teeth used for ground sections should not be allowed to dry out after extraction, because drying makes the hard tissues brittle and the enamel may chip off in the process of grinding. Extracted teeth should be preserved in 10% formalin until used.

Precision equipment for making ground sections with much greater accuracy is available. The method described here is one in which equipment at hand in almost any laboratory is used. The technical literature contains a number of articles on the preparation of sections of undecalcified tissues.

PREPARATION OF FROZEN SECTIONS

Fixed soft tissues or fresh unfixed soft tissues may be cut into sections 10 to 15 μm thick by freezing the block of tissue with either liquid or solid carbon dioxide and cutting it on a freezing microtome. Frozen sections can be quickly prepared and are useful if the immediate examination of a specimen is required. Frozen sections are also useful when the tissue characteristics to be studied would be destroyed by the reagents used in paraffin embedding.

Details of the preparation of frozen sections can be obtained from books on microtechnique.

TYPES OF MICROSCOPY

A thin tissue section has the property to modify the color or intensity of light passing through it. The modified, light-containing information from the section is amplified through the lens system of a microscope and transmitted to the eye. Since the unstained tissues do not absorb or modify the light to a useful degree, tissue staining is used to induce differential absorption of light so that tissue components may be seen.

Many types of microscopes are used for the study of tissues. The most common is the bright-field microscope, which is a complex optical instrument that uses visible light. Modifications of this instrument have provided the phase-contrast, interference, dark-field, and polarizing microscopes. The optical systems that utilize invisible radiations include the ultraviolet microscope, roentgen-ray, and electron microscope. Each of these instruments has been a valuable tool in the study of oral tissues.

REFERENCES

Bodecker CF: The Cape-Kitchin modification of the celloidin decalcifying method for dental enamel, J Dent Res 16:143, 1937.

Brewer HE and Shellhamer RH: Stained ground sections of teeth and bone, Stain Technol 31:111, 1956.

Davenport HA: Histological and histochemical technics, Philadelphia, 1960, WB Saunders Co.

Fremlin JH, Mathieson J, and Hardwick JL: The grinding of thin sections of dental enamel, J Dent Res 39:1103, 1960.

Gatenby JB and Beams HW, editors: The microtomist's vade-mecum (Bolles Lee), ed 11, Philadelphia, 1950, The Blakiston Co.

Guyer MF: Animal micrology, Chicago, 1953, University of Chicago Press.

Koehler JK: Advanced techniques in biological electron microscopy, New York, 1973, Springer-Verlag.

Krajian AA and Gradwohl RBH: Histopathological technic, ed 2, St. Louis, 1952, The CV Mosby Co.

Mallory FB: Pathological technique, Philadelphia, 1938, WB Saunders Co.

Morse A: Formic acid–sodium citrate decalcification and butyl alcohol dehydration of teeth and bones for sectioning in paraffin, J Dent Res 24:143, 1945.

Nikiforuk G and Sreebny L: Demineralization of hard

tissues by organic chelating agents at neutral pH, J Dent Res 32:859, 1953.

Pearce AGE: Histochemistry, ed 3, vol 1, Baltimore, 1973, The Williams & Wilkins Co.

Sognnaes RF: Preparation of thin serial ground sections of whole teeth and jaws and other highly calcified and brittle structures, Anat Rec 99:134, 1947.

Sognnaes RF: The organic elements of the enamel, J Dent Res 29:260, 1950.

Weber DF: A simplified technique for the preparation of ground sections, J Dent Res 43:462, 1964.

Yaeger JA: Methacrylate embedding and sectioning of calcified bone, Stain Technol 33:229, 1958.

INDEX